The
Addiction
Spectrum

The
Addiction
Spectrum

A Compassionate, Holistic
Approach to Recovery

PAUL THOMAS, MD
and
JENNIFER MARGULIS, PhD

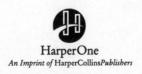

HarperOne
An Imprint of HarperCollins*Publishers*

HarperOne

This book contains advice and information relating to health care. It should be used to supplement rather than replace the advice of your doctor or another trained health professional. If you know or suspect you have a health problem, it is recommended that you seek your physician's advice before embarking on any medical program or treatment. All efforts have been made to assure the accuracy of the information contained in this book as of the date of publication. This publisher and the authors disclaim liability for any medical outcomes that may occur as a result of applying the methods suggested in this book.

All but two of the addicts who shared their stories in this book chose to remain anonymous and picked their own pseudonyms. Because of the sensitive and personal nature of this topic, every effort was made to give them the opportunity to review their stories for accuracy. Names and some personal characteristics of patients have been changed to disguise their identities. Any resulting resemblance to persons living or dead is entirely coincidental and unintentional.

Some of the material in chapters 3 and 8 first appeared in a different form in *The Jefferson Monthly* and *The Jefferson Journal*, respectively.

FIRST EDITION

Designed by Ad Librum
Illustrated by Han Sayles

Library of Congress Cataloging-in-Publication Data

Names: Thomas, Paul, MD, author. | Margulis, Jennifer, author.
Title: The addiction spectrum : a compassionate, holistic approach to
  recovery / Paul Thomas, MD, and Jennifer Margulis, PhD.
Description: First edition. | New York, NY : HarperOne, 2018
Identifiers: LCCN 2018014674 | ISBN 9780062836885 (hardback)
Subjects: LCSH: Substance abuse—Alternative treatment. | Integrative
  medicine. | BISAC: SELF-HELP / Substance Abuse & Addictions / Alcoholism.
  | SELF-HELP / Substance Abuse & Addictions / Drug Dependence. | HEALTH &
  FITNESS / Alternative Therapies.
Classification: LCC RC564 .T48 2018 | DDC 362.29—dc23
LC record available at https://lccn.loc.gov/2018014674

18 19 20 21 22   LSC   10 9 8 7 6 5 4 3 2 1

To Paul's wife, Maiya,
and
Jennifer's mother-in-law, Susan,
and
every reader who's ever done battle with addiction—
may this book guide you on your journey.

Contents

Authors' Note

It is abundantly clear to anyone who watches or reads the news that the world is in the midst of an addiction crisis. Opioids steal most of the headlines. Whether it is from heroin, meth, or another substance, thousands of people have died, and sadly more will die in the coming months and years. Many of you reading this book are terrified that someone you love will be a casualty of this crisis. If that is your fear, and you are reading this book to prevent that from happening, you are in the right place. But I want you to stop and take a breath before you dig in to what I hope will become a valuable life-giving resource for you. This book does not address politics or policy, the legal or penal system, or the "first responder" issues involved with drug overdoses. As critical as all these factors are, we see them as the end result of a broken approach to addiction. If addiction is a tree, these are the leaves on the tree. In this book, we will address the entire tree—the roots, the trunk, the branches, even the soil in which the tree is growing, as well as many of the leaves.

Addiction is a chronic condition, not a broken leg that can be fixed by setting the bone and putting the limb in a cast; nor can it be "solved" by throwing someone in jail or even in a hospital detox unit. Chronic conditions have a multiplicity of causes, but also a multiplicity of factors that can promote healing. Everything that you do to support that healing decreases the chances that you will someday receive the nightmare phone call that your loved one has overdosed. I sincerely hope that within the pages of this book you find all the support, strength, and resources that you need to deal with this terrifying and difficult condition.

Introduction

My name is Paul, and I'm a recovering alcoholic. My wife, Maiya, is a recovering opioid addict. Five of our nine kids (we have three biological and six adopted, all of whom are young adults now) have struggled with substance use. As much as addiction has affected my life on a personal level, it is also one of the most critical health problems of our time.

We are in the midst of a devastating addiction crisis in the United States and around the world—one that is affecting each and every one of us. You picked up this book because you or someone you love is struggling with addiction. That addiction probably involves opioids or even heroin, though it may be an addiction to another hard drug like cocaine or meth, to alcohol or marijuana, or to something more seemingly "benign," like gaming, the internet, or that brand-new smartphone you can't stop yourself from checking over eighty times a day (the national average).[1]

Not a day goes by without public-health officials, doctors, politicians, and even the president calling attention to this crushing crisis of addiction. There's a reason the Office of the Surgeon General now names addiction a top public-health priority:[2] more people are dying from drug overdoses than from traffic accidents in the United States.[3]

The numbers are grim and are getting worse.[4] Over 20 million Americans (more than the entire population of New York) are addicted to drugs or alcohol.[5] Some 12.5 million people over the age of twelve report misusing prescription opioids in the prior year,[6] and the Centers for Disease Control and Prevention says that **115 people a day are dying from opioid overdose** in the United States alone.[7] Next time you're at a party or a family gathering, look at the people around you—1 in 7 of your friends is expected to become addicted at some time in the future.[8]

According to data compiled by the *New York Times*, drug overdose is now the leading cause of death for Americans under fifty and touches people from every socioeconomic background and every region of the United States from Texas to Virginia to California.[9] More Americans were killed last year by drug overdose than died in the entire Vietnam War.[10] At the same time, over 15 million adults in America[11] are abusing alcohol and over 88,000[12] people are dying each year from alcohol-related deaths. Addiction is an unsustainable tragedy of epic proportions. We need to fix this problem, and we need to fix it now.

In 2016, more people died from drug overdoses[13]
than from motor vehicle accidents.[14]

I'll put it bluntly: I wrote this book because I don't want you to die. I don't want addiction to ruin your life. I don't want addiction to steal your loved ones from you. I want you not only to survive, but also to thrive. Which is why the book you're holding in your hands is literally a matter of life and death.

While the mainstream media has been relentlessly reporting on the *problem* of addiction, no one is offering real *solutions*. Alcoholics Anonymous works for some—myself included—but we know that Narcotics Anonymous is less effective. Other programs like Self-Management and Recovery Training (SMART) are making great strides but haven't been able to move the needle. The life expectancy of a person with an opioid or heroin addiction is abysmally low, and relapse rates are sky high.

That's the bad news. It's overwhelming.

My name is Paul, and I'm a medical doctor. I am board-certified in addiction medicine and pediatrics. I have spent my entire professional career finding effective and lasting ways to help people addicted to narcotics as well as to alcohol, stimulants, pot, and even screens. I've been practicing medicine for over thirty years with an open mind, a keen interest in the most recent science, and a willingness to adapt my treatment techniques based both on the latest research and on what is working and what isn't for each patient. I have a thriving integrative addiction treatment clinic called Fair Start and a busy pediatric practice, which now has over thirteen thousand patients, six doctors, eight nurses, and four nurse practitioners.

With a team of the best, most forward-thinking, and most compassionate doctors, nurse practitioners, and nurses by my side, I work day in and day out to help young people at risk of becoming addicted improve their mental and physical health and to help adults who are addicted get out of the clutches of drug abuse and get into recovery. I have also spent much of my life struggling to overcome my own demons.

Like you or your loved one, I have battled addiction. I spent twenty-seven years of my life abusing alcohol and eleven of those years addicted to nicotine. Though I've been sober for over fifteen years, I still struggle with overeating and other unhealthy behaviors, which I'll tell you more about later in this book. At the same time, I've been blessed with a tremendous amount of energy and a stubborn determination to change the world by improving people's health. Mine is an optimistic—and highly effective—approach to treating what has proven itself to be one of society's most challenging health problems. I have developed a recovery plan that *actually works*, not only to help you avoid addiction when you think you may be sliding into it, but to support every aspect of your health as you struggle to beat the habit, subdue your cravings, and redirect the destructive behavior that may be ruining your life.

In 2009 I opened my addiction clinic in Portland, Oregon. Its mission, from the beginning, has been to help young adults kick addiction and take back their lives. I treat mostly millennials who are hooked on heroin, opioids, cocaine, methamphetamines, marijuana, alcohol, or some combination of these. In the past nine years, we have treated over five hundred patients struggling with addiction, including teens and even some tweens. We have also helped opioid-dependent young women navigate pregnancy and deliver healthy babies.

Although conventional doctors may protest that a pediatrician is not qualified to treat addiction, the sad truth is that *every pediatrician* in America needs to be more aware of and more educated about how to prevent addiction in young people and how to help them once it starts. In the past twenty years, America has experienced an explosion of brain disorders, mental illness, and addiction among children and young adults. Anxiety, depression, and focus challenges—including ADD and ADHD—put young people at greater risk for addiction. Fifty-four percent of my Fair Start patients report having anxiety, depression,

ADD, or ADHD prior to becoming addicted. To practice pediatrics in America today is to practice mental-health and addiction medicine.

Why are people struggling with mental-health issues and addiction more today than ever before? Policymakers and doctors dodge this question with long-winded jargon-filled answers, but I am going to tell it to you straight: **You are stressed out, undernourished, vitamin D deficient, and sleep-deprived. You are not getting enough exercise, time outside, or community support.** Courtesy of your handheld computers, you feel more disconnected than ever before. At the same time, your immune system is under constant assault from the chemicals in your food, your water, and even your medications. **Add to all this a medical system that profits from patients' poor health, and you have the perfect addiction storm.**

Sometimes it is family history that puts you at higher risk for addiction; other times it is as simple as a bout of anxiety or a dental procedure. But **we are all vulnerable to becoming addicted**. I want to stop for a moment and reiterate that truth: every single one of us is a potential addict—you, your partner, your friend, your parent, your child. If you yourself have struggled with addiction, think of the sober people in your life who have judged or dismissed you and remember that within them is a potential addict. If you have never had a problem with addiction, recognize that, given the wrong circumstances, you too could become addicted. Our unhealthy lifestyles and exposure to toxins make us more vulnerable to addiction than we have ever been before. Understanding this is the only way to make sense of the explosion of opioid addiction in this country and explains why my solutions, which you'll learn about throughout this book, are so effective.

Many of my patients who spiral out of control with drug addiction were first prescribed opioids after an injury, an accident, or a wisdom-tooth extraction. Their doctors often *insisted* on doling out prescriptions for these highly addictive painkillers, even when my patients (or their parents) said they preferred to stick with something milder, like aspirin or ibuprofen! Just last month a young person in my practice who was off to college in a new city was hospitalized for severe stomach pain. The hospital doctors tried to put her on a morphine drip even before they had a diagnosis (it turned out to be appendicitis). Knowing her family history, she said, "No, thank you," opting for a nonaddictive pain medicine instead. If the doctors had asked before they offered, they would have found out that this eighteen-year-old has alcoholism and addiction on both sides of her family. Exposing her to a highly addictive opioid could have had disastrous results.

We know from science that the earlier young people are exposed to drugs, the more likely it is that they will get addicted.[15] Early and repeated exposure to opioids can even cause addiction in young people who have no other obvious risk factors. I've seen this happen in my practice. Yet medical doctors irresponsibly continue to expose even the youngest patients.

We also know that untreated mental- and physical-health problems can catapult people into addiction. For those of you who suffer from attention deficit disorders, anxiety, and depression, self-soothing with alcohol or drugs feels like a solution. It *is* a solution! You use substances to self-medicate without ever realizing that is what you are doing. At the same time, your doctors fail to recognize and treat the underlying causes of your poor physical and mental health, prescribing you medication to mask the symptoms instead. When you are already struggling with mental- and physical-health issues—as so many of us are—and you are then prescribed highly addictive medication, is it any wonder you succumb?

Opioid-induced euphoria is enticing for everyone, and irresistible for some. Usually with a doctor's blessing, you get your prescription refilled many times, long after the initial need for the medication is gone. And when those same doctors finally notice there's a problem and refuse to write another script, you turn to street drugs like heroin for relief. It sometimes takes only months, or it may take several years, but eventually the drugs stop working, the anxiety gets worse, and you find yourself in a downward spiral of self-loathing, pain, and despair.

Addiction has no regard for wealth or status. Though the heaviest users who come to Fair Start are often unemployed or underemployed, I also have many full-time college students and many professionals working in occupations like medicine, engineering, law, and education. My patients reflect the demographics of the greater Portland area. They are mostly white; some are Hispanic, Asian American, African American, and Native American. Although many are not married, nearly all have partners. Their significant other may also be struggling with substance abuse. About a quarter have children and arrive for visits with a baby or toddler in tow. Many, however, have lost primary custody of their kids because of their drug use. Some have had run-ins with the law.

In the past nine years of scheduling hundreds of patients at Fair Start, I found that 15 percent never showed up to the first appointment. This reflects one of the biggest challenges facing addicts who want treatment. Your life is disorganized, and you may not be thinking straight. You want help today—so you make an appointment with a doctor like me who takes insurance, is here to help you, and has a supportive, compassionate, and well-trained staff. But by the time the appointment comes, your motivation to stop using is already gone. Why go to the doctor for help when your solution of choice is within arm's reach?

If you're not an addict, you probably think this can't and won't happen to you. You're mistaken. **Our high-stress lives, unhealthy lifestyles, and lack of community leave us all vulnerable. To be human is to be prone to addiction.** The rate of full-blown addiction has tripled in the United States in the last twenty years. The only way to understand this incredible rise in addiction statistics is to fundamentally change the way we think about, talk about, and treat addiction.

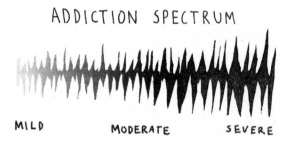

Addiction is a spectrum. Most people think the world is divided into two kinds of people: addicts and nonaddicts. You're either an alcoholic or you're not, with no in between. But that is not how addiction works. In reality, we are all somewhere on the addiction spectrum. When you are on the mild end of the spectrum, you have little problem with alcohol, drugs, or addictive behaviors. You are able to enjoy alcohol, experiment with addictive substances, take opioids for a limited amount of time and for their intended reason, or engage in highly pleasurable addictive behaviors without it becoming a problem. You may overuse once or twice, but you learn from your mistakes. You stop if you are worried, often for good. You don't want to live life in an altered state, so for the most part you stay away from anything that you could become addicted to.

Others of you are at moderate risk. Like those on the mild end of the addiction spectrum, you often can and do restrain your use, at least at the beginning. You manage to keep yourself under control, though you may overindulge from time to time. You may wake up feeling miserable, guilty, or ashamed, but you are usually able to conquer the urge to use too much. You would not necessarily be diagnosed as an "addict," but if you told a knowledgeable mental-health professional the truth (which you don't, because you're too ashamed or too private to admit what you are actually doing), you would likely be diagnosed with a substance-use disorder. You are using more than is healthy and are always at risk of developing a more severe use disorder, but because your use is not ruining your life, you remain somewhere in the middle of the spectrum.

And some of you, like me and my wife and my patients, are or have been on the severe end of the addiction spectrum. You experience unbearable and often uncontrollable cravings. Once you start, you don't seem to have an off switch. Your addictions take over your life.

You have the power to change your destiny. Your place on the addiction spectrum is always changing. Although you may feel as if you're climbing an insurmountable mountain as you struggle to recover, don't despair. You can't change certain factors that put you at risk, which I'll talk about in the next chapter, but the more you improve your eating habits, make lifestyle changes, reduce your exposure to toxins (including stress), and seek out and find connectedness, the more you will move toward the mild, healthy end of the spectrum, creating for yourself a steadier, more manageable, and more joyful life.

The opposite is also true. You may be in perfect health and look down on all the addicts whom you secretly think of as poor saps who lack willpower and moral fiber. But being on the mild end of the spectrum today does not mean you may not be moving toward the severe end of the addiction spectrum tomorrow. You are most susceptible to addiction after a traumatic event like an unwanted divorce, unexpected loss, or physical injury. Understanding that addiction is a treatable condition that happens on a spectrum is crucial to preventing addiction and helping you heal.

If you're holding this book in your hands, you have likely lost much to addiction. Maybe you've been told addiction is an intractable problem with no real solution, a sign of moral failing or weak character. You're embarrassed, tired, and discouraged. Perhaps you've tried on your own to conquer your addiction and failed. You picked yourself up and tried again—only to fall flat on your face. You may be suffering from other chronic or acute health problems. Left to fend for yourself, you have fallen victim to isolation and pain. You self-medicate and feel trapped in a vicious cycle of drinking, drug use, or unhealthy behaviors. Unable to handle the withdrawal symptoms that occur when you try to stop, you're in prison and you are your own jailer.

Or perhaps it is your loved one who is suffering, and you have no idea how to help. You feel out of answers.

That's where I come in. You are the reason I wrote this book. I don't have all the answers—no one does—but **I do have an implementable, individualized plan of action that is going to help you begin to enjoy better health, today, as you work to beat back addiction**.

The best part about my treatment approach? It has worked for hundreds of addicts, and it will work for you too.

I am here to tell you that you are not alone. And you don't need to suffer any longer. Addiction is not intractable. Addiction is not a moral failing.

You do *not* need to be exhausted. You do *not* need to be stressed out. You do *not* need to be miserable. You do *not* need to be ashamed.

In this book you are going to learn **the key strategies you need to overcome addiction, prevent future relapse, and feel better in literally every aspect of your health and your life**. They include how to:

1. Eat real food as it comes from the earth.

2. Reduce stress in all forms, including from television, news, social media, toxic people, and toxic environments.

3. Increase your level of vitamin D through lifestyle intervention and supplementation.

4. Improve your mental and physical health with daily exercise.

5. Discover high-quality sleep that refreshes and rejuvenates.

6. Fix your broken gut microbiome (if you don't know what that is yet, you soon will!).

7. Find and build connectedness, replacing the false connection of addiction with true relationships.

Some of these interventions may seem obvious; others may be ideas you've never heard of before, let alone considered trying. You don't have to be perfect. You don't have to do it right every time. **In my approach it's okay to fail.** I want you to embrace your imperfections instead of feeling ashamed of them. But don't underestimate the revolutionary power of making what may seem like simple health and lifestyle changes. Throughout this book I'm going to walk you through all of these strategies and more, explain the science behind them, and give you detailed advice about how to implement them successfully in your life.

There seems to be a growing lack of true connection in our culture—genuine connection to ourselves and to each other. But to beat addiction you must build connections with other people. Lasting, sober, healthy connections are an essential component to good health for everyone. This is, after all, the elusive thing that so many of you are looking for when you drink or use. You feel socially inept, so you drink and the awkwardness goes away. You feel lonely and alone, so you use in order to bond with other people who are also using. You believe you're having a rip-roaring good time, and you feel profoundly connected to your addict friends.

The paradox, of course, is that the high is a lie. As you spiral from the moderate to the severe end of the addiction spectrum, you start to realize that the false sense of connection you have been getting from your addiction is actually cutting you off from other people and crippling your ability to connect. Recovery is so painful because it involves waking up to the fact that you are disconnected. If that sounds hard, it's because it *is* hard. But millions of others have gotten drug-free and sober. If you follow my program, you can and you will get sober too. But you can't do it alone. Luckily, you don't have to.

The Failed Conventional Medical Approach

The problems addicts face are physical, behavioral, and emotional. You often lack a sense of purpose. You often feel profoundly alone. But when you seek help from the medical system, rarely do you find answers that address all the facets of your addictive tendencies. Instead, you're met with disapproval from doctors who may believe you are just not trying hard enough. You know what I'm talking about, because you've lived it. Conventional medicine treatment options often feel more like judgment than help and frequently come laced with insinuations, accusations, and hostility.

Doctors are taught to focus on physical symptoms. Medical doctors have very little, if any, training in anything else. Can't sleep? There's a pill for that. Depressed? Here's some medication. Overcome with anxiety? I've got a pill for that too. Side effects from all those meds you're on? There are pills for those as well! I have patients whose doctors have put them on thirteen different medications *at the same time*, despite the fact that no studies exist showing that the combination of those medications is safe or effective.

Don't misunderstand me—I use pharmaceuticals in my practice every day. I am grateful for them. Sometimes a pharmaceutical intervention is the first and best step to helping a suffering addict. There is often benefit to using controlled prescription medication to support a brain that has been chronically flooded with harmful drugs in order to begin the process of allowing the body to heal.

But as an integrative physician, I strive to give my patients the tools to recognize the underlying health conditions that contribute to their struggles. These tools can be applied to many different kinds of addiction, not just to heroin and opioids, which is why this book deals with the origins of addiction and with so much more than just "hard" drugs. Most drug abusers also drink, smoke cigarettes, and find themselves with behavioral addictions as well. Most alcoholics or heavy drinkers also do a lot of drugs. And, as I said earlier, many of us who are not ostensibly addicts—as hard as it might be to admit—have addictive tendencies that negatively affect our lives and that we often unwittingly pass on to our children.

Although "integrative medicine" is a household term in most of my circles, unless you're already a progressive-minded doctor or have been studying alternative health, you may have never heard this term before. Integrative medicine is healing-oriented, taking account of the whole person and including every aspect of her or his lifestyle. It emphasizes the relationship between practitioner and patient, is informed by the most current scientific research as well as a doctor's own clinical experience, and makes use of many different healing modalities and therapies that more conventional, mainstream doctors may dismiss as "crazy" or "woo-woo" (without bothering to research or try them).

Just as every human fingerprint is a unique pattern of whorls and lines, every person's brain offers a unique challenge. As an integrative physician, I look for root causes of addiction instead of just treating symptoms. I combine the best of modern medical practices with a more holistic approach. I gather information from the patient about genetic vulnerabilities, food and nutrition, and other lifestyle choices and then use this information to devise a plan that integrates alternative healing practices designed specifically for the patient.

Your particular addiction is unique to you and therefore requires a unique integrative medical approach. Addiction treatment is not one-size-fits-all. So the first thing we need to do is locate the root causes of your addiction, which is what I talk about in part I. It is important to begin at the beginning—together we will figure out where you are now on the addiction spectrum, explore the risk factors that got you there, and discuss the myths about addiction that you need to let go of in order to heal. In part I, I also help open your eyes to how the medical establishment, the food industry, and pharmaceutical companies have primed you for and profit from your addiction. I also help you figure out how your genetic vulnerabilities, sleep habits, food choices, and stress levels contribute to the problem.

Once you know better, you can do better. Armed with information about who is benefitting from your addiction and how you are being encouraged to take more drugs that you don't actually need, in part II, I walk you through the best ways to set your body up for success. Because every addiction has a different effect on both your mental and physical health, part II covers major addictions in separate chapters and offers ways to heal your body and your mind from the abuse it has received courtesy of your drug or behavior of choice, whether it is opioids, meth, alcohol, marijuana, or even screens. In each chapter in part II, I give you an individual treatment plan, which includes lifestyle changes, nutritional intervention, and the supplements you need to support your best health. In part III, I explain my integrative health program in more detail, giving you advice on how to navigate a sometimes hostile medical system and providing inspiration on how to embrace your recovery journey. I explain why I believe you need mind, body, and spirit to work together to heal.

There are stories, suggestions, and solutions in every chapter, so I recommend you read this book from cover to cover, though you may be tempted to start with the chapter in part II that tackles your or your loved one's most pressing addiction and then circle back to the other parts of the book. My goal is to get you far, far away from the severe end of the addiction spectrum, regardless of your drug of choice.

If you take only one thing away from this entire book, here's what I hope it will be: **The journey to health is so much more than a pill or some counseling.** To find your true exuberance, real potential, and lasting good health, you must rebuild the basic cornerstones of your brain and body. This requires a change to your entire approach to recovery. You must understand that you are on a spectrum of addiction, and that **the power to heal is in your hands.**

Will You Benefit from Reading This Book?

Chances are a medical assistant has asked you some or all of the questions below while he or she was sitting in front of a computer typing away, checking off boxes on a list and not making eye contact. Chances are you didn't even know that person's name. And I'd be willing to bet you didn't answer truthfully. Why should you? None of us feels comfortable revealing intimate details about our personal struggles to someone we've just met, who isn't looking at us, and who we'll probably never see again. But you are safe here with this book in the privacy of your own space. I want you to be straight with me now—and, more important, with yourself. You have nothing to lose, and everything to gain. So here goes. If your answer to the question is yes, mark the box:

- ☐ Do you ever drink or use drugs more than you planned to?

- ☐ Do you ever have remorse about drinking, using drugs, or any other potentially addictive behavior, including but not limited to playing video games, surfing the internet, gambling, or watching porn?

- ☐ Do you ever hide your alcohol use, drug use, or other addictive behaviors from your family and friends?

☐ Have you ever had a blackout?

☐ Are you struggling to make commitments or tackle new things because you're more interested in drinking or using?

☐ Are you having problems at work or at school because of your drinking or using?

☐ Have you lost interest in activities that were once important to you?

☐ Are you feeling unwell or unhappy?

☐ Do you feel tired all the time?

☐ When you don't drink or use drugs, do you feel sick, or suffer anxiety, cravings, or shakes?

☐ Have you ever thought, "I should cut back," but then pushed that thought out of your mind?

☐ Do you have family members or friends who would answer yes to these questions for you, even if you're sure the answer is no?

Maybe you know full well you have a problem, which is why you're here. Or maybe you don't consider yourself an addict or an alcoholic, but you're worried that your substance use or other addictive behavior may be getting out of hand. Or maybe it's not you, but a loved one who is struggling. Or perhaps you're an educator, public-health worker, or addiction specialist working with people who would answer yes to some of the questions above, and you are looking for more information to help your patients.

In any case, *if the answer to even just one of these questions is yes, for yourself or for another, you've come to the right place.* I am here for you. If the yeses are your own, I will help you identify your demons and free yourself from the stranglehold your addiction, dependence, or troubling behavior is having on your life.

Together we will build health and wellness into your life starting now. Start today, regardless of your age. Start before you get addicted. Start after you've already succumbed. Start before you get pregnant. Start as you cradle your newborn in your arms. **It is never too late and** it's never too early to implement a wellness plan that will help you take control of your addictions, your health, and every aspect of your life.

The Addiction Spectrum explains the factors that prime the brain for addiction, gives you the information you need to avoid addiction before it starts, and offers an approach to help you become physically and psychologically healthy, well grounded, and addiction-free. It's a compendium of everything I've learned in the past nine years of treating addicts and the last thirty years of practicing medicine. Filled with stories of recovery and hope, the book you are holding in your hands may be the most important book you will ever read.

PART I

The Addiction Epidemic

CHAPTER I

Where Are You on the Addiction Spectrum?

ALL MY CHILDHOOD MEMORIES are of Africa. I was born in Oregon, where I live and practice medicine today, but my parents were missionaries with the United Methodist Church. My family moved to Rhodesia, the country we now call Zimbabwe, when I was about to turn five and my sister Mary was three.

Our home in the village of Arnoldine was made of sun-dried bricks. We had no electricity or running water; the kitchen was a detached round hut. There were about fifty families total in our village and just one three-room schoolhouse. The nearest store was eighteen miles down a rugged dirt road.

No one in our village smoked or drank. I'm not sure if it was because cigarettes and alcohol were forbidden by the church, culturally unacceptable, or both, but I never saw anyone in my family—or anyone with whom my family came in contact—light up a cigarette or take a drink of alcohol. The exception was at weddings and funerals, when village men would share a thick fermented cornmeal drink, a foul-smelling homemade concoction called *maheu*.

High School: Starting Along the Addiction Spectrum

When it came time for high school, I went to a boarding school in Mbabane, the capital of Swaziland. I was away from my parents and the

United Methodist Church for the first time in my life, and it was then that I tried my first drink. My buddy Mark and I snuck down to the little store four miles from school, and we each bought two large bottles of Kronenbourg. Sitting on a large rock overlooking the valley, we chugged our beer. I honestly didn't enjoy the taste; I wasn't used to fizzy drinks. But I didn't care. I was excited and purposeful. I was a young man on a mission, focused on the warm feeling in my belly. A sense of well-being washed over my brain. There was no doubt in my mind that I would be doing this again.

Drinking filled me with euphoria. I did not just *like* the feeling—I loved it. The pleasure was a whole-body sensation. For the first time in my life I put my guard down. "Ah, that's better," my whole body sang. "*This* is how I'm supposed to feel." I was relieved of the anxiety I had been carrying around with me, an anxiety I didn't even know existed.

Unknown to me at that time, that was the beginning of my journey along the addiction spectrum. But I was stuck on a mountain in Swaziland, highly supervised, and with no disposable income, which meant I had no access to alcohol throughout high school. Imagine if I had grown up attending an inner-city school with an open campus, as my own children did. I would have had access to liquor stores, convenience stores, and adults eager to make alcohol purchases for me for a few bucks at any time. Given my instant love for the mellowing effect of alcohol, there is no doubt in my mind that I would have gone careening along the addiction spectrum toward the severe end much more quickly. Our environment plays a powerful role in our progression along the spectrum.

Looking at my parents, family, and background, you would hardly think I was "at risk" for addiction. I was a high-energy, creative, and highly motivated teenager—and the class clown. I was also restless and easily distractible—I'm sure I would have been labeled ADHD if I were a child today—but I was also a good student and a hard worker.

I got plenty of exercise in high school. I was on the soccer, field-hockey, squash, and track teams. We were outside all the time, for sports and for work duty, soaking up the African sun. Although I hated the food at boarding school, it was made from fresh produce and free-range animals. We drank mountain spring water, and the air was clean. I had almost no exposure to toxins. These protective lifestyle factors—enough vitamin D from time outside, organic real food, ade-

quate sleep and exercise, a lack of exposure to toxins, and a supportive community of friends and teachers—were all a natural part of my
boarding-school life. All of this, combined with my lack of access to
alcohol, was highly protective at that time, keeping me from progressing along the addiction spectrum.

All of that would quickly change.

So What Is the Addiction Spectrum?

When you are in pain and go to the doctor, you are asked to quantify
your pain. Zero means you have no pain, and ten means you are in the
worst pain of your life. The addiction spectrum works like that as well.
On one end you have no symptoms; you are healthy and addiction-free.
On the other end, you are unable to stop drinking or using and you're
suffering major health consequences; you may even feel as though
you're dying.

Everyone begins addiction on the mild end of a spectrum. Physiologically, you do not get addicted to a substance or behavior right away,
but you enjoy it—so you continue doing it with increasing frequency
and intensity. But as you get deeper into addiction, you move along
the spectrum, and your addiction symptoms and health consequences
become more severe. By understanding that addiction happens on a
spectrum and by implementing the lifestyle and integrative medicine
solutions I offer you throughout this book, especially in part III, you
can tame your demons and move from the severe back toward the mild
end of the spectrum.

Once you understand the biological, physical, emotional, social, and
environmental factors that have pushed you toward the severe end of
the addiction spectrum, you now can do something about it. **You have
the power to change your place on the spectrum, to lessen how addiction impacts your life, and to improve your health.** In a sense you could
say you always have the potential to move along the spectrum of addiction at any time. Either you are improving your diet, your vitamin D
status, your sleep, exercise, and gut microbiome and you are reducing
stress, surrounding yourself with a supportive network of sober people, and learning the skills needed to keep you from relapsing, or you

are ignoring these important keys to recovery and allowing yourself to stay at or move toward the severe end of the spectrum.

There are things that make it more likely that you may begin drinking, using, or excessively engaging in addictive behavior patterns. These are your risk factors, which I talk about more below, and they can speed your progression along the addiction spectrum. If you have a strong family history of alcoholism or addiction, you are more likely to progress along the addiction spectrum more quickly than someone with no family history. If you grow up surrounded by alcohol and drugs, you are more likely to start using at a younger age. All children and young adults have people in their lives who are modeling either healthy or unhealthy relationships with alcohol or drugs. When you lack good role models and see people overusing, you are also more likely to mimic that behavior and end up with a severe addiction.

As I mentioned earlier, the sheer number of addicts has grown exponentially in the last decade. Why such a steep increase? Why are so many millions of us now struggling with addiction? What is the thread that connects us all? The truth is that we are all vulnerable to harming ourselves by our own poor choices. We have all felt lonely and isolated. We have all at one time or another disappointed ourselves, our friends, and our loved ones. Can you honestly say you never get obsessed, overeat, or engage in behavior you know is unhealthy? That you always get enough sleep, exercise, and time outside? We all have areas of our lives—often many—that could use improvement. When you compromise your mental and physical health with an overexposure to toxins, a sedentary lifestyle, poor eating habits, disconnection, and a lack of a sense of purpose, you put yourself at risk of moving from the mild to the severe end of the addiction spectrum.

Relapse is not gradual; it's all or nothing; you either use again or you don't. If you relapse, the trip back to the severe end of the spectrum can happen at lightning speed. Addicts who have been on the severe end of the spectrum for most substances and behaviors may need to abstain completely. I certainly can't drink alcohol, and I won't be able to for the rest of my life. I will never be a "social drinker."

But you can and will have an easier, more lasting, and more hopeful recovery when you implement the ideas in this book and consistently keep yourself moving toward the mild end of the spectrum. Every day doesn't need to feel like a slow climb up a steep cliff. You have the potential to increase your emotional stamina, resiliency, and capacity for change. You can improve your ability to withstand internal and external pressure, to feel optimistic about your future, and to live a life in which your addictions aren't front and center.

Where Do You Fall on the Addiction Spectrum?

Dr. Paul's Self-Test

Check all the boxes that apply to you:

- ☐ I frequently feel irritable.
- ☐ I'm tired all the time.
- ☐ I have sleep problems.
- ☐ I suffer from anxiety and/or depression.
- ☐ I have ADD/ADHD.
- ☐ My brain often feels foggy; I have trouble thinking.
- ☐ I feel lonely a lot.
- ☐ I've lost interest in activities I used to enjoy.
- ☐ I have difficulty starting new projects.
- ☐ I'm drinking or using drugs more than once a week.

Give yourself 1 point for each checked box. **Total points:** _____

- ☐ I crave my substance or behavior of choice.
- ☐ I drink or use to relax, to sleep, or to perform.
- ☐ I drink or use when I tell myself I won't.
- ☐ I feel remorse about drinking or using.
- ☐ I lie to my family or my friends about how much I drink or use.
- ☐ I am increasingly drinking/using more to get the desired effect.

Give yourself 2 points for each checked box. **Total points:** _____

- ☐ I've blacked out as a result of drinking or using.
- ☐ I experience withdrawal symptoms (irritability, depression, despair) when I don't drink or use.
- ☐ I drink or use more than most people and at times when others don't.
- ☐ I try to stop or cut back, but I can't.
- ☐ I've driven a car under the influence of drugs or alcohol in the last month.
- ☐ I've lost a job or a relationship over drinking or using in the last year.
- ☐ I've been cited for driving under the influence once.

Give yourself 5 points for each checked box. **Total points:** _____

☐ I've been cited for driving under the influence two or more times.
☐ I've been in a treatment program for my addiction in the past year.
☐ I've been hospitalized for my addiction in the past year.
☐ I know I'm addicted.

Give yourself 10 points for each checked box. **Total points:** _____

Scoring

0–9 points: Good news. You are on the mild end of the addiction spectrum. There may be areas of your life that you want to improve, but addiction is not overwhelming your life or compromising your health. You will still benefit from the advice and tips in this book, but you're on the right path. The key for you is to stay the course.

10–20 points: Not such good news. You are approaching the middle of the addiction spectrum. You may be struggling with some mental- and physical-health issues, even though they seem to be *mostly* under control. You may be headed toward the severe end of the addiction spectrum, and now is the best time to address these issues and get help. Good for you for reading this book before things spiral out of control. Read on.

More than 20 points: Cause for concern. Either you're approaching the severe end of the addiction spectrum, or you've been there in the past. Your addiction may be overwhelming your enjoyment of life, your mental health, and your physical well-being. It may feel impossible to stop. But you can move toward the mild end of the spectrum and find lasting recovery. This book will show you how. If your high score is due to your recent past, but you are now in active recovery and free of destructive substance use, keep it up. You will also benefit from ideas in this book.

Why Did I Marry an Addict?

When you're struggling with addiction, or when you even just love to drink or use drugs, you gravitate toward people who drink and use. When it comes time to pick a partner, you don't pick someone healthy who would have concerns about your alcohol or substance use or make it difficult for you to carry on with it. I was in medical school when I first met my wife. I was twenty-five years old and drinking too much. She was a brown-eyed, curly-haired cutie who, as a neonatal intensive-care nurse, was saving the lives of babies born prematurely. We shared wine from a bota bag skiing down the slopes near Dartmouth Medical School. I could tell she enjoyed the warm buzz as much as I did. There would be no judgment from her.

Maiya needed multiple surgeries for a degenerative jaw condition. She was prescribed opioids after each operation. Prescription opioids are powerful—they create feelings of pleasure and relaxation, mimicking the brain's natural endorphins. They're also highly addictive. Some 92 million Americans are prescribed opioids by their doctors for pain management, about one-third of the population. Like the 2 million of these folks who then became unable to function without them,[1] Maiya got addicted. Maiya started getting more and more into her addiction and becoming less and less functional and available in the rest of her life. I'll be sharing her story (with her blessing) throughout this book. I was attracted to Maiya because she was fun-loving, nonjudgmental, and spontaneous. Neither she nor I had any idea that she would ultimately end up on the severe end of the addiction spectrum, but that's what happened.

What Are the Risk Factors for Addiction?

Though we had very different childhoods, Maiya and I both succumbed to addiction. Unlike mine, Maiya's early childhood was spent in an authoritarian-style home, and she had ample access to marijuana and alcohol in her early teens. She ate sugary cereal for breakfast and was not athletic growing up. When she was sixteen, she worked at Jack in the Box in San Diego. Her manager brought alcohol to work and put it in the soda cups of his teen employees. They all got drunk together. They were "having fun."

We know that genetic vulnerabilities and certain childhood factors can predispose people to become addicts. Physiological and emotional factors also enter in. But even those who have several significant risk factors can stay on the mild end of the addiction spectrum. Some people simply have no predilection for drugs; others are afraid to experiment because they have seen how their loved ones suffered from addiction. We all know people who are teetotalers, who avoid all addictive substances, and never develop a problem. Unless some stress, like a major surgery or divorce, pushes them further, they usually stay at the mild end of the addiction spectrum their whole lives.

Genetic Vulnerabilities

I graduated from high school in December 1974. My parents arranged for me to fly back to the United States through Austria and spend New Year's Eve with family friends. The beer flowed endlessly during that two-hour meal. To ring in the New Year, each of us was given our own bottle of champagne.

I recall a whole pig roasting over an open fire, lots of dancing, and throwing up after the party. The rest of that evening is absent from my memory. That was my first blackout. Sadly, it was not my last.

Alcohol was the friend I turned to when celebrating success, when I was feeling anxious, and when I needed relief from stress. I became a binge drinker. Drinking helped me calm down, distracting me from my fears and problems. During college and medical school, I either didn't drink at all, or I drowned myself in alcohol.

After my drinking spun out of control and I was struggling to recover, I was surprised to learn that I had a great-uncle who died of complications due to alcoholism. I had had no idea, until my mother shared this family secret (it was her uncle), that I was genetically predisposed to becoming an alcoholic. If you have a strong family history of alcoholism or addiction you are at higher risk of ending up on the severe end of the addiction spectrum.

I also found out through genetic testing that I had verifiable genetic defects that increased my risk for addiction. It turns out there are genetic differences, called single-nucleotide polymorphisms (SNPs), that put us at increased risk for addiction and for problems with our neurotransmitters. It can be enormously helpful to identify these genetic vulnerabilities to addiction. But these are *vulnerabilities*, not inevitabilities. This is all complicated and fascinating. You can have your SNPs tested by companies like 23andMe, which give you raw data that you can then have analyzed.

Childhood Factors That Lead to Addiction

Early use: The younger you are when you try alcohol and drugs, the more likely you are to get hooked. Just ask fifty-six-year-old Calvin, a friend of mine from Alcoholics Anonymous. Calvin is a recovering heroin addict and alcoholic. Growing up in Happy Camp, California, in a family with thirteen kids, Calvin had his first drink when he was five. He smoked pot, which he and his sister stole from their older brothers, when he was eight; smoked cigarettes before he hit his teens; and also started huffing gas. He tried heroin for the first time when he was sixteen. It may sound extreme—the idea of a child drinking alcohol—but most of my patients started drinking or using drugs in their early teens.

Child abuse: Children who grow up in abusive homes are much more likely to turn to addiction to escape. Maiya spent much of her early childhood cowering in a closet for fear of her father's belt or to get away from the screaming going on between her parents. Many of my female patients (and some of my male patients as well) have experienced physical and sexual abuse at the hands of relatives or family friends. Research from Harvard University has shown that early child abuse can alter important parts of children's brains, making them more susceptible to addiction.[2] José, now in his mid-twenties, was repeatedly sexually abused by his high-school coach in his teens. A court case in which he will be asked to testify looms in the future, and for the past three years this has been the most significant stress in his life. Nicholas became a male prostitute in his mid-teens, surviving on the street the only way he could at the time. Bit by bit he is slowly taking back control of his life. Far too many of my patients were abused by a relative, someone who should have been safe to be around.

Chaotic home life: When you grow up in a family that does not set clear expectations for behavior, with parents who are not paying much attention to what their children are doing, you are at higher risk of addiction. Parents in chaotic homes may dole out severe or inconsistent punishment, which just makes things worse. Young people exposed to a lot of family conflict, including acrimonious divorce, are also statistically more likely to become addicts.[3] In our house, with nine children and two parents working full-time, supervision was often less than ideal.

High anxiety and depression: Children with high anxiety are more likely to suffer from addiction as adults.[4] Forty percent of the patients in my addiction practice had previously been diagnosed with anxiety or depression. I suspect most of my patients struggle with some level of anxiety, though it has not been diagnosed as a disorder. These anxious or depressed young people start using as a way to self-medicate and keep their emotions under lock and key. One thirteen-year-old in my practice who was suffering from post-traumatic stress, depression, and difficulties in school started smoking marijuana every day because, as he told me, "It's my medicine."

Positive feelings toward drugs: Studies show that if you come from a family with favorable attitudes toward drugs and alcohol you are also at higher risk.[5] Your parents' attitude matters. If your parents tend to look positively on drugs and alcohol, it is more likely you will use. When your friends and peers are using and you believe it's "no big deal," you are also more likely to become addicted. A straight-A student in high school and president of the Honor Society, Anita grew up in a family where alcohol was everywhere. "It was very normal at our house to get drunk," she recalls. She had her first blackout in eighth grade. "That is what celebration was to me. You have a party. You get drunk." Anita, whose drinking problem worsened while she was attending an Ivy League university, and her sister both became alcoholics.

Easy access: Ease of availability of drugs and alcohol is one of the most important risk factors for early initiation into drinking or drug use.[6] As I mentioned earlier, the complete absence of drugs, alcohol, and cigarettes in my childhood delayed my progression along the addiction spectrum and protected me from the dangers of early brain exposure. My kids have had much easier access to drugs and alcohol than I did growing up in the southern part of Africa. In the United States, where my children spent their adolescence, drugs

Some Factors That Move You Along the Addiction Spectrum

- Family history of addiction
- Epigenetics—how your individual genes are expressed
- Lack of nurture, protection, and sober mentors
- Lack of nutrients in food
- Lack of diversity in the GI tract (a depleted microbiome)
- Inadequate vitamin D and time outside
- Early exposure to drugs and alcohol
- Exposure to toxins in food, air, water, and the environment
- Overuse of pharmaceuticals
- Opportunity and availability of drugs and alcohol
- Feelings of loneliness, social anxiety, and disconnectedness
- Boredom, lack of a sense of purpose
- Stress
- Poor-quality sleep
- Not enough exercise
- Divorce, death, or other serious loss
- Serious injury or chronic, debilitating pain
- Overprescription of highly addictive drugs

are ubiquitous. Our fair city of Portland, Oregon, has the fourth highest drug-use rate in the United States[7] despite being twenty-seventh in population.[8] With genetic predisposition, parents battling their own addiction issues, and such easy access, perhaps it's not a surprise that five of my children have also struggled with substance use.

Oppositional personality: A tendency toward oppositional behavior also predisposes people to drug use and addiction. That certainly describes Josh, a patient of mine being treated for heroin and meth addiction, whose story I share in chapter 5. Josh frankly explains that he's always had an issue with authority. "I'm like a petulant child," he says. "If someone tells me, 'You can sit anywhere, *except* that chair,' I'm like, 'I want to sit in *that chair*, dude.'"

Nutrient Depletion and Stress

Most Americans are eating food not only lacking in nutrients but also loaded with pesticides, herbicides, and artificial dyes and colors. You're not getting enough sunshine or vitamin D, time outdoors, or exercise. You're stressed out, being constantly bombarded by social media and screen time, and sleep-deprived. Your gut health, which is linked to brain health, is compromised.

Disconnectedness

Despite feeling connected via your smartphones, you are actually feeling more isolated than ever. This lack of human-to-human connection, along with exposure to so many toxins, may be the last straw, pushing you along the addiction spectrum. Not only are you self-medicating the loneliness and emptiness you feel, you are trying to overcome the physical problems you have because of an unhealthy lifestyle.

So What *Is* Addiction?

The question of what addiction *is* isn't as easy to answer as you might think. Even the experts in the field of addiction medicine aren't always clear on the differences between addiction, dependence, and bad habits.

Except for the small number of babies born to moms who were actively drinking or using drugs, we all start life as nonusers. As a teen you're excited about the thrill, you're having fun and feeling cool. There is something very enticing about the forbidden, especially when it is a drug or a drink that helps you feel carefree. But this drug use, even though it's sporadic and seemingly harmless, primes your brain, which is especially vulnerable the younger you are. You start to progress along the addiction spectrum. You make yourself sick by overusing, or you put yourself or others in danger with destructive behavior, like driving drunk or having unprotected sex.

Your use might have started as a way to mask your pain, but then the use itself starts to generate more pain. You're attracted to drugs or alcohol because you are seeking relief—from a painful past, from anxiety, from thoughts and feelings that you don't know how to deal with. Some honestly just love the effect that alcohol or drugs produce; you simply want more. Then you experience more psychological problems because of the addiction.

Just to be clear, I'm not interested in judging anyone for illegal or illicit behavior, even if this behavior concerns me because it's harmful to your health. What I am interested in doing is helping you better understand what is leading you to the severe end of the addiction spectrum, so you can turn it around. I want to help you move in a positive direction in your life and provide you with the tools you will need to find freedom, serenity, and a sense of purpose.

So when I am talking about addiction, I am talking about a **chronic relapsing condition that involves an unhealthy relationship with drugs, alcohol, or other behaviors.** This unhealthy relationship includes:

- An irresistible compulsion
- An inability to limit the use or behavior
- Physical and emotional withdrawal symptoms

Addiction is when your repetitive drinking, drug use, or behavior—and your extreme preoccupation with it—gets beyond your control. You can't stop even if you want to. When you try to quit, you experience overwhelming cravings and severe withdrawal symptoms. You need more and more of the substance or behavior to get the same effects. Your only relief from withdrawal comes from indulging again. Every cell in your body tells you, "I need this." You suspect or even know that you're in trouble, but you ignore the warning signs. Your addiction is your best friend. You can't conceive of life without it. You are now on the severe end of the addiction spectrum.

Addiction Is Dangerous

Many addicts don't make it out of adolescence. They may die from a drug overdose or alcohol poisoning or from an accident related to addiction. Sadly, we all know someone. A young man in treatment with my son Noah died four months after completing the program from a heroin overdose. Maiya's roommate was a heroin addict and committed suicide. Our friend's eighteen-year-old daughter, drunk and high on the back of her boyfriend's motorcycle, died in a crash. Two of the seven friends in Maiya's process group also died. One, Lydia, was in her late thirties when she killed herself because she could not stop drinking. The other, Stephanie, was in and out of treatment but continued to relapse on opioids. Stephanie died from use-related health complications when she was in her early thirties, leaving two little kids and a devastated husband behind.

Take a quick look at the headlines, and you'll see hundreds of other tragic stories: thirteen-year-old Nathan Wylie, who overdosed on what was suspected to be his father's heroin,[9] in Ohio; fifteen-year-old Ryleigh Ackles, who nearly died of alcohol poisoning while at a sleepover with her friends,[10] in Massachusetts; sixteen-year-old Sirena Lawson, who took five Xanax, paid a neighbor for heroin, and overdosed, in Michigan.[11] If you survive your teens and young adulthood, you often face a litany of physical and psychological problems later—everything from liver damage, endocrine disruption, and high blood pressure to anxiety, depression, and suicidal thoughts. In extreme cases you lose everything—your job, your home, your family.

Common Addictions

Most of us are familiar with alcohol; nicotine (the addictive agent in tobacco); prescription medications like fentanyl and oxycodone, used by doctors to treat both chronic and acute pain; cocaine; and heroin. Though they aren't in the news as often, there are many other highly addictive drugs—some legal, some illegal—that people find themselves abusing. These include benzodiazepines ("benzos") like Valium, Xanax, and Ativan, which are prescribed to treat anxiety, insomnia, and alcohol withdrawal. There are the rave drugs like MDMA (Ecstasy, Molly), sedatives like barbiturates and sleeping pills, hallucinogens like LSD and mushrooms, and stimulants like methamphetamine. There are inhalants, like solvents, paints, nitrites, and anesthetics, that people also abuse; and there are, of course, marijuana and ADHD medications.

Certain behaviors—like gambling, playing video games, and watching porn—can also be highly addictive for some. Gabor Maté, a medical doctor based in Canada who worked for twelve years with drug addicts on the east side of Vancouver, British Columbia, describes being addicted to buying classical music CDs. Although buying Mozart and Liszt may seem so benign that it's almost comical to consider it an addiction, Maté details how obsessed he became, how he lied to his wife about it, spent thousands of dollars on CDs, and felt great shame about a behavior that started to control his life.

Maté points out that Imelda Marcos, First Lady of the Philippines for twenty years, was addicted to shopping, spending lavishly while her country experienced extreme poverty. She amassed as many as three thousand pairs of shoes. Many high-achieving corporate executives and businessmen become addicted to money.

I don't want to leave the impression that all addictions are equal in their severity or in how they impact your life. Some addictive substances are so physically toxic that they will destroy you if you keep using them. The average life expectancy for a heavy meth user is thought to be between five and seven years[12]—if you begin using heavily at twenty, you may be dead by the time you are between twenty-five and twenty-seven. Other addictions—like shopping or gambling—usually don't put your life in jeopardy. But they do compromise the quality of your life, your relationships with other people, and your general health and well-being. No one is perfect. And I would even argue that we don't need to try to be perfect. If we remember that the goal for all of us—whatever our vices—is optimal health and wellness, that helps put things in perspective.

Why Are Humans So Prone to Addiction?

I'm simplifying a little here, but nearly all addiction works on the brain in the same way. As a human being you are hardwired to seek out pleasure. Put a newborn baby on the mother's body, and the baby will slowly find the way to her nipple and start suckling. Breastfeeding fills a baby's brain with nutrients and with pleasure—as do all of the activities and behaviors essential to the baby's survival, including being held skin-to-skin, cuddled, and kissed. The more secure an infant feels, the more the brain and body are filled with positive chemicals. One of the main chemicals involved in helping the brain feel pleasure is dopamine, a neurotransmitter that sends chemical signals to cells throughout the body. Anything pleasurable—reading a book, drawing, walking in nature, going for a bike ride, making love—can increase dopamine levels in the body, but addictive drugs, especially, give the brain and body a huge dopamine rush, leading to that telltale euphoric feeling. And once you get that rush, you want it again and again.

People who are boosting their dopamine with one substance will turn to other substances if their substance of choice is removed. My colleague Marvin Seppala, who is a medical doctor, addiction special-ist, and the chief medical officer of one of the largest recovery pro-grams in the United States, gives a lecture entitled, "My Dopamine Made Me Do It." Although for some people positive dopamine-derived feelings may not trigger a desire for more, for those moving toward the severe end of the addiction spectrum, once this reward pathway is sufficiently established and stimulated, a craving develops that drives you to seek more of your substance or behavior of choice.

My Progression Along the Addiction Spectrum

In college and medical school my diet was poor, I was vitamin D defi-cient, I was getting almost no exercise, and I was sleep-deprived. As I juggled work and school to make ends meet, my life was filled with stress and a feeling of disconnectedness. My family was still in Africa, so I had very limited social support. I was now in the moderate range of the addiction spectrum and binge drinking on the weekends, but I still didn't know I had a problem with alcohol.

By 1989 I was working as a pediatrician in Portland at Randall Chil-dren's Hospital. I was teaching residents and medical students. I was in charge of the pediatric after-hours clinic, and I established and led the Friday morning case conferences, where residents, medical stu-dents, and pediatricians from all over town would come to hear the cases I presented. I was at the top of my game. I was also addicted to alcohol.

I followed self-imposed rules. I would only drink after work, usually in the evenings, and never on nights when I was on call. But as I progressed along the addiction spectrum, I started to break even these rules. I would wake up hung over, remorseful, and ashamed. "I did it. I drank too much. I'm done. I'm going to quit," I'd say. Then I'd get drunk again.

I had a tradition of taking time to reflect on my life each New Year's Eve. I would make a colorful poster with pictures cut from magazines of goals for the coming year. Goal number one at the top of my pyramid on that 1989 poster, and for many years after that? *Stop drinking.*

But despite my resolve, it took me thirteen more years to get sober. In 2000 I sat in my first meeting as a participant in Alcoholics Anonymous. I stayed sober for three months. Even though I knew then that I was an alcoholic, felt highly motivated to stop drinking, and even found a sponsor, it wasn't enough. I had proven to myself thousands of times that I couldn't just have one or two drinks. I told myself I would stop, only to find my car heading to the liquor store on the way home after work. That car seemed to have a mind of its own.

In meetings I listened to Brandon, my sponsor, repeatedly talk about how alcoholics have no effective mental defense against drinking,[13] but I didn't really believe it. I felt I wasn't like the other people in the meetings: I wasn't really an alcoholic. *I* was a successful doctor. *They* got out of control; *I* just went a little overboard once in a while.

If I had known about the addiction spectrum and integrative medicine, I would have become aware that I could have stopped my progression from mild to severe with lifestyle and other integrative interventions. I could have learned how to heal my body and my brain and reduce my craving for alcohol by addressing the underlying causes that were making me want to drink. Had I known earlier how to clean up my diet, practice better self-care, and follow the other protocols in this book, I could have saved myself and my family years of suffering and pain.

When I was recovering from my addiction, I didn't know the things you'll learn in this book. What I want to give to you is the knowledge I wish I'd had, so that your recovery is smooth and you are primed for success. I'll tell you the rest of my recovery story in chapter 6 as we take the next steps toward recovery together through the pages in this book.

Maybe you've heard the story of the old man and his hound? An old man was sitting on his front porch with his hound dog. His hound dog was always howling and making a racket. One day a neighbor walked by and asked, "Why's your dog always howling?"

"Oh," the man answered, "he's sittin' on a nail."

"Well, why doesn't he get off the nail?" the neighbor asked.

"I guess it doesn't hurt bad enough," the old man said.

I don't want you to spend your life sitting on nails, hurting so badly you're howling but not hurting badly enough to seek help. Recovery is a journey of action that begins with getting off the nail. Throughout this book, I give you the tools to make the changes that will lead you to freedom, serenity, and a sense of purpose.

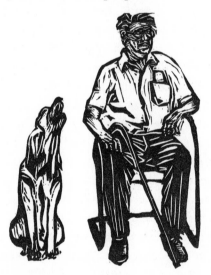

Now let's talk about why some of our most basic beliefs about addiction are actually wrong.

CHAPTER 2

Myths and Facts About Addiction

MORE THAN HALF of all adults in America today struggle with chronic health problems.[1] Besides full-blown addiction, adults suffer from attention deficit disorders like ADD and ADHD; mental illnesses like anxiety, depression, and bipolar affective disorder; and endocrine disruption that manifests as obesity, weight issues, and thyroid disorders. Then there's chronic fatigue and fibromyalgia (a widespread pain disorder) as well as allergies and autoimmune conditions—asthma, diabetes, eczema, inflammatory bowel disease, celiac disease, and rheumatoid arthritis, to name just a few. And nearly 15 million of us are living with cancer.[2] What your doctor is not telling you is that the first line of defense to better manage and sometimes even completely reverse your chronic health problems is right outside your window—in the garden—and right there in your dining room— on your breakfast, lunch, and dinner plates. The choices you make about what to eat, how much to eat, and even how you eat your food determine first and foremost how well your body and your brain will work. The second line of defense is your lifestyle choices—how much exercise you do throughout the day, how much sunlight you get, how much time you spend outside, how you manage your stress and anxiety levels, how many other environmental toxins and harmful chemicals you're exposed to (in your air, water, homes, cosmetics, hygiene products, and elsewhere), and the people you choose to have in your lives.

But don't expect your conventionally trained addiction doctor to ask you *any* questions about your eating and lifestyle habits. In fact, if you suggest that changes to your diet and an increase in exercise and non-toxic living might be the first steps toward conquering your addiction and health problems, your doctor will likely scoff.

A quick look at the food in your doctor's own refrigerator and cupboards will reveal why. American physicians—just like the rest of us—don't eat real food anymore. They eat highly processed faux food, which is loaded with pesticides and herbicides and full of fillers, additives (like mold inhibitors), and petroleum-based "food" dyes. Glyphosate (the main ingredient in the weed killer Roundup), which you may already be concerned about because of the mainstream press it has gotten of late, is just the tip of the iceberg. Decades of hybridizing wheat for higher gluten content along with other food-science technology that has led to genetically engineering crops to withstand pesticides and herbicides, splicing together genetic pieces of different species to grow everything from chickens to tomatoes faster, and creating artificial flavor enhancers—all of this has produced Frankenfood, which is taking a heavy toll on our health because it affects our moods, our energy levels, and our brains. **Addiction is primarily a brain disorder.** When we feed our addict brains with Frankenfood, while simultaneously leading a sedentary lifestyle, which is known to cause depression, and experiencing stress and anxiety on top of all that, is it any wonder that for many of us our condition gets worse?

Eating real food grown without chemicals and as close to its natural state as possible is the most radical step you can take for any of your health issues, including addiction. And there's more that you can do to jump-start the healing process, including reducing gluten and dairy in your diet, eating naturally fermented foods with every meal, taking high-quality probiotics, and getting enough vitamin D, preferably from sunshine. But most addiction doctors have almost no training in nutrition, no time to keep up with the scientific literature, and no interest in helping support the body to heal itself naturally when it's quicker and easier to prescribe medication, make a referral to therapy, and move on to the next patient.

Most conventional docs are not even aware that **healing gut inflammation has the potential to heal the brain and reverse autoimmune conditions and chronic health issues**. Mention this to them, and they will give you that all-knowing smile of contempt or might even ridicule you for being so gullible as to fall for all that natural alternative "nonsense."

Over 100 million nerve cells line your gastrointestinal
tract.[3] Your brain is in your gut. So is almost 70 percent of
your immune system.[4] Healing the gut strengthens the
immune system and heals the brain.

The approach conventionally trained doctors take to almost every condition is to make a diagnosis and then write a prescription. If that doesn't work, they make a referral to a specialist. When patients push back, they label them—often in writing in their charts—as difficult or noncompliant. The saddest part of all of this is these doctors are too blind to even know what they don't know. They refuse to admit that the human body is a whole package and to fix any part of it we must pay attention to *every* part of it. These doctors don't want to admit they don't have the training or knowledge to treat the whole person, which is what integrative and functional medical practitioners strive to do. They just don't have the bandwidth or the desire to embark on their own journey of discovery to figure out what works best for an individual patient. Doing so is time consuming, highly individualized, and sometimes difficult. It is much easier to make blanket recommendations, offer one-size-fits-all "solutions," and insist that there is only One Right Way.

Doctors also feel defensive. They feel threatened by new ideas or new ways of thinking, threatened by the thought that they themselves might be eating poorly or too much, living too stationary or even too sanitary a lifestyle, and being exposed to too many toxins. They find it easier to just dismiss anything that does not lend itself to a pharmaceutical fix.

Addiction Is Complicated

Your place on the addiction spectrum is not static. You can go weeks or even months without your substance of choice, but then start using again, going from mild to severe in a matter of hours. The truth is that each person's struggle with substance abuse is unique. At the same time, **it is not weak character that causes addiction, just as it is not weak character that leads to breast cancer, asthma, atten-**

tion deficit disorder, or any other health problem. It is our genetic vulnerabilities along with environmental toxins (stress, unhealthy food, and early neglect, abuse, or chaos are included in this definition of environmental toxins) that create the fertile ground within which addictions develop. Vibrant health requires embracing a new lifestyle that starts with eating real food as well as avoiding toxic foods, people, and environments.

Doctors working in the field of addiction medicine and you yourself may have negative stereotypes about what causes addiction and what it takes to beat it. Yet many beliefs about addiction are not, in fact, true.

Now that I've convinced you that **you must take an integrative approach to addiction** (I have convinced you, haven't I?), I want to examine—and dispel—some of the common myths about addicts.

Myth #1

"Addiction is the addict's fault." Most people used to believe, and many still do, that it's *your fault* that you became an addict or an alcoholic. All you had to do was say no.

Addiction is much more complicated than that. Since 2011 there has been a profound shift in how the medical community understands addiction. It was then, after four years of study and consultation with over eighty experts, that the American Society of Addiction Medicine (ASAM) released a new definition of addiction characterizing it as a chronic brain disorder: "Addiction is a primary, chronic disease of brain reward, motivation, memory, and related circuitry. Dysfunction in these circuits leads to characteristic biological, psychological, social, and spiritual manifestations. . . . Like other chronic diseases, addiction often involves cycles of relapse and remission."[5] Once considered a moral and spiritual failing, addiction, as most doctors understand it now, is actually a disease, a chronic brain disorder that, in its most extreme forms, will cause cognitive decline, organ failure, and premature death.

There is ongoing controversy about the disease aspect of addiction. Many consider addiction to be primarily a behavioral disorder, something we learned as we tried to adapt to the stresses in our lives. I believe that the psychological, spiritual, and social aspects of this condition are as important as the medical ones. **Addiction is actually a *public-health crisis*, a symptom of our failure as a society to protect those at risk.**

We can craft better treatment plans when we remember that a young person who is addicted or on the road to addiction is not weak, but rather is someone who has been failed by the educational system, the medical system, and our public-health institutions, as I'll be talking more about in the next chapter. In order to help that young person reverse course, we have to pay attention to both his or her individual case and the ways in which society is responsible. Addiction is not someone else's setback. It is our *collective problem* and one that can only be solved when we all take responsibility for it.

Myth #2

"Successful people don't get addicted." Many people believe that intelligent, highly educated people with integrity and willpower do not become alcoholics or addicts.

This simply isn't true. The truth is that anyone can become addicted to drugs or alcohol. In fact, gifted children—those out-of-the-box thinkers who have unique ways of learning and looking at the world—are actually overrepresented among illicit drug users and addicts.[6] Addiction is not something that happens to losers; addiction is something that can happen to anyone. People struggling with addiction are not stupid.

Charles Dickens was addicted to opium. *Star Trek* star Leonard Nimoy struggled with alcoholism, as did the nineteenth-century painter Vincent van Gogh. First Lady Betty Ford was addicted to painkillers, which is why there's now a center named in her honor. One of America's most accomplished literary giants, Ernest Hemingway, was also an alcoholic. Science fiction writer Philip K. Dick had a problem with amphetamines (he died of a stroke when he was fifty-three years old), and horror writer Stephen King, one of the world's bestselling authors, needed a cocktail of drugs to get him through the day before he got sober. Your doctor, your child's teacher, your favorite YouTuber, blogger, actor, or singer may also be an addict.

I'm not giving you these examples to glorify addiction. There is nothing glorious about abusing drugs. There's nothing glorious about dying of alcohol-induced cirrhosis of the liver. But I think it is important for all of us to remember that addiction is often a hallmark of misdirected intelligence and underserved creativity, not of laziness, moral failings, or stupidity.

Myth #3

"All it takes is willpower to stop addiction." Millions of Americans use mind-altering drugs every year, but only one in every ten of those who try them actually becomes addicted. Millions more gamble, watch pornography, play video games, and enjoy sex. All of us must eat to survive. Most of us have smartphones. So who ends up an addict? Why can one young man engage in a highly pleasurable experience—like gaming or sex—and walk away from it without a backward glance, while another, perhaps his own brother, finds himself addicted?

"Why do you have to drown yourself?" was my mom's question one day after I had nearly killed myself with alcohol. I was eighteen, our family was building a house in Monroe, New Hampshire, and I had been invited to a garbage-can party by some local friends. Fresh-faced from boarding school in Swaziland, I didn't know that inside that black plastic garbage can was mostly hard liquor mixed with just a little Kool-Aid. It tasted like Kool-Aid to me. It was a hot day, and I gulped down three or four 20-ounce glasses of the stuff like it was water. That's all I remember.

When I woke up at 3:00 p.m. the next day, I had the worst headache of my life; angry elves with sharpened knives were hacking at the inside of my skull. I felt terrible. I didn't want to ever get that drunk again, and I told myself I never would. The next time I had a drink I didn't intend to black out. And I certainly didn't enjoy the headaches and hangovers that followed. But, despite my strong resolve not to, at any opportunity to drink too much that was just what I did.

For the alcoholic or addict, it is not a matter of willpower. Willpower is the exact thing that leaves the second you put a drink to your lips or take that first dose of your drug of choice. It is at that moment that your craving kicks in, and you lose the power of choice. If you aren't an addict, this is one of the hardest things to understand about your loved one's behavior. There are some exceptions to this rule, but most of us have little or no defense against the overwhelming urge to have another drink or take another drug. Our subconscious wiring and learned behaviors become so automatic that they create an inability to see clearly and remember what happened last time.

Virtually all addicts or alcoholics who have become aware of their condition, aware that they need to stop, aware that the alcohol, drugs, or behavioral addiction is destroying their lives and hurting not just themselves but others, want desperately to stop. But because addiction has affected and altered your brain, you have lost the power of choice.

Can you have one or two drinks and stop? Once you start to feel buzzed, can you walk away? If you can't, it's not because you have no willpower; it's because you have an illness. There is no human power great enough to keep you from using. No, willpower alone will not stop addiction. What you need to do is heal your brain, which will enable you to take control of your life.

Myth #4

"The cause of alcoholism is alcohol. The cause of drug addiction is drugs." It is important to understand that the bacteria in our gut ferment sugars into alcohol, so we are always exposed to tiny amounts of alcohol even if we don't drink a drop.[7] We have opioid receptors, cannabinoid receptors, and numerous other receptors in our brains that provide us with a system of pain relief and feelings of pleasure, which is all perfectly natural. Seeking out good feelings, enjoying the natural endorphins and adrenaline that our bodies produce, and looking for ways to relax and have fun are all part of being human, as I mentioned in the last chapter. It's when we abuse drugs, alcohol, or pleasurable behaviors that we have a problem.

Different cultures tolerate different drugs, considering some "bad" and others perfectly acceptable. In Peru ayahuasca, a hallucinogenic brew made from a vine that grows in the Amazon, is legal and used in traditional healing. In Muslim countries like Somalia and Yemen, chewing qat or khat (a leafy plant that contains cathinone, a Schedule I drug in the United States) is a widely accepted national pastime, but drinking alcohol is considered taboo.[8] I agree with Andrew Weil, MD, one of the founding fathers of integrative medicine. "Any drug can be used successfully," Weil writes, "no matter how bad its reputation, and any drug can be abused, no matter how accepted it is. There are no good or bad drugs; there are only good and bad relationships with drugs."[9]

I'm not a big fan of drugs, to be honest. I'd rather you never try any and stay away from people who are using them. But I also recognize that tremendous creativity and healing have come from the use of both drugs and alcohol.

Opioids are being overprescribed and abused, but they are also important for some pain management, as I'll explore more in chapter 4. It would be brutal indeed to have major surgery without morphine or another opiate for pain relief. But continuing to use morphine once the pain has passed can get you addicted, not because of the drug itself—at least not at first—but because you start abusing it.

As Gabor Maté, MD, has noted, if it were the substance or behavior itself that causes the addiction, everyone who goes shopping would become a shopaholic and everyone who eats food would become a food addict. Your alcoholism or drug addiction is but a symptom of a larger problem of compromised psychological and physical well-being.

Myth #5

"It's okay for kids to experiment with drinking and drugs—they're just being kids." Walker and his friends started smoking dope in the bushes after school freshman year. Lisa started stealing wine from her parents' liquor cabinet when she was fourteen. Sam, an eighth grader, dismissed her mom's concerns about her drug use. *"Everyone* at school is doing drugs!" Sam said. "Lighten up." So what if her uncle died of a cocaine overdose in his thirties? She's sure there's *no way* that would happen to her. "Mom, you know *I* would *never* try cocaine."

Most parents in my practice believe that it's harmless for teenagers to experiment with drugs. They laugh it off, shrug their shoulders, and say, "It's no big deal. Kids will be kids." Since our friends' children are experimenting too, we tell ourselves it's normal. At the same time, we are all bombarded with advertisements glorifying the use of alcohol and, more recently, marijuana, which serve to reinforce the idea that these potentially addictive substances are just good old-fashioned fun.

But the more we learn about the vulnerabilities of the developing brain, the more we discover that early drug and alcohol use is the opposite of harmless. It's really *not* okay for kids to experiment with drinking and drugs. It's anything but harmless. And it's not "just being a kid."

We know without a doubt that the earlier you start drinking or using drugs, the more likely you are to succumb to addiction later in life. The fact is that the younger you start, the worse it is for you. Young brains are more vulnerable to addiction. Young brains also experience pleasure in a more heightened way. Kids really do have more fun than adults. But what that means is that when children expose their brains to drugs, they are at higher risk of addiction. "Having fun" is more like playing with fire, as that "fun" can lead to a lifetime of struggle. You have a six times greater chance of being an alcoholic if you start drinking before age fifteen than if you start at or after age twenty-one.[10] Those who start using marijuana at an early age are nearly twice as likely to become addicted.[11]

My own children have struggled with addiction, in part because my wife and I didn't give this enough thought and did not know how to keep them from early exposure. My younger brother, Bruce, has genetics similar to mine, obviously, and had a similar upbringing. Yet Bruce has two amazingly bright girls who have never struggled with substance abuse. Bruce and his wife, Michela, were more open about sharing the family's struggles with addiction, more vigilant about keeping drugs and alcohol away from their daughters, and careful never to make using drugs or drinking seem "cool," "fun," or "harmless." They kept their daughters busy in after-school activities and didn't allow them to spend the night at anyone else's house. Sleepovers were at their place, where they always knew where the girls were and what they were doing.

We can argue all day about overscheduled kids or overvigilant parenting, but the truth is that kids who are involved in lots of extracurricular activities; who have positive, healthy outlets for stress and anxiety; and whose parents are keeping closer tabs on what they're doing, where they are, and who they're with are less likely to become addicts. Using drugs in your teens is not harmless. It's potentially devastating.

Myth #6

"You have to hit rock bottom before you can climb out of addiction." Most people believe that you have to "hit bottom" or "bottom out" to conquer your addiction. That simply isn't true. You can jump off the addiction train at any station; you don't have to wait for it to be going so fast that it derails and falls into the ocean.

As we mentioned in the last chapter, people on that train toward self-destruction usually progress from being fully functional to becoming desperate and nonfunctioning over the course of months or years. The challenge is that the farther along you are, the less likely it is that you have any choice in the matter. But the truth is that you can—and should—stop the train at any point. You don't have to hit bottom. It's possible you won't be successful at first, but then you try again. Wherever you are in the process, you can use the techniques in this book to help yourself.

Myth #7

"If an addict doesn't want to be treated, there's nothing you can do." Maiya was days away from an overdose. Her doctor hadn't realized that she was hiding IV morphine and injecting herself with it. I hadn't realized it either. But the kids and I had noticed that Maiya was falling asleep at the dinner table, slurring her words, and walking unsteadily. I was scared we were going to lose her. I arranged for an intervention. Our family counselor was there, along with three of her closest friends, her younger sister, and me. I had already contacted her doctor, who had secured a bed at a local treatment center and gotten it preapproved by our insurance plan. Shocked and resistant, Maiya reluctantly went into treatment.

Maiya wanted to be well, but she did not want to stop using. She was scared that she would die if she didn't have access to her opioids, a feeling many addicts share. Withdrawal from opioids is very intense and painful, and the reason Maiya had started taking them in the first place was because she had been genuinely in terrible pain. She was also still in denial about her use. "I have real pain—you don't understand!" was her defensive response to all of our questions, no matter how gentle, about her use. But with her loved ones gathered together, along with our family counselor, we were united. We did not offer her any other choice. So Maiya got in the van, crying, shaking, furious, but surrounded by those who loved and cared about her most. She now has over fifteen years of sobriety, sponsors other women who are suffering, and is a shining example of a life saved.

Most of you are told that if you don't want it badly enough, your treatment will fail. You are shamed and scolded and exhorted to care more and try harder. Although it's true, and I'll talk more about this, that willingness can help you move from the severe toward the mild end of the spectrum, it's not true that you have to *feel* ready for treatment. You can get treatment even if you aren't ready. You can be helped even if you know, deep inside yourself, that you don't want it. Who wants to lose their crutch? Their most faithful companion?

It is often more difficult to convince teenagers they have a problem than adults. But legal guardians, depending on state laws and the age of consent, can force treatment on children under a certain age. It gets trickier for adults. In some states, including Ohio and Kentucky, there are laws in place allowing family members to petition for court-ordered involuntary treatment. I never want to talk to another parent or partner who regrets not intervening or who wishes they insisted on treatment the minute they discovered the problem. If your loved one is sick, you must help him or her get well. If an addict in your life does not want treatment, do everything in your power to help him anyway.

Myth #8

"Drinking and drugs are fun. Being sober is boring." The human brain thrives on stimulation. We all want to feel good. As I mentioned above and as I will remind you throughout this book, there's nothing wrong with seeking out pleasurable experiences. You are hardwired to look for pleasure and do everything you can to diminish pain. That makes sense. It becomes a problem when the pleasure you have found—which you mistake for your best friend—is actually a wolf in sheep's clothing bent on destroying you.

Maybe you're worried that once you stop using, you'll never have fun again. Using gives you an instant group of friends to party with

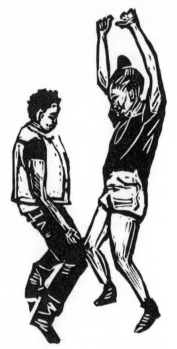

SOBRIETY IS **NOT** BORING!

and feel close to, and the drugs and alcohol you enjoy with others gives you a sense of intimacy and urgency that was lacking when you were sober. But the most effective addiction programs teach you to replace unhealthy pleasure-seeking behaviors with healthy, nonaddictive, pleasure-producing activities. You can get high as often as you want in sobriety! And feel good! But the ways you find your high will change.

Last Christmas my AA friends rented a bus with an amazing sound system. Our group, about twenty-five squarely sober adults, drove through the streets of Portland looking at the Christmas lights, bedazzled by the displays, and singing at the top of our lungs. Some of us got up from our seats and danced our hearts out. You would never have guessed there was not a drop of alcohol or drugs on that bus. Pure and simple clean sober fun. No, we are not a glum lot. Sobriety is not boring.

Myth #9

"It's all in your genes. You're hardwired to be an addict." When we're looking for something to blame for addiction, genes make a good punching bag. Some scientists still believe that genes are *everything* when it comes to addiction and that succumbing to addiction for some unlucky souls is as unavoidable and inevitable as having blue eyes or blond hair. Based on studies that looked at addiction in siblings, particularly twins, it appears that 50 to 60 percent of addiction is hereditary.[12] Does that mean you will be an alcoholic or an addict if one or both of your parents is one? Of course not.

When my wife was in treatment for opioid addiction, she asked her physician if he was an alcoholic.

"No idea," he said. "I've never had a drink." Alcoholism ran in his family. He chose not to tempt his genetic fate.

In the right environment—like Maiya's doctor's total abstinence—it is not a problem to have this or that genetic tendency. In the wrong environment—stress, childhood neglect, nutrient deficiencies, drug or alcohol use during gestation, or a toxic chemical overload dumped on you during your early years—your genetic tendencies become a recipe for trouble. You may have been told that your addiction is genetic and that you have no control over your diagnosis and your treatment. But don't let anyone dupe you into believing that you have "bad" genes. We know now that it is actually possible to activate or deactivate your genes through lifestyle decisions. This is exactly what Maiya's doctor did: he chose not to activate his genetic risk for alcoholism.

Although DNA does play a role in addiction, human behavior is much more complicated than simple on/off genetic switches. Where you are on the addiction spectrum at any given time in your life depends on your unique combination of genetic vulnerabilities and current life circumstances. The less you are paying attention to your nutrition, vitamin D levels, gut microbiome, stress, sleep, exercise, and connectedness to a supportive network of other people, the greater your chance of moving toward the severe end of the spectrum.

How your potential gene expression interacts with your environment is called epigenetics. Although both your genetics and your epigenetics affect the pain and pleasure receptors in your brain, how quickly you metabolize drugs, and how well you respond to different medications, it is becoming increasingly clear that epigenetics matters more. This is good news. You are not chained to your genes, and you can choose how your genes manifest in your life. You have the power to influence how the genes you have that put you at risk for addiction are expressed.

Your genes are not your destiny.

Myth #10

"Making lifestyle changes cannot help you as an addict." In the same way that conventional medical thought leaders dismiss the idea that we can reverse autoimmune disorders, heal from cancer, and improve our brain functioning through lifestyle interventions, doctors often dismiss the idea that we can reverse addiction through lifestyle changes. Although it is true that we have identified some genetic risk factors for addiction, your genes are not your destiny. Your early exposures are not your destiny either. Addiction does not have to be a death sentence. From the most benign behaviors that have somehow gotten out of hand (like Gabor Maté's obsession with classical CDs) to the most full-blown and seemingly intractable addictions, where patients are on the verge of death, addiction can be conquered, as I've seen with my own eyes.

Lifestyle changes are actually the key to both overcoming addiction and mitigating the poor health outcomes resulting from substance abuse. As I talk about throughout this book, nonmedical interventions, including better eating habits, more exercise, reduced stress, and finding other ways to produce natural, healthy, sustainable feelings of euphoria (as opposed to potentially lethal drug-induced highs), are crucial when it comes to treating addiction.

Lifestyle changes have literally saved my life and supercharged my ability to live in recovery. Because I stay connected to a recovery program, committed to a healthy lifestyle, and am constantly vigilant, there is no way I would go back to the severe end of the addiction spectrum. I look back on that time of bondage and say, "Hell, no!"

You too can implement the changes in this book and experience peace and serenity as never before. The more sunshine you get, exercise you enjoy, pain relief you seek from natural sources, and stress you reduce; the better the foods you eat, the restorative sleep you get, and the support you get for your gut microbiome; and the more connected you become to people in a positive drug- and alcohol-free way of living, the less your risk for relapse. Not only that, but you will be healthier in every way.

If you continually assess your place on the spectrum, you have a better chance of keeping life's difficulties from getting the better of you. If there is a devastating life event like a death in the family, illness, or injury, you no longer feel destined for failure or relapse. You've built up strength and a capacity for resistance. You pause before impulsive action and decide in each situation which action leads you in the healing direction along the spectrum. You no longer blindly react to life; you control your responses to what happens to you with intention.

Will you make lifestyle changes and stick to them perfectly? No. Is it worth starting the journey back toward the mild end of the addiction spectrum? Yes.

As you work through this book, I will be giving you healthy healing strategies to integrate into your life. Start doing them now. Start with one or two things you know you can do and do them today. Do them again tomorrow. By the end of the week you'll be feeling better and that good feeling will keep you going. But the only way to make it manageable is to concentrate on this moment and this day. One day at a time.

Your journey along the addiction spectrum—like mine, like everyone's—is uniquely your own. Take ownership of where you are now. You make hundreds of little choices each day that impact your place on the addiction spectrum. Armed with the information in this book and the deep knowledge that you can heal your life, you are now in charge. You are not a victim of circumstance. Your hardest challenges become your greatest strengths.

At the same time, big business—from the pharmaceutical companies to the food industry—*purposefully* promotes, cultivates, and nurtures your addictions. Every day you're bombarded with enticements that encourage you to take drugs, drink in excess, make bad food choices, and stay in poor health. In the next chapter I'll explain how medical doctors and corporate America are peddling addiction and how you can keep from being deceived.

CHAPTER 3

How Medical Doctors, Pharmaceutical Companies, the Food Industry, and Our Stressed-out Lives Push Us Toward Addiction

L IKE ALL MEDICAL DOCTORS, I was trained to *diagnose and treat dis-ease*. As I mentioned earlier, most conventional medical doctors—probably most of the doctors you know—think this is the right model to follow. A patient has a problem? Write a prescription and move on to the next patient. Problem solved. Or is it?

What if, instead of *solving* health problems, our current medical system is *creating* problems where they might not otherwise exist? What if medical doctors are actually partially responsible for peddling addiction?

Even before birth, you were probably being exposed to pharmaceuticals. The entire medical profession once cautioned *against using any medication* during pregnancy, but doctors today now aggressively promote insulin injections for gestational diabetes (dismissing lifestyle and nutrition improvements as ineffective), recommend Tylenol (even though we know now acetaminophen is damaging for all age groups, as I discuss in chapter 6), and insist on influenza and pertussis vaccines (despite once insisting expectant women avoid vaccines and currently having no long-term safety studies). Most doctors also encourage epidural anesthesia to ease labor pains without ever telling patients that one of the main ingredients in this drug cocktail, which will enter the baby's bloodstream, is fentanyl, a highly addictive opioid.

Where Addiction Begins

Like fans around the world, I was stunned when the musical genius Prince, who was only fifty-seven, was found dead in his home on April 21, 2016. Then, on June 2, there was more surprising news: Prince, a well-known teetotaler who did not allow drugs or alcohol at his 65,000-square-foot, $10 million Paisley Park estate, died from an accidental overdose of fentanyl.[1]

Fentanyl is a drug that is thirty to fifty times more potent[2] than its illegal cousin heroin and *fifty to a hundred times more potent than morphine.* It is a highly effective, fast-acting, and addictive opioid, a class of drugs I'll be talking more about in the next chapter. Because fentanyl, which goes by the street names China White, China Girl, Apache, and many others, is cheaper and more potent than heroin, dealers cut it into heroin to give the heroin more kick. Fentanyl is so powerful, warned CNN's Sanjay Gupta, MD, during a newscast, "that just a quarter of a milligram can be fatal."[3]

I was glad to see the dangers of fentanyl discussed on the news. But although much was made of Prince's death, most people don't realize that **fentanyl is one of the ingredients in the epidural anesthesia given to women for pain management during childbirth.**

Epidural anesthesia is a localized anesthesia injected into the spine, numbing sensation from the waist down. Epidurals are tremendously popular among women in labor in America: over 60 percent of women in labor in hospitals in America every year, nearly 2 million moms, have epidurals.[4] Epidurals usually contain an anesthetizing agent, such as bupivacaine, chloroprocaine, or lidocaine, along with an opioid like fentanyl or sufentanil. We know that some fentanyl will reach the baby, as will any medication taken by the mother to relieve pain.

The Food and Drug Administration actually cautions against the use of fentanyl during delivery, citing a lack of safety studies: "There are insufficient data to support the use of fentanyl in labor and delivery. Therefore, such use is not recommended." The FDA also points out: "There are no adequate and well-controlled studies in pregnant women."[5]

Colorado-based Louana George, who first worked as a labor and delivery nurse and then practiced midwifery for over thirty years, attending over one thousand births, started researching the effects of epidurals on breast-feeding when she was studying for a master's degree. "Fentanyl rapidly crosses the placenta,"[6] she explains. "Since neonates do not have the blood–brain barrier for opioids, the drug rapidly binds to receptors in the brain. The result is depressed neurobehavioral and breast-feeding in the newborn. This explains why my clients who had epidurals seemed to have trouble initiating breast-feeding."[7]

George found that babies in her clinical practice born to women who had had epidurals were often too sleepy to nurse, couldn't seem to coordinate their suck, and often did not even reach for the breast. She noticed that the difference between epidural babies and babies birthed without medication was striking.

Researchers in Sweden have observed the same phenomenon, which they captured on videotape: infants born to mothers who had been given epidurals had trouble beginning breast-feeding, had higher temperatures, and cried more in the first hours of life.[8] Scientists at Wichita State University have also found that labor pain–relief medication interfered with suckling reflexes.[9]

It makes sense that exposing babies to opioids during the birth process is not a good idea. "While parents may be told that labor medications and epidurals have no effect on newborns, the literature reports significant neurobehavioral effects of these medications on the newborn and the mother-infant relationship,"[10] concludes Marsha Walker, a nurse and lactation consultant who served on the board of directors of the Massachusetts Breastfeeding Coalition.

But could newborn exposure to very small amounts of opioids have a lasting effect? We don't definitively know. But, disturbingly, a 2015 study by a team of researchers at Columbia University found that the use of epidurals was associated with measurable changes in the volume of parts of a newborn's brain.[11]

My colleague Gregory Smith, an addiction and pain-management specialist, producer of the film *American Addict*, and a doctor in private practice in Beverly Hills, California, has administered thousands of epidurals in his thirty years of clinical practice. But Smith now does as few as possible and even advises women against them. "It's not a benign procedure," says Smith. "I would avoid epidurals altogether if you can."[12]

Midwife Louana George thinks we should be talking more about the fentanyl in epidural anesthesia and the role overmanaged and over-medicated childbirth may be playing in the nation's current opioid epidemic. "Maybe it's time, in this era of recognition of the problems with addictions, to look at what could be influencing the onset of addictive behavior," George says. "Maybe it starts with the epidural."[13] I agree.

Peddling Pills

Medical professional organizations give doctors instructions and insurance plans add financial incentives and doctor-rating systems to ensure aggressive pharmaceutical intervention from the first day of a human baby's life. If your baby develops eczema, we prescribe a steroid cream. If your toddler gets asthma, we recommend an expensive inhaler. We prescribe antibiotics for everything from mild ear infections to lung-compromising pneumonia, whether your child needs them or not. Though I would never treat an infant with psychoactive drugs, over 26,400 American infants from birth to age one are prescribed antidepressants and over 227,000 are given anti-anxiety drugs.[14] That's just when they are babies.

By school age, one in six children is struggling with an attention disorder. So then we dose them with stimulants like Ritalin or Adderall, drugs that are just a step removed from meth, as I'll talk about in chapter 5. It gets worse from there. One in four to five teens ages thirteen to eighteen struggles with a mental-health disorder such as anxiety or depression,[15] but, never fear: we have more brain-altering drugs, selective serotonin reuptake inhibitors (SSRIs), for that.

By the time individuals reach adulthood, if they're not dependent on some pharmaceutical drug to stay focused, keep alert, or treat their anxiety, chronic eczema, asthma, insomnia, or other health problem, they're the exception. Indeed, research published in the *Journal of the American Medical Association* in 2015 found that almost 60 percent of Americans are now taking prescription drugs.[16]

Doctors are taught—actually encouraged—to foster an attitude of drug dependence in patients right from the start. We are trained that we must practice what is called the standard of care, which means practicing medicine the way every other doctor practices medicine.

Often referred to as "best practice," the standard of care encourages doctors to continue outdated and sometimes dangerous approaches to medical care, sometimes for decades, stifling innovation and scaring them away from introducing newer, safer, and better practices.

Doctors who practice the standard of care are considered good doctors. But doctors who practice medicine according to their own extensive clinical experience, recent scientific information revealed in peer-reviewed medical journals, and the individual needs of their patients are "deviating" from the standard of care and risk getting reprimanded, blocked by insurance companies, and even sued. Is it any wonder so many patients become addicts? Children and teens start first with doctor-prescribed drugs and then begin self-medicating with illegal substances. The same doctors who helped them along the addiction spectrum are often the first to judge and dismiss addicts, without paying attention to the way addiction fits into the modern agenda of using pills to solve problems.

The medical establishment as well as the drug companies, the food industry, and Silicon Valley work around the clock to push and promote addiction, encouraging the overuse of prescription medication, overeating, excessive screen time, and even substance abuse. That's the bad news, and it's pretty disheartening.

But the good news is that knowledge is power. Realizing how addiction is being peddled and promoted is the first step to resisting it.

I became a doctor to promote lasting health and wellness. But in my obstetrics rotation in medical school we were actually told to treat young women who were having an abortion roughly in order to "teach them a lesson," so they would not have future unwanted pregnancies. As awful and jarring as that sounds, it's true. We also learned that pregnancy was a problem we doctors had to solve by C-section and were told that abdominal birth was the safest method most of the time (which I know now is completely untrue, though many of my colleagues still believe this). In my psychiatry rotation more than 95 percent of the curriculum focused on pharmaceuticals: for anxiety, depression, borderline personality disorders, and bipolar and suicidal patients. There was no concept that the whole person was important, that your underlying health could affect your brain, that what you were eating and how much you were exercising mattered, or that *any* treatment beyond pills or surgery could be of benefit.

It took me, as a practicing physician, a long time to realize that I had become a prescribing machine, that I had been duped by a pharmaceutical industry that cared more about selling pills and promoting sickness than about lasting good health, and that we doctors had actually been contributing to the decline in America's health and the increase in America's addictions. At first I was defensive: like many of my colleagues, I made the mistake of believing that doing something the same way as everyone else was doing it the right way. I didn't want to admit I had been making mistakes. I didn't want to change. But once I realized what was happening, and once I was willing to look honestly, openly, and critically at my own prescribing habits, my way of practicing medicine changed for the better and my patients got healthier.

Diana's Story

Diana, who is in recovery from heroin addiction, has light hair, green eyes, and a wide smile. White and middle class, she had no heroin addicts in her family before she and her sister both started using. Diana's story of how she got hooked is one I hear over and over in my clinic. She had meningitis when she was eighteen, which caused painful headaches. The doctor prescribed opioid pain medication. Finding the root causes of her migraines never crossed his mind.

At first the medication helped. But a few years after she started taking prescription narcotics, Diana couldn't say for sure if she still had migraines or if she just liked the way the pills made her feel. As Anna Lembke, MD, explains in her book *Drug Dealer, MD*, even if you have no history of addiction and no risk factors for it, you can become addicted to opioids in the course of routine medical treatment. "The prescription drug epidemic is first and foremost an epidemic of over-prescribing,"[17] she says. Even today, doctors continue to hand out opioids to children and adults without a backward glance.

Diana was soon hooked. After a few years she couldn't function without medication, and she found she needed higher and higher doses of the opioids to take away her pain. Diana is a good example of how doctors catapult their patients from the mild to the severe end of the addiction spectrum. She had few risk factors and no active addiction issues until those first opioids were prescribed.

> *"I wasn't actually sure that I really had migraines or whether it was something I convinced myself of because I liked how I felt when I took the drugs. But I didn't want to explore that possibility. After a while, I realized I didn't like to function without my medication. I'd sit and do nothing, waiting for that feeling, because I didn't want to be busy and miss that feeling. I didn't want to 'waste it.'"*
>
> —DIANA, TWENTY-SIX, WHO BECAME AN OPIOID ADDICT IN HER TEENS AND A HEROIN ADDICT AS A YOUNG ADULT, AFTER FIRST TAKING OPIOIDS FOR SEVERE HEADACHES

That Diana's doctors continued to prescribe highly addictive opioids to such a young mom—by then she was in a stable marriage to her high-school sweetheart and they had three small children—without even considering the consequences is irresponsible and infuriating. You could say they didn't know better, and that may be true. But it is also true that it is lamentably easy for doctors to fall into prescribing habits that are lucrative for them and harmful for their patients. Healthy people with no need to visit the doctor besides a yearly physical put pain physicians (and everyone else) out of business.

Diana was addicted to pain medication for seven years. At the same time that her addiction was becoming increasingly unmanageable, Oregon doctors started coming under more scrutiny for overprescribing opioids. State public-health officials who had basically been asleep at the wheel finally started paying attention. They were shocked and concerned by what they saw. Doctors—from pain specialists to general practitioners—were irresponsibly encouraging the use of highly addictive and dangerous drugs in a state that has one of the highest rates of opioid misuse in the country[18] and where overdose was sharply on the rise. This is still the case, by the way. As I mentioned in the introduction, these days more people die from drug overdoses than from traffic accidents in Oregon and thirty-five other states.[19]

In light of all this, Diana's doctors were still supplying her with prescription pain medication like Vicodin and Percocet, but more reluctantly and in smaller amounts. So Diana started supplementing her habit by illegally buying prescription medication off the street. At that time she was living in Ashland, Oregon, an upscale tourist town known for its theater, outdoor recreation, and "boho chic" hippie culture. She got pregnant again. She used throughout her pregnancy to help her with the pain, with the approval of her doctors (though they didn't realize she was taking more than they were prescribing), and she left the hospital where she gave birth to her fourth child with a prescription for Percocet.

A few weeks later Diana smoked black-tar heroin for the first time. It was easy to get and cheaper than illegally buying pain meds, and she loved how it made her feel:

> After that I knew I wasn't going to go back to pills. At the time you're just excited you've found a more direct way to get your high. You don't realize the implications of it. Your heart is racing, you get a rush, you get a lot of endorphins. You feel pretty invincible. You feel you can do anything you want to do. Nothing is gonna hold you back, no pain, no illness. . . . It seems like a good thing. And you overlook all the negative things like, "I'm falling asleep while I'm trying to cook," or "I'm putting off other things so I can go get a bag." And your sense of time gets to the point where you say, "I'll be back in five minutes," and you come back the next day. It gets that bad. I don't even know how I didn't see that at the time.

As I talked about in the last chapter, drug addicts face a tremendous amount of social stigma. The blame for addiction is placed squarely on their shoulders, and it is seen as a character defect or a lack of willpower.

But where does the blame really lie? Is an eighteen-year-old following her doctor's orders who then becomes addicted really the person to blame? What about an eleven-year-old?

Recently a mom wrote to me on Facebook:

> My son just had a cervical fusion and is in a halo [brace]. They sent us home with Dilaudid [the brand name for hydromorphone, a highly addictive opiate], which I weaned him from within ten days. At our two-week checkup with the local pediatrician, she said he must still have pain, so he was [to] take all of these. I said "No,

he doesn't even say 'ouch' anymore and is on a muscle relaxer to help his neck relax in the halo. He is fine." She said, "No, he must still be in pain," and gave us a prescription for 120 oxycodone!!! My son is eleven.

Have you heard of pill mills? These are clinics run by unscrupulous medical doctors who usually don't take insurance, make patients pay in cash, falsify medical records (one undercover police officer reports that he successfully used the X-ray of a dog to get a prescription for pain medication and muscle relaxants from a pill mill),[20] and write prescriptions for highly addictive narcotics to literally hundreds of people a week. One such doctor was Mohammad Derani,[21] who was arrested in August 2017 at the Dearborn Medical Clinic in Michigan, where long lines of people would wait to see him at all hours of the day and night. Derani had allegedly prescribed more than five hundred thousand opioid pills since January of that same year, handing out on average forty-three prescriptions for controlled substances a day!

Then there's Dr. Henri Wetselaar, who switched from family medicine to pain management in 2008 despite having no training or certification. Convicted of illegally prescribing oxycodone in March 2017, the Las Vegas physician ran a lucrative pill mill. Information that came out during the trial showed that he had patients who came from as far away as Kentucky and Ohio, that he rarely performed a physical exam, and that he only accepted cash. Dr. Wetselaar was banking as much as $90,000 a month in cash, depositing a little less than $10,000 at a time so he would not tip off the Feds.[22] It's easy to dismiss these as unusual cases of extreme medical misconduct, but these are just the doctors who got caught. Doctors around the country routinely and irresponsibly prescribe highly addictive synthetic opioids without thinking twice. After all, it's within their standard of care.

The P-*harm*-aceutical Mission Is to Make Money

It's time to tell it like it is. The pharmaceutical industry does a lot of worthless research, spends a fortune on advertising in every media (television, radio, newspapers, magazines, YouTube, online) to get you to "Ask your doctor for . . .," and turns a blind eye to human suffering. They hire "scientific" researchers who are experts in designing studies to get the projected outcomes they want, ignoring data that doesn't fit their paradigm and even falsifying information to ensure the desired result. "Tobacco science" at its finest, folks. I could write a whole book about corruption in the pharmaceutical industry. Indeed, many have already been written. Instead, I'll give you a couple examples that are emblematic of how this industry behaves.

Mylan increases the price of EpiPens 500 percent. You may have heard about the EpiPens scandal, since the media did a good job investigating and reporting on it in 2016 and 2017. EpiPens are a simple but lifesaving medical intervention. They reverse the symptoms of anaphylactic shock through an injection of epinephrine, usually shot into the thigh. They cost about $30 to make.[23] But as the rates of food allergies among children have risen,[24] the pharmaceutical giant Mylan, which owns EpiPens, has marked up its product over 500 percent. In 2009 a two-pack of EpiPens cost $100; in 2016 the company charged $608 for the same product.[25] Families with children with life-threatening allergies struggle to pay this outrageous price, while the CEO of the company makes nearly $19 million a year.[26] As if that's not bad enough, Mylan's CEO is Heather Bresch, whose father is a US senator[27] and whose mother oversaw a national school-board group that launched a campaign to require schools to buy EpiPens.[28]

Is it a good idea to have EpiPens in schools? Absolutely. But Mylan rigged its contracts to specify that schools could only buy Mylan's pens, potentially violating antitrust laws. This isn't only unethical; it's illegal. Don't be fooled into thinking any of this outrageous behavior has been punished. In March 2017 CNBC reported that Mylan's stock had been climbing.[29]

Insys Therapeutics fakes cancer patients to sell its drug. Insys Therapeutics, an Arizona-based pharmaceutical company, got FDA approval in 2012 for a sublingual spray pain reliever made from fentanyl. The drug is very expensive and requires prior authorization from insurance companies. When sales weren't satisfactory, Insys took matters into its own hands by falsifying patient files (to make it look as though patients who did not have cancer had cancer), having their drug salespeople phone insurance companies pretending to be calling on behalf of doctors' offices while never revealing they were working for the company, and bribing doctors to prescribe it to patients who didn't need it. All of this has come to light thanks to an investigation led by Missouri senator Claire McCaskill.[30]

Tobacco Science

We seem to forgive and forget when it comes to big business, but a quick look at the cigarette scandal should be enough to convince any thinking person that industry-sponsored "science" is often little more than bought advertising. Though tobacco companies knew since as early as the 1950s that their products were carcinogenic, they spent millions manipulating scientific research to create doubt about the host of health problems that were clearly linked to smoking.

Drug companies continue to use "science" to promote their products in the most duplicitous ways. It turns out it's very easy to design a study with confirmation bias if you want to "prove" the outcome you desire. You minimize side effects by designing short-term studies that won't reveal long-term health issues or by simply excluding any real side effects that would be expected from the drug or product. Compare lung cancer rates for one year in those who smoke one pack a day with those who smoke two packs a day, and—presto, change-o—cigarettes are safe! It takes decades for lung cancer to develop, and no nonsmokers are included in the study, so of course there is no difference.[31]

We've seen drug companies do this with Vioxx, a pain reliever that was finally recalled for causing heart problems, as well as antidepressant medications, attention-deficit drugs, and even vaccines before they have been withdrawn from the market.

Like tobacco and drug companies, Big Alcohol funds and promotes flawed scientific studies to manipulate consumers. According to an investigation by *Mother Jones*, the industry has spent millions of dollars funding hundreds of biased studies. At the same time, at least half a dozen government officials—including the director of the Division of Metabolism and Health Effects of the National Institute on Alcohol Abuse and Alcoholism—have left jobs in Washington to work for Big Alcohol.[32] Though the health problems with excessive drinking have been replicated in well-designed scientific studies, and alcohol is identified as a known carcinogen by the World Health Organization,[33] most Americans have been effectively duped into believing that alcohol has tangible and lasting health benefits. I also have some swampland in Florida for sale and some rights to land on Mars, if you're interested.

Food Matters

Maiya and I like to unwind in front of the television in the evenings. No matter what show we watch together, we see advertisements for edible foodlike substances full of flavors and additives manufactured in a laboratory—everything from potato chips to the latest fast-food gimmick. TV viewers are led to believe this crap is actually food, and

AMERICA'S WEAPONS OF MASS DESTRUCTION.

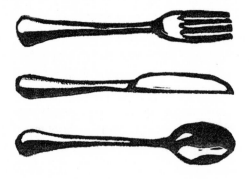

they become convinced that it is the gateway to happiness. A gorgeous young woman closes her eyes in sensual delight as she bites into a sandwich; a deep manly voice narrates as a hamburger is piled with toppings. These ads, like the "food" itself, appeal to our most primitive brain. They give us the message that all we need to be slim, beautiful, and sexually appealing is to eat like the good-looking women and men in the ads.

Which is one of the reasons why so many of us do. We eat a Standard American Diet that's not only SAD (get it?)—it's actually making us sick. Those packaged foods full of chemicals and endocrine disruptors may taste good while you're eating them, but don't be fooled. SAD eating negatively affects your mood, your ability to concentrate, your digestive system, and even your self-confidence.

I recently attended a lecture on children's health by a nationally known pediatrician who performs a specialized kind of surgery. The first slide my colleague showed was to underscore the "beauty" of the city hosting him. Click: a picture of a burger, fries, and a soft drink from a fast-food chain. The audience laughed boisterously. The doctor boasted he had gone to the chain for dinner the night before and breakfast that morning and was planning a stop there for lunch on his way back to the airport. Giving kids highly processed fried foods and sugar-laden drinks flies in the face of everything we know about how to raise healthy children, yet here was a pediatrician, someone who advises parents every day, championing fast food to a group of health professionals!

Many—if not most—of the health problems that we face today are a direct result of our SAD diet. Yet this is how we eat.

Maiya and I both worked when our kids were little. We were busy and stressed-out. We honestly didn't understand how important food was to our children's developing brains and lasting good health. Maiya breast-fed but not for long and not exclusively. We gave the babies artificial milk substitutes and store-bought baby food.

Why wouldn't we? Neither of us realized at the time that this jarred, canned, and pouched "food" had been sterilized at high heat for optimal shelf life and was pretty much devoid of nutrients. These products were endorsed by our doctors, and we were fooled by the advertisements we saw on TV. Besides, everyone was feeding their kids boxed breakfast cereals, toaster pastries, and frozen waffles for breakfast; canned soup, ramen noodles, and Lunchables for lunch; and Shake 'n Bake chicken washed down with Crystal Light iced tea for dinner. And, wow, the kids loved it all and ate well. Brightly colored sugary cereals were especially popular at our house, as were cookies, muffins, apple juice, and soda. To say nothing of candy at the movies, candy at Halloween, candy on birthdays, and candy the other days of the year. And I honestly thought we were being healthy!

I now know one reason Maiya and I struggled for so long with our addictions was that we were eating so badly. In order for you to be mentally and physically healthy, you must eat real foods—plants from the garden grown without harmful pesticides, fruits and nuts that come from trees, high-quality protein that comes from animal and plant sources. The Food and Drug Administration recommends three to five servings of vegetables a day.[34] How well are you doing with those recommended vegetables? Do you eat about a cup of leafy greens or half a cup of other veggies with every meal? Bet you don't. Most of the time, though I know better now and I try hard, I don't either.

If you have a tendency toward addiction, are actively addicted, or are in recovery and you fill your bodies with edible crud disguised as food, your body becomes more vulnerable to pain and infection, making it more likely that you will slip back into addiction. Highly processed foods, especially refined sugar, create inflammation throughout the body. Inflammation in the body causes pain. If it's in the brain, it causes headaches; if it's in your intestinal tract, it causes stomachaches; and if it's in your joints or muscles, it causes them to ache. When your body is inflamed because of bad food and too much stress, you don't feel well. And then you turn to drugs and alcohol. It becomes a vicious cycle.

Everyone benefits from a healthy, fresh, whole-food diet—of course!—but **addicts need real food even more than other people**. You've spent so many years abusing your body and your brain and making yourself more susceptible to illnesses and mood disorders that when you don't eat right, you are in trouble.

To be well nourished, you need macronutrients (protein, fat, car-

---

Food for Thought

Is your food improving your health or causing health problems?

Is your food providing you with all the nutrients your brain and body need?

Is your food bathing your brain and body in toxins?

The best way to find out is to keep a food journal. For three days write down everything you eat and drink. For any processed foods or snacks, include the list of ingredients as well. You may be surprised by how much refined sugar, food dyes, and additives are in what you've been told your whole life is "food."

bohydrates) and micronutrients (vitamins, minerals, phytonutrients). Even if you eat well, you could be poorly nourished because your body is not absorbing nutrients effectively. Although it's best to get your micronutrients from real food, you may still benefit from taking vitamins, minerals, and other supplements. Specific supplements can be particularly helpful for recovering from addiction, supporting your brain, liver, lungs, and detox pathways, and helping you with your mood, sleep, anxiety, and fatigue.

Have you ever gone shopping and brought something to the cash register only to find that it's on sale? You know that boost you feel at saving money? Your brain suddenly feels a jolt of happiness. You think you're making a good decision when you buy cheap, fast food or conventional packaged food on sale at the grocery store. Your brain gets a rush of dopamine, and you feel less stressed—saving money makes life feel more manageable. What you don't realize is that it's worth paying more up front for real, whole, fresh foods to avoid paying a fortune down the road to manage chronic diseases and addiction. Organic food tends to be more expensive, but you can find affordable options, including beans and rice, on-sale frozen organic vegetables, and wild-caught canned salmon (which is a cheaper and healthier alternative to tuna).

Highly sweetened foods full of additives and technologically enhanced flavors are designed and packaged to entice us to eat and crave more. One study found that Oreo cookies were as addictive to rats as cocaine and morphine.[35] Corporate America has us exactly where it wants us. The foods we eat make us sick, so we spend a lot of time at the doctor. The doctor prescribes meds and more meds, so we spend a lot of time at the pharmacy. We don't change our eating habits or our lifestyles, and we keep getting sick. Who wins? Big Food, Big Pharma, and medical professionals. Who loses? We all do.

POPULAR FOODS THAT WREAK HAVOC ON OUR HEALTH

Anything containing artificial colors or flavors

Anything containing flavor enhancers like MSG and "natural" flavors (which are usually anything but)

Anything containing trans fat or partially hydrogenated fat (like margarine, vegetable shortening, and coffee creamers)

Anything containing unnecessary additives (including emulsifiers like polysorbate-80 and cellulose gum and stabilizers like mold inhibitor)

Artificial sweeteners, especially aspartame

Butter flavoring

Diet and regular soda

Highly processed grains, including "enriched" white flour

Processed meats

Sweetened drinks

The Addiction Spectrum X Factor: Stress

Combine doctor ignorance with corporate greed, add our Standard American Diet, and mix in a large helping of stress, and you've got a prizewinning recipe for addiction.

What's stress got to do with it? I believe stress is the X factor in addiction.

Sometime in your teens, maybe just at puberty, the total weight and magnitude of your task at hand—growing up—probably started to sink in. Your body was changing, your hormones were raging, and you were trying to make sense of the world, become independent from your parents, and learn to take care of yourself all at the same time. Even if you were born into a very loving family and grew up in the happiest home, transitioning from childhood to adulthood is hard. You may not have come from a happy home. Maybe you were belittled. Maybe you were spanked, or shamed for your nightmares, fears, or hurts. Maybe you were exposed to things you shouldn't have been, like sex or drugs, when you were too young to understand.

All parents make mistakes, usually not on purpose. So even though your parents probably did their best, you end up feeling unworthy, unloved, unlovable, and unwanted. You may have been exposed to more stress at a young age than you could handle, which can create lasting challenges for the rest of your life.

Poverty; dysfunction at home; addicted parents; sexual, physical, or emotional abuse; tragedies like the loss of a sibling, parent, or friend—all these circumstances can cause overwhelming stress. As a tween, teen, or young adult, you look for relief. You feel alone, scared, and misunderstood. You feel exhausted. At this point cannabis, alcohol, opioids, stimulants, or any number of other substances fill the void.

Whether from illness, fatigue, inflammation, poor sleep, anxiety, or depression, stress disrupts your hormones and neurotransmitters. The pituitary gland in the brain, also known as the "master gland," initiates the release of hormones. These hormones direct the production of testosterone, which gives you energy and libido; adrenocorticotropin (ACTH), which stimulates the adrenals to make cortisol (cortisol helps with everything from blood sugar, to stress management, to blood pressure); and thyroid-stimulating hormone (TSH), a hormone that tells your thyroid gland to make thyroid hormone, which is needed for brain development, energy, and so much more. With chronic stress the system starts to fail.

Maybe you've heard the expression "adrenal fatigue"? Adrenal fatigue happens when the hormone messages overload the pituitary, resulting in lower levels of these hormones. You may experience fatigue, blood-sugar problems, weight gain, depression, and anxiety. Some conventional doctors quibble about whether adrenal fatigue is real. But we all feel tired, and you can bet your bottom dollar that stress and hormone disruption have a lot to do with that exhausted feeling. Stress can lead to fatigue, which in turn makes you want to drink or use in an attempt to feel better and improve your energy.

So Now That You Know You're Being Duped . . .

What do you do about it? The philosopher René Descartes tells us that we have to examine everything we do, everything we feel, and why we hold fast to certain beliefs. We have to take our beliefs out of the box where they're held, spread them on the table, and look at them. This isn't something we do once or twice in our lives in order to substitute one rigid set of beliefs for another, but something we do as often as possible, keeping some, rejecting others. Being willing to grow and change and reconsider makes us more alive, more engaged, and more interesting.

Once you know better, you do better. We've all been duped, we will all change our minds sometimes, and we will all get new information that will help us improve our lives. So when you're with your friends or family watching TV and manipulative ads come on the air, either mute the tube, turn away, or relentlessly critique the advertisements you see for pharmaceutical products, edible foodlike substances, and alcohol. Talk about why they're misleading, Tweet about what you don't like, or share your frustration on another social-media outlet. Identify the hidden messages that appeal to your primitive desires, and mock the false promises and lies you're being fed in the ads. You'll find this is a great conversation starter.

Does it feel as if the whole system is profiting off you? That you've been manipulated by the pharmaceutical industry, conventional medicine, and Big Food? Part of the process of recovery is seeing the truth that so many people are getting rich off your addiction and suffering. It's time to send them to the poor house.

There are all sorts of grassroots social-justice, responsible-medicine, medical-freedom, and organic-food movements you can join. These are groups of passionate people who want to educate others and change the world. It feels good to be part of something like this, to attend rallies and get involved. Two birds with one stone: as I'll be talking about throughout this book, strong social ties and connectedness protect you against relapse. It's exciting to attend conferences, TED Talks, and seminars where activists and experts come together to talk about integrative medicine and reducing toxic exposures. My favorite conferences include the Wise Traditions, Preventing Overdiagnosis, and the Medical Academy of Pediatric Special Needs (MAPS). I also recommend attending conferences where you can hear some of today's smartest and most articulate thought leaders on medical topics, like Anita Devlin, Joel Fuhrman, Sara Gottfried, Zen Honeycutt, Sayer Ji, Ray Lozano, Ben Lynch, Gabor Maté, Deanna Minich, David Perlmutter, Marvin Seppala, and Andrew Weil. If you decide to attend one, you may see me there!

I think it's always better to attend in person, but there are also many free summits that happen online as well as dozens of documentary films and miniseries that will open your eyes to how you are being systematically misled, including *The Addiction Summit,* that I hosted, *Super Size Me, The Truth About Cancer,* and *GMOs Revealed.* Make some popcorn, cut up some vegetables and throw them on a plate, and watch these films with your friends and family. Visit addictionspectrum .com for my latest updates on resources.

What else do you need to do to stay in recovery and in charge of your health?

Choose your doctor wisely. Always remember that your doctor works for you, not vice versa. It makes sense to visit prospective doctors' websites, talk to their other patients, and read their books and articles, if they've written any. Many doctors in America, unfortunately, take unadvertised kickbacks from the pharmaceutical industry. These gifts can influence their prescribing behavior in the worst ways. Medical-device and pharmaceutical companies are required by law to disclose the dollar amounts they pay docs (for promotional talks, travel, "research," consulting, meals, and other activities), which is available online at openpaymentsdata.cms.gov.

Even if your doctor's not taking payments from drug companies, is he or she committed to your lasting good health or are you being treated like an item on an assembly line? Does your doctor talk to you about natural healing and how to recover through lifestyle changes? Your best bet may be to fire your conventionally trained medical doctor and seek out a doctor trained in integrative or functional medicine who treats your addiction and other health challenges by identifying the root causes and devising an individually tailored healing approach to overcoming them. The goal is to be healthy and drug-free and to work with a doctor who wants to help you get off pharmaceuticals, not one who throws pills at you.

> *"Most of the things worth doing in the world had been declared impossible before they were done."*
>
> —LOUIS D. BRANDEIS, SUPREME COURT JUSTICE

Fight Big Pharma. I hope I've convinced you by now that pharmaceutical companies profit when they ply you with as many drugs as they can. As I've already mentioned, many patients in my addiction clinic who come directly from an inpatient or doctor-run outpatient program usually arrive on a laundry list of medications. They have an SSRI or two for depression, a stimulant for ADD and focus, gabapentin for pain or anxiety, one or two medications to help with sleep, buprenorphine or methadone for their opioid dependence, and more. Maybe you do too. Like my patients, maybe you believe you need each and every one of these. But my patients quickly realize after we start working together that they don't. And you don't either!

Fight Big Pharma by being skeptical of their promises, advertising, and the doctors on their payroll. Wean yourself off of their products while finding natural and safe alternatives. Figure out ways to treat your addiction and other health issues by giving your body what it needs to boost your neurotransmitters naturally and by keeping most, if not all, of your money out of the hands of the pharmaceutical industry.

Fix your food habits. There honestly isn't anything more important than what you eat. It's easy to get bogged down with a million questions about food and get hooked on fad diets, but let's keep it simple and real. You need to be eating real, fresh, whole foods that are as organic (pesticide- and herbicide-free) as possible. This means avoiding GMOs (genetically modified organisms) and shopping the outside aisles of grocery stores—buying fresh produce and herbs, eggs, fish, and grass-fed meats. Stay away from the aisles of boxes and cans. Moving from a SAD diet to a nutrient-rich, fresh, real-food diet takes time and persistence. Rome wasn't built in a day, and your improved diet won't be either. Start by making small changes (add a vegetable to every meal, choose a snack of organic dates or raisins over candy bars, eat an apple instead of a pastry), and keep on changing for the better.

There's a worldwide movement to promote organic farming called WWOOF (which stands for Willing Workers on Organic Farms or World Wide Opportunities on Organic Farms). If you can come up with the money to get yourself there and back, you can create your own residential detox program by becoming a WWOOFer, where you work on an organic farm either in the US or abroad in exchange for free room and board. I have known many friends of Bill W. who have volunteered on organic farms in exchange for nutritious produce.

Whether you do a monthlong stay or spend half a day volunteering on the weekends, exchanging your time for healthy, fresh organic food is a win-win for everyone. You get to be outside in the sunlight soaking up the vitamin D, being out in nature, and feeling purposeful as you work side by side with others. At the end of the day you have a basket of health-giving, life-altering fresh produce to take home. If you're not ready to do some volunteering or commit to a longer stay, you can start visiting farmers' markets. Most gladly accept government food stamps. I also recommend you befriend an organic gardener, plant some fruit trees in your or your landlord's backyard, and grow herbs like basil, chives, and parsley in a sunny window in your home or apartment. The key is to become committed to eating real food instead of edible foodlike substances, which I'll be talking more about throughout this book.

Free yourself from stress. Life is always going to throw you curveballs. Though you can minimize stress, you can't, unfortunately, rid yourself completely of either day-to-day stress or life-altering trauma. But it's how you handle the stress that matters most. Turn off the anxiety-inducing commercial-laden nightly news, lock yourself out of the internet at night (more on that in chapter 8), and distance yourself from the toxic stressed-out people who enable your addictions.

Try taking a yoga class at a place where they also teach meditation. Some yoga studios will let you volunteer at the front desk in exchange for free classes, which is a great way to find out if you like yoga or meditation without the stress of spending money (which you may not have right now). Volunteering has given my own children and my patients a chance to find out what they like and don't like, who their tribe is, and the best ways to lessen their stress.

Volunteering is also a great way to eventually get a job, if you've been struggling to find employment. If you love animals, volunteer at an animal shelter or a local veterinary clinic. If you want to take a gym class but can't afford it, offer to do some grunt work before and after class like taking out the trash or cleaning the equipment in exchange for lessons. Staying busy, thinking about how you can help other people, and giving the gift of your time to others will reduce your stress and move you in the right direction on the addiction spectrum.

Getting enough sleep, eating real foods, and exercising daily are also incredibly effective ways to deal with stress. I'll be getting on my stress-busting soapbox and giving you more tried-and-true relaxation techniques throughout this book.

Diana, the mom of four who was hooked on heroin, takes long bicycle rides and goes running to de-stress. Life has presented her with some serious challenges—including her husband briefly relapsing and her bicycle getting stolen—but she's dealing with them. Raising her family, working full-time, and going to community college, she always makes sure to schedule time to have fun. She's found her tribe in many ways, including by doing volunteer work on behalf of medical freedom and attending rallies and Senate hearings to champion parents' rights. She currently works as a community health worker with recovering addicts. The pay isn't great, but she has a lot more money now that she is not spending it on drugs.

Now that we understand how the pharmaceutical companies, medical professionals, and food industry play a large role in creating our addictions, let's think about this with regard to your place on the addiction spectrum. Anyone who is struggling with any kind of addiction always has the potential to move one direction or the other on the addiction spectrum. There are times in your life when everything is good and you are stable. But even then, if you are eating junk food loaded with toxins or taking a slew of pharmaceuticals, you are priming yourself to move toward the more severe end of the addiction spectrum.

To stay at the mild end or move back there, you need to be active in your food choices, free yourself from pharmaceutical products as much as you can, and fill your body with the bioavailable nutrients that come from organic, whole, fresh foods. I know this will sound strange coming from a doctor, but to be totally honest with you, being anti-addiction (desiring to move to the safe end of the addiction spectrum) requires us to be anti–junk food, anti-drugs, anti-Pharma, anti–false advertising, and, for the most part, anti-doctor!

Do you want to join the growing army of health-freedom activists?

We have a strong sense of purpose. We are fighting for the very lives of our children and our families, for the very survival of the human race and the promotion of a healthy society. Take care of yourself first.

Get back to the mild end of the addiction spectrum. Then come join the heroes of our time and fight for health freedom.

Freedom to decide what goes into our bodies.

Freedom from Big Agriculture, with all its pesticides and herbicides and engineered "food."

Freedom from pharmaceutical companies that want you to depend on their products for life.

Freedom from the medical system and doctors.

Either we are living in harmony with the environment, or we are destroying it.

Now let's take a closer look at specific addictions Americans are facing. How do major addictive substances and behavior impact your life and the lives of your loved ones? More important, perhaps, what can you do about it? Part II will empower you and start you on your journey to health freedom, whatever your or your loved one's addictive substance of choice. As I remind my patients all the time: **The goal is not to feel perfect. The goal is to be free.**

PART II

A Closer Look at the Addictions

CHAPTER 4

How to Keep Opioids
from Destroying Your Life

MYLINN, twenty-four years old, is with her dad, who gave her a ride
today. He sits in the waiting room, leafing through a magazine
and looking at his phone, while Mylinn comes into the exam room. The
sunglasses pushed on the top of her head hold back her long brown hair,
dyed blond at the ends. She and her boyfriend, a stocker at a wholesale
electrical supply distributor, have an eighteen-month-old son. Mylinn's
mother-in-law watches the baby when they are both at work.

When Mylinn was eighteen, she was rear-ended on her way to beauty
school. She had mild whiplash from the accident—and says she wasn't
in much pain—but the urgent-care doctor prescribed her an opioid.
Her regular doctor renewed the prescription for a year. Two years later,
by the time she was twenty, she had started smoking heroin.

As author David Sheff, who wrote *Beautiful Boy*, a book about his
son's addiction, explains, when he was a teenager experimenting with
all sorts of drugs including cocaine and LSD, he avoided heroin at all
costs.[1] Heroin wasn't a drug that seemed fun, and heroin junkies—
even to Sheff's eager-to-party group of friends—didn't seem cool. They
seemed pathetic. The idea of using heroin was bleak and depressing.

But as heroin has become cheaper and easier to obtain in the United
States, the face of the heroin addict has changed. Like Mylinn and
Diana, whose story I shared in the previous chapter, the majority of
my patients seeking treatment for heroin addiction got their start from
prescription pain medications. Opioids (the term I use throughout this
book)—whether natural or synthetic—are any drugs, including morphine, codeine, fentanyl, oxycodone, and heroin, that work by binding

to opiate receptors in the brain. Many people use the terms "opiate" and "opioid" interchangeably, but technically "opiate" refers only to a drug derived from opium. "Opioid" is the more modern, all-encompassing word. If you are prone to addiction because of the factors I talked about in chapter 1, you may respond very strongly to opioids and quickly start to crave more.

Opiates are derived from the opium poppy, a plant that does well in warm, dry climates. The top opium poppy–producing countries (in order of amount of land devoted to cultivation) are:

1. Afghanistan   5. Laos

2. Myanmar   6. Pakistan

3. Mexico   7. Colombia

4. India   8. Iran[2]

Opium poppies are also grown in Australia, Thailand, Turkey, and elsewhere around the world.[3] Although it is illegal to purposefully grow opium poppies in the United States, farms have been discovered by federal agents in California,[4] North Carolina,[5] and Washington State.[6]

There are opioids that are street drugs, like heroin, and others, like Vicodin, that are legal with a prescription from a doctor and also available on the black market. Opioids are prescribed to treat pain as well as coughs.

PRESCRIBED OPIOIDS[7]

codeine (only available in generic form)

fentanyl (Abstral, Actiq, Duragesic, Fentora, Onsolis)

hydrocodone (Hysingla ER, Zohydro ER)

hydrocodone and acetaminophen (Lorcet, Lortab, Norco, Vicodin)

hydromorphone (Dilaudid, Exalgo)

meperidine (Demerol)

methadone (Dolophine, Methadose)

morphine (Astramorph, Kadian, Morphabond, MS Contin, Oramorph SR) oxycodone (Oxaydo, Oxecta, OxyContin, Oxyfast, Roxicodone)

oxycodone and acetaminophen (Endocet, Percocet, Roxicet)

oxycodone and naloxone (Targiniq ER)

OTHER OPIOIDS

heroin   kratom   opium   poppy tea

Every form of opioid, whether legal or illegal, synthetic or natural, eases both physical pain and mental angst. Taking opioids fools you into feeling you're better able to cope with your life and your problems, even as the opioids themselves may start to destroy your health, damage your brain, and compromise your well-being. If opioids are your drug of choice, you know that feeling. The process of how they work is complicated, but opioids basically act by attaching to receptors in the cells in your brain, spinal cord, gastrointestinal tract, and other organs to reduce the perception of pain and increase feelings of pleasure.

A Public-Health Crisis

Unless you assiduously avoid the news and social media, you already know that opioid abuse is one of America's fastest growing public-health problems. In just seven years, the number of emergency-room visits related to the nonmedical use of pharmaceuticals more than doubled, from 500,000 to around 1.25 million. Specifically, opioid-involved emergencies rose 183 percent, with over 315,000 more opioid-related trips made to the ER in 2011 than in 2004.[8] In 2015, 2.1 million Americans ages twelve or older misused pain relievers for the first time. Today the majority of drug-overdose deaths involve an opioid. From 2000 to 2016, about 400,000 people died from opioid-drug overdoses. On average, 115 Americans die every day from them.[9]

A tragic shift that has escalated since 2015 has been the introduction of fentanyl into street drugs seized by the Drug Enforcement Administration (DEA).[10] I talked about fentanyl, a fast-acting opioid that is a hundred times more potent than morphine, in the last chapter. Fentanyl kills you by shutting down your breathing center. I suspect that neither dealers nor opioid users are aware of just how potent fentanyl is.

At a recent addiction conference, I learned about another drug that is even more worrisome. **Carfentanil is a new opioid that is *ten thousand* times more potent than morphine.**[11] The trade name is Wildnil. It's used by veterinarians to sedate elephants. An amount smaller than a grain of salt can be fatal. I thought to myself, "Surely they are not putting *that* on the market to give to people?" Guess what? In the preliminary findings of one hundred accidental drug overdoses in the Dayton, Ohio, area in the first two months of 2017, 99 percent tested positive for fentanyl and three deaths were from carfentanil.[12]

Nicky's Story

Nicky, who is thirty-three years old and Mexican American, was a cheerleader in high school, sang in the church choir, and was always the one her six siblings (two biological and four adopted) looked up to the most. Nicky tried smoking marijuana at age eleven at her older sister's urging. Then she did inhalants. She and her friends would buy cans of spray paint or potpourri, put a rag over the top and over their heads, and inhale the fumes until they got high or passed out, whichever came first.

When Nicky was fifteen she started dating a guy whose family grew marijuana. Pot was easy to get and free. She got pregnant, and they got married. Wanting to give her baby the best start, Nicky stayed sober for four years. Then she relapsed, first with a capsule of meth that her sister (who has since died from an overdose) told her was a diet pill, and then with heroin. Smoking led to injecting. She was scared at first, but her new boyfriend and his friends encouraged her. Soft-spoken and articulate, Nicky speaks sadly when she talks about this period of her life. She sounds ashamed—and even a little incredulous—about some of the things she's done.

"They kept saying it's a waste of money to smoke it," Nicky remembers. Her jet-black hair is pulled back in a tight ponytail today, and she's wearing a gray hoodie. Her dark brown eyes look serious. "You get higher quicker when you inject it. I was a phlebotomist. I knew how to find a vein."

Every morning before work (she always had a job, even at the height of her addiction), she would get up and have a shot of heroin the way other people have a cup of coffee. With the heroin running through her veins, she was ready to start the day. Most of today's heroin addicts don't fit the stereotypes of what we think of as junkies. These are regular folks like you and me who usually start buying opioids from friends on college campuses, at work, or at the gym. They aren't buying from drug dealers in dark alleyways. They aren't poorly dressed strung-out street dwellers committing petty crimes to get their next fix. At least, not at first. And often not for years.

Are You at Risk for Opioid Addiction?

Doctors often prescribe opioids for pain without asking you *any* questions about your risk factors for or previous history of addiction. The overall picture from multiple data suggests that most people prescribed opioids for pain management use them responsibly,[13] but it is important to be aware of the risk. Remember that we all fall somewhere on the addiction spectrum; taking an opioid can very quickly get you addicted.

The key to responsible opioid use is to wean yourself off them as quickly as possible. If you need surgery, ask the doctor about what kind of pain you should expect to feel afterward and the time it usually takes for the pain to diminish. Write down everything your doctor tells you. Put the date of the surgery and the date you should expect to feel better on your calendar. If the pain hasn't gone away by that time, talk to your doctor. Try not to use opioids beyond the projected recovery period. If you do, you risk addiction.

Maiya's Progression Along the Addiction Spectrum

My wife, Maiya, was twenty-eight years old when her jaw locked shut. Her condition has a long and unpronounceable name—temporomandibular joint disorder. The joints that connect the jawbone to her skull essentially froze. When steroid injections to reduce the swelling didn't work, her doctors decided to operate. Maiya underwent major surgery to implant her jaw with artificial plastic joints, followed by excruciatingly painful physical therapy that lasted for months.

Skip these details if you don't like to read about pain. After the oper-

Lifesavers or Life Destroyers?

If you've been in an accident or had a broken bone, you probably know that opioids can be a lifesaver for acute pain. Opioids can also be tremendously helpful in some cases of severe chronic pain.

Using opioids for mild chronic pain can be tricky. People who use them longer than just a few weeks can develop a tolerance. This means you need an increasingly higher dose to have the same pain-relieving effect. As your tolerance continues to rise, your brain adapts accordingly. With continued use, you may actually start experiencing more severe pain from something that might previously have caused mild or moderate pain.[14]

I've seen this phenomenon play out in my practice many times. First let me say that my patients are often in terrible and very real pain. They are understandably scared to taper off opioids. But nine times out of ten my patients are surprised to discover that their pain actually starts to go away as we wean them off the drugs. As counterintuitive as this may seem, the lower the opioid dose, the *less* pain they feel.

My clinical observation is backed up by peer-reviewed science. A 2017 study revealed that patients on higher-dose pain medication experience worse outcomes when it comes to pain. They feel greater pain intensity and have worse quality of life.[15]

If doctors want to continue prescribing opioids to manage pain, they must do so more responsibly. It is unethical to prescribe opioids to people at risk for addiction or on the addiction spectrum for any substance. Doctors must do everything possible to avoid triggering a physiological dependence. Doctors should offer alternative pain management techniques, prescribe opioids much more judiciously, closely monitor patients who are taking them, and help patients stop as soon as possible.

ations, a physical therapist would put an expander in her mouth and force open her jaw. This caused tearing and scarring and led to more pain. It was torture for her. She had to take opioid pain pills all the time just to be able to function. As if all that wasn't bad enough, the Proplast joints that the doctors had surgically implanted turned out to be defective and were recalled, because they were leaching microscopic particles that triggered chronic inflammation, joint destruction, and pain. But since Maiya had moved from California to Oregon, she was not notified that the joints in her mouth were malfunctioning.

Over the course of a decade she endured multiple surgeries: surgery to remove the Proplast joints, then surgeries to try an ear-cartilage transplant, a temporal-muscle transplant, and then finally radical bilateral toe-to-jaw intact joint transplants. The first surgeries failed, but the final one, miraculously, worked. A little-known fact: my wife has only four toes on each foot and is one of the first people to have living toes successfully implanted into her jaw. Every time she wiggles her toes, it moves her jaw! (Running joke.) Fighting the pain, holding a job, raising a family, and dealing with the dark parts of her childhood, Maiya found herself addicted to the pain meds.

She couldn't make it through the day without opioids. Every day, as the painkillers were wearing off, she experienced severe withdrawal symptoms. This pain was hard to distinguish from the jaw pain she had originally been treating. Maiya was a nurse—she worked in intensive care at a trauma center. She had easy access to opioids, which her doctors were always happy to prescribe. This built up her tolerance and kept her on the severe end of the addiction spectrum for years.

Why Are Doctors (and Other Humans) So Afraid of Pain?

I was a newly minted doctor when the pharmaceutical industry did its masterful rollout of prescription opioids, duping us into believing that *prescription* opioids were not addictive. Pharma-sponsored magical thinking spread like wildfire among physicians, who started prescribing opioids for even the smallest aches and pains. If the pain didn't improve, we simply prescribed more. This is the kind of attitude that leads to giving an eighteen-year-old like Mylinn an opioid for mild whiplash.

Extended-release OxyContin was first made available in 1995.[16] I read in several articles in Pharma-supported magazines distributed free to doctors that OxyContin was safe, effective, long-acting, and not addictive.[17] This was a lie that, in retrospect, any thinking doctor should have seen through right away. But none of us did. Addiction doctors—and the general public—now understand that any opioid can trigger addiction.

When I opened my addiction clinic in 2009, more than 50 percent of my patients were addicted to OxyContin. Many swallowed it, but most crushed it to snort or inject. My patients compared the high to heroin. That same year, according to government statistics, there were half a million new nonmedical users of OxyContin aged twelve or older.[18] OxyContin was reformulated in 2010, making it impossible to crush, so Oxy addicts switched to heroin.[19] Today opioid addicts who come to my clinic for treatment are usually using heroin.

How did doctors get so hoodwinked? Why do doctors to this day—despite the fact that every shred of evidence shows that opioids are addictive and must be carefully controlled—continue harmful pre-scribing habits? Doctors are trained to defer to "experts." They have to be smart and work hard to make it through medical school. But as intelligent as doctors are, they seem to park their brains at the door when "renowned experts" start spouting nonsense. Doctors truly believed they were doing the best they could to treat patients' pain.

In the early 1990s, backed by the pharmaceutical industry, the US Department of Veterans Affairs and the Joint Commission rolled out the "Pain Is a Vital Sign" campaign. This big push trained medical professionals to assess each patient's pain level, so that pain could be medically managed. Hospitals and doctors not assessing pain were considered negligent. This resulted in a massive increase in the use of opioids for pain.

At the same time, doctors were actually sued for not adequately treating pain. In one high-profile case in the medical community, *Bergman v. Chin*, a jury in California awarded the adult children of William Bergman, an elderly man experiencing severe back pain as he was fighting lung cancer, $1.5 million for the undertreatment of pain. William Bergman died in 1998. Three years later his doctor, Wing

Chin, was found guilty of elder abuse. A bioethics scholar at the Medical College in Wisconsin told the *LA Times* that the verdict was "exciting," given the "sad history of inadequate pain management in this country."[20] American doctors are terrified of lawsuits. Is it any wonder that opioid prescriptions for both severe and mild pain have escalated ever since?

The takeaway from the "Pain Is a Vital Sign" campaign should have been that pain is useful information: a body's signal to itself that something needs adjusting. To be in the business of healing and wellness, doctors' first job should be to identify the underlying health problems, so they can be fixed and the body brought back into balance. Instead, conventional doctors have become prescribing automatons, treating pain with highly addictive drugs and ignoring the consequences. Most of my colleagues are completely unaware or in adamant denial that they are creating an opioid dependence for their pain patients.

My wife's story says it all. Watching somebody progress along the addiction spectrum and feeling helpless to do anything about it, I swore to do my utmost never to create this kind of problem in a patient. Over the past ten years, in a pediatric practice that has grown to care for over thirteen thousand children, I have written a prescription for opioids only twice. **If my patient is experiencing severe pain, I want to get to the root cause, not just treat the symptoms.** The last thing I want to do is prematurely mask the pain and potentially miss an important diagnosis (like meningitis, appendicitis, or a serious joint injury), which needs further evaluation or immediate treatment.

Pain is information—a body's signal to itself
that something needs adjusting.

Jessica's Story: Finding the Root Cause of Pain

Jessica, a thirty-six-year-old advertising executive, suffered from terrible headaches. She had them on and off for years, but it felt as though they were getting worse. She had a CAT scan (to rule out the possibility of a brain tumor), consulted several specialists, and tried three different pain medications. The painkillers helped, but she was concerned about getting addicted and didn't like the brain fog she felt when she took them. She noticed that every time she skipped a dose, the headaches returned full force. It was bad. She was having difficulty concentrating, making mistakes at work, and starting to despair. Her regular doctor wanted Jessica to keep taking opioids and start an anti-anxiety medication. Jessica agreed that she felt depressed and anxious, but she told her doctor she thought the anxiety came from the increasingly painful headaches. He spent all of fifteen minutes talking to her, wrote her a script for a benzodiazepine (a psychoactive, highly addictive anti-anxiety medication), and went on to his next patient.

As a last resort, Jessica went to a colleague of mine, a functional physician who was trained to dig deep for underlying causes of health problems and not just treat the symptoms. Known as a doctor who took the time to solve unsolvable health problems and who was always excited by challenging cases, my colleague herself took an exhaustive medical history, asking Jessica dozens of questions beyond any traditional medical questionnaire and listening closely to the answers. She did not follow a script and she did not type the answers into a computer, looking at the screen instead of making eye contact while Jessica was talking, as Jessica's regular doctor did. That first appointment lasted almost two hours. My colleague asked Jessica to keep a food diary for a week and also to track the timing of every headache, something no doctor had suggested before.

Together they identified two root causes of the headaches. Stressed about work and in too much pain to cook decent meals, Jessica had been eating an increasing amount of packaged and fast food. She grew up in a conventional family, and fast food—like burgers and fries—was comfort food for her. A stir-fry seasoned with soy sauce was one of her favorite "home at six, dinner by six-thirty" meals. Nearly all the foods she was eating regularly, including nacho-flavored corn chips, boxed macaroni and cheese, fried chicken, pizza, and certainly that soy sauce in her stir-fry contained monosodium glutamate (MSG, also called "Chinese salt"). Because no doctor had ever suggested she look at her diet as a root cause of the headaches, no doctor had ever told Jessica that it is well established that MSG can trigger headaches and even migraines. MSG is often a hidden additive in foods, disguised as "natural flavors," so you often don't know you're eating it.

The other culprit my colleague suggested was Jessica's choice of undergarments. The straps of the underwire bras Jessica wore were so tight they were putting pressure on her neck and shoulders. At first Jessica was totally skeptical. She knew theoretically about "healthy eating" (everyone knows it's important to eat "healthy," right?), but she had grown up on the food choices she continued to make and she hadn't had headaches as a child. Even though she was big-breasted and had had trouble playing sports in high school, needing to wear two sports bras at a time, she also didn't really believe her choice of bras could be contributing to her health problems.

My colleague recommended that Jessica change her diet, revisit her wardrobe, and also start seeing a therapist to deal with her emotional eating. With the therapist and her doctor's help, Jessica had the support she needed to make what for her were radical lifestyle changes. She stopped the processed foods, switched to MSG-free tamari, committed to making fresh whole foods the bulk of her diet, and started reading ingredient lists to avoid food additives. She exchanged her tight underwire bras for natural fiber ones and started taking her bra off as soon as she got home from work.

Success! Jessica's headaches completely disappeared. If she had continued to follow her conventional doctor's advice, she may have ended up on the severe end of the addiction spectrum. It turned out she did not need highly addictive prescription medication—she needed a refrigerator, wardrobe, and anxiety overhaul.

> *Some lifestyle changes that will help you move*
> *toward the mild end of the addiction spectrum and*
> *take back every aspect of your health are simple*
> *to understand, but not easy to implement.*

What Motivates You to Seek Help?

Sometimes you seek treatment when forced to by an employer, spouse, or parent. The possibility of losing your job, your marriage, or your place to live can be a powerful motivator. But in my experience that is the exception, not the rule. Mostly you seek help because you're sick and tired of being sick and tired. You've come to realize, for whatever reason, that the euphoria and positive effects of your drug of choice are short-lived and elusive and your life has become an endless and meaningless search for more drugs. The misery of withdrawal is always lurking around the corner; you're tired of lying to friends and family; either your money is running out or you can no longer live with the shame of spending other people's money on drugs. You feel as though you're in bondage to the very thing you once worshipped. Even if you still worship it, long for it, dream about it, and look forward to it, you just want to be done.

My patients have watched opioids, particularly heroin, kill people they love. Close friends or family members, who are on the severe end of the addiction spectrum, accidentally overdose, deliberately commit suicide, or get into drug-fueled accidents. Perhaps it's counterintuitive, but in my experience losing a loved one, as devastating as that is, doesn't usually motivate you to be more committed to recovery. Often it's the opposite—unable to cope with the pain sober, you relapse after finding out a friend has died.

If you're reading this, you probably know what it's like to try to quit and fail. You probably know what it's like to feel that life is too overwhelming to live sober. Maybe you were actually able to stay off drugs for a few months—or even a few years—but then something sent you back. You may feel ashamed, demoralized, or hopeless. Stay with me. Don't give up. You can do this. Be kind to yourself. Embrace imperfection. And keep reading.

All You Need Is Willingness—and Honesty

A key question I ask addicts is about their motivation to change. The more willing you are to change, the more likely you are to succeed. But even if you're very motivated, it's not easy to give up a life of getting high.

I am willing to work with anyone who is committed to being honest with me. My only real expectations are honesty and a willingness to try to better your life.

Question: *There are three frogs sitting on a log, and one decides to jump in the pond. How many are left on the log?*
Answer: *Three. Making a decision doesn't change anything until you act.*

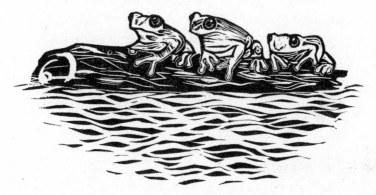

DECIDING TO ACT IS NOT ENOUGH.

YOU HAVE TO TAKE THE LEAP.

Is Harm Reduction Right for You?

Harm reduction, sometimes known as the methadone model, works by giving you daily doses of methadone or buprenorphine as a safer substitute for the other opioids you have been using—in order to reduce the chance that you will overdose or share needles. In this way you are causing less harm to yourself and to society. Both these opioids prevent withdrawal symptoms. Since they are administered in high doses, they allow for a doctor-prescribed "high" that is controlled and closely monitored.

You may have heard methadone—administered as a pink drink in a sugar solution—called "liquid handcuffs." You are chained to that clinic and that doctor and the need to go daily for the foreseeable future. Many recovering addicts feel they will be stuck taking it for the rest of their lives. They go to a clinic desperate for help to get off heroin only to find themselves pushed to take high doses of methadone and actually discouraged from weaning themselves off opioids.

The standard harm-reduction approach of giving high-dose methadone or buprenorphine indefinitely essentially turns people into lifelong state-funded addicts. I do not think it makes sense to prescribe high doses daily and use a one-size-fits-all approach, especially on teenagers and young adults, many of whom have not been using opioids for very long. This approach also has the unintentional consequence of suppressing a patient's pituitary function, which results in lowered thyroid and sex hormones and suppression of the adrenal gland. It has been sharply criticized in other countries because of the rise in methadone overdoses. According to the CDC, methadone overdoses alone took five thousand lives in 2012.[21]

Michael's Story

If you're actively using opioids, even heroin, and having trouble getting free, don't let anyone tell you you've served yourself a death sentence. I've seen even the most down-and-out heroin addicts turn their lives around.

"I know you're kicking me out," Michael said, tears rolling down his face. The skin around his nostrils was almost as red as his eyes. Michael had been snorting meth and was also shooting heroin. "I'm just going to die."

The last time I saw him, Michael seemed to be responding to treatment. But then he disappeared for several months. Today he was wearing a threadbare T-shirt. It was cold outside, and I remember noticing he had no coat.

"Why did you come back?" I asked gently. Michael was twenty-four years old, the same age as one of my sons. Like my son's, his arms were covered with tattoos. He had silver rings in both eyebrows, a ring in his nose, and one in his upper lip. And he was in so much pain.

He hung his head and didn't answer.

"It's Christmas Eve," I said after a pause. "You're here, which means you want to fix this, and you aren't afraid to ask for help. There's no way I'm kicking you to the street today. We all make mistakes. I know you can do this. I believe in you."

We reviewed his chart together. Blood work revealed that his vitamin D levels were low. It's nearly impossible to get enough sunlight in Portland in the winter, and Michael had been so strung out on drugs that he had stopped taking a supplement. People with low levels of vitamin D, which is important for both brain function and mood, are at high risk for depression. Michael had also stopped taking the buprenorphine I had prescribed to keep him off heroin. It goes without saying that he was no longer exercising and hadn't eaten a proper meal in weeks. He was also having trouble sleeping, a problem common for so many addicts.

We talked about how this was a setback, not a death sentence. We talked about how failing gives you space to try again and how tough the holidays can be. I wrote Michael a one-week prescription for buprenorphine, got him a refill of vitamin D, recommended he try adding kava-kava to lemon-balm tea, an herbal remedy that is nonaddictive, and drink one to two cups before bed and throughout the night as needed, and urged him to start that night to get his sleep back on track. Together we figured out a plan to avoid contact with his drug dealer and get him back to exercising. I also had him commit to keeping a food diary for the following week, so when he came back into the office we could review it together.

"Might be kinda short, Doc." Michael laughed.

Michael's drug use had gotten so extreme that it was destroying his will to live.

I asked him to commit to coming to our weekly appointments and told him I wanted to see him even if he started using heroin again. He didn't have to be ashamed, and he certainly didn't have to disappear. He promised he would try. After four months of regular visits, Michael came into the clinic for his appointment smiling, joking with my office manager, and making himself at home. He has stayed drug-free since Christmas Eve. He had needed someone to believe in him then and a concrete plan to help him through the hardest time of the year.

Michael and I sat together on the couch in the treatment room and reviewed the timeline we'd created to finish tapering him off buprenorphine. He was so motivated to taper down that we both agreed we could lower his dose more quickly than other patients, if he was able to tolerate it. He was scared and excited. I was too.

We were both quiet for a moment, realizing that if all went well,

Michael would be off the buprenorphine sometime in the next few months. Though I would still see him for a follow-up visit—probably in six months—we might not be working together much longer. It was a bittersweet feeling. Michael had rebuilt his life to the point where he didn't need our office any more. That's exactly where we wanted him to be, but at the same time he'd be missed. He'd become family.

Kicking the Opioid Habit, the Dr. Paul Way

I hope I've convinced you by now that doctors need a more comprehensive method to combat addiction. My approach addresses addiction from an integrative perspective. I use a specific protocol that combines a taper-down-slowly prescription with identifying and healing the physical and emotional health problems addicts are facing.

So how do I get you off opioids? Tried and tested over the past decade,

Why Buprenorphine?

Buprenorphine is a partial agonist, which means it acts on your opiate receptors, and a partial antagonist, which means it also blocks them. Think of it as activating only half the opiate receptors and blocking the other half. You cannot and will not get high on buprenorphine if you have been using high doses of opioids when you start taking it. You won't feel the intense pleasure you feel from a full opioid. For some of you this will be an issue, as you are still seeking that feeling, and not being in an altered state may create anxiety and despair. You cannot overdose on buprenorphine if you're already opioid dependent, which makes it the safest drug available to help addicts. You also won't have overwhelming withdrawal symptoms if you take your buprenorphine and slowly taper down. Some doctors are prescribing much higher doses, which I think is a mistake, as it makes it more difficult to wean yourself off this medication. At a dose of 16 mg. we are covering over 90 percent of your opiate receptors (half blocked and half activated), so you almost never need to take more.

my method begins with buprenorphine. I have found that most who have been using daily opioids for between three to five years will require a starting daily buprenorphine dose of 16 mg. After one to four months at that dose, you can usually decrease the dosage to 12 mg. I want you to be at a high enough dose that you do not have withdrawal symptoms. This dosage will prevent you from getting an effect if you use heroin or other opioids while you are on it. At the same time, I will work with you to manage any accompanying anxiety, depression, sleep issues, attention disorders, or other underlying medical conditions.

A 16-mg. daily dose of buprenorphine usually results in improved mood and increased energy. You're no longer on the addiction roller coaster, where you get tired from taking too many opioids and then experience overwhelming withdrawal when you run out. Buprenorphine may not take all your anxiety away, but it will help. Your neurotransmitters have been hammered for . . . how many years? Be kind to yourself and patient with the process. It takes time for balance and healing to occur.

When you first lower the dose from 16 to 12 mg., you may experience mild withdrawal symptoms, including less energy, some trouble sleeping, and some anxiety. This usually lasts only a few days. Within a week or two, your brain readjusts to the smaller dose, and you start feeling as good at 12 mg. as you did at 16. Success! After you are stable at 12 mg. for at least a couple months, I start lowering the dose by 1 to 2 mg. every one to three months.

Getting lower than 4 mg.—which means you're in the homestretch of being completely opioid-free—is the hardest. My patients sometimes feel the most discomfort when we are lowering their dose to 2 mg., then 1.5 mg., then 1 mg., and finally to 0.5 mg. a day. On average this takes over a year. Often at this point in the journey, loved ones are eager for you to be completely off buprenorphine. At the smallest doses I need to support my patients the most—using natural sleep aids, intensive emotional support, and clonidine (a nonaddictive medicine for anxiety). It's common when you are decreasing your dose to experience muscle twitches, which can sometimes be painful. Some addiction doctors prescribe muscle relaxants for this. I have patients in my clinic take vitamin D with K_2 and a calcium and magnesium supplement. This combination usually solves that problem.

I currently have about forty patients who came to my clinic as chronic daily users of high doses of heroin and have now tapered down to low doses of buprenorphine over the course of two to four years. It took an average of seven months for them to taper down from 16 to 8 mg., an additional four months to lower to 6 mg., and another four months to get to 4 mg. These patients have all been able to work or go to school, and they have all done well throughout this process.

I've come to appreciate that there are some recovering addicts whose brain chemistry has been so compromised that they cannot recover enough to function well if they are completely buprenorphine-free. I no longer force these patients to reduce their dose on a rigid, prede-termined schedule. We do our best, tapering as much as appropriate and as they have the desire and support in place. I think this is a big reason I've had so few deaths and relatively few failures with addicts in my care.

I imagine some readers shaking their heads. Before you throw this book across the room, I will agree with you that it's not perfect. The goal is getting completely drug-free, not taking maintenance doses. But I will also remind you that part of recovering from addiction is embracing imperfection and being kind, gentle, and patient with our-selves.

This whole process of weaning off drugs requires you and your doc-tor to be engaged in the recovery journey together. You no longer see yourself going back to the life of using drugs, you've embraced the goal of being drug-free, and you have a doctor who supports and believes that you will succeed.

More honest disclosure: most of my patients also use cannabis daily when they start treatment. I have found that to institute an absolute no-cannabis policy discourages patients from getting help. But I am usually able, over time, to encourage many to reduce or completely stop. When this happens, you can see the lights come on in their eyes. More about cannabis in chapter 7.

My taper-down approach to opioid recovery works hand in glove with embracing lifestyle improvements and integrative solutions that support your recovery. Here are seven steps to follow:

1. **Eat real food.** It's best if the food you eat is organic and unprocessed and does not contain any additives or added refined sugar. You want to eat some high-quality fats, like avocado, olives, or coconut, every

Withdrawal Symptoms

When you or someone you love is in withdrawal from opioid addiction, expect the following symptoms:

Agitation	Joint pain
Anxiety	Muscle pain
Diarrhea	Poor appetite
Dilated (larger than normal) pupils	Restlessness
	Runny eyes or crying
General discomfort (one addict described this as feeling crawled over by biting ants)	Runny nose
	Shakes
Goose bumps	Stomachaches
Insomnia	Sweating

day as well as high-quality protein. You also want to make sure you are eating more vegetables than you ever have before, especially colorful veggies and green leafy ones, which are high in iron and fiber. More on my food cure for pain below.

2. **Get enough vitamin D.** Vitamin D plays a crucial role in the immune system and is vital for proper brain function. Unless you live close to the equator and work outside with your shirt off, it is very difficult to keep your vitamin D level in the optimal range of 50–80 ng/dL without a supplement. I recommend 5,000 IU a day of vitamin D_3, maybe more, especially in the winter. Get your vitamin D_3 level checked and supplement accordingly.

3. **Work on your worry.** I know you're stressed. I am too. Getting off opioids is stressful, to say nothing of the problems that got you into opioid addiction in the first place! But that stress compromises your immune system, causing pain and inflammation. Financial worries, problems at work, and unhealthy relationships as well as the news and your smartphone alerts can all stimulate stress hormones in your body. As I talked about in chapter 3, stress is the X factor in addiction. You must address both your

daily stress and the stress you may be carrying with you from your childhood in order to recover. You can't rid yourself of stress completely, but you can find ways—big and little—to reduce and better cope with stress.

4. **Seek quality sleep.** Sleep is restorative, allowing your body to get back into balance and heal itself. Most of us need between seven and nine hours of sleep a night, but few get that much. See my sleep solutions on pages 124–25 and 257–61.

5. **Say okay to exercise.** You're tired. You're sore. Everything hurts. The last thing you want to do is move. You'd rather pop a pill. But exercise—even slow, quiet, calm exercise—will help every ache and pain, as I talk about more below.

6. **Heal your gut microbiome.** You have trillions of microbes (bacteria, viruses, and other microorganisms) living in you and on you (your biome), especially in your intestines and colon (the gut microbiome). Chances are you grew up being told that germs were bad, when in fact some bacteria and other symbiotic organisms are not only helpful but even essential for your survival.

   We know now that good diversity in the gut microbiome reduces inflammation and can even reverse autoimmune conditions. Some of our essential vitamins are actually produced by the beneficial bacteria in the GI tract. Many nutrients are released from food because bacteria help break them down. Many of the neurotransmitters essential for good brain function and mood, including dopamine and serotonin, are affected by your microbiome.

   Healing your gut microbiome is part of the process to heal your brain. Help your microbiome heal by taking probiotics, eating fermented foods like kombucha, sauerkraut, and kimchee, and adding probiotic yogurt (sheep, goat, cow, or coconut) to your diet.

7. **Surround yourself with a supportive network of sober people.** Humans thrive in community. In addiction you feel isolated and alone. You may be with a group of "friends" acting as though you're having fun, but deep down you feel empty and alone. Developing a support system is a key to enjoying life without opioids. Chances are most of your friends—and maybe even family members—are also users. So when you're in the early part of your

recovery journey, you have to develop a whole new set of contacts and friends.

Spend a little time with elementary school kids, and you'll see that it's hard to make friends *at any age*. It's even harder for addicts, because you are often awkward in social situations (one of the reasons you started using in the first place), so without opioids you feel even more uncomfortable. You can and will find your new tribe. As a wise friend used to remind his daughter, "It only takes one." One friend who is kind, understanding, and supportive will help you change your life. Just one.

Your new support system can also include a therapist who will counsel you one-on-one, an outpatient group at a hospital or sobriety clinic, 12-step meetings, our office (of course), and your old friends who are not users and who are willing to accept you the way you are, warts and all, without judgment.

More on Integrative Ways to Treat Pain

After surgery a few years ago, my doctor asked me to rate my pain level as the anesthetic was wearing off.

"Oh, about a three or four out of ten," I said.

"Nonsense," he said. "We can do better than that." He told the nurse to give me a push of IV morphine. In an instant I felt the most amazing sense of calm and well-being flood my body.

"I think my pain was a ten!" I told the doctor.

I had been suffering from a chronic sinus infection. The total absence of pain for perhaps the first time in over a decade felt amazing. I was already in recovery from alcoholism, and I could see how someone would start to crave that incredible opioid-induced sensation.

In my experience, being in pain is often what starts you along the addiction spectrum. That pain can be physical or emotional. Physical pain, often the initial trigger that led you to use opioids, is usually due to inflammation. If you have headaches or migraines, your brain is inflamed. If you have joint pain like arthritis, your joints are inflamed. The key to reducing that inflammation is integrating the basics discussed in this book into your everyday life—not using drugs or alcohol.

My patients describe the feeling of using heroin and other opioids:

"All my problems disappeared."

"A calm feeling of peace."

"Every painful experience gone."

"Bathed in warm sunlight."

"I was surrounded by love for the first time in my life."

"I thought, 'If this is how I'm supposed to feel, sign me up.'"

Are you in physical or emotional pain? Of course, you don't want to feel bad. You can't ignore your pain. Masking it with opioids doesn't work either. My patients never believe me when I tell them that their physical pain will improve as we taper down the dose of opioids, but it does. When you first used an opioid for pain, it worked like magic. Then it stopped working, and your doctor increased the dose, leading it to help again. Then it stopped working. So you increased the dose again, either with your doctor's blessing and a prescription or with pain pills, heroin, or fentanyl acquired illegally. Your developing tolerance resulted in the activation of new opiate receptors in your brain. Opiate receptors are pain receptors, so now you feel even greater pain from things that you normally would have handled just fine. When you stop taking opioids, you will start to feel less pain! Regardless of the underlying reason for the pain, your experience of that pain will improve as you decrease the dose and implement my seven strategies (pages 94–97).

You need to address the underlying causes of your pain. Pain, as I mentioned, is usually triggered by inflammation, which is the body's natural response to injury. Inflammation usually helps us heal, but we can also have too much of a good thing. Sometimes our bodies become chronically inflamed. When that happens, our immune system mistakes our own tissue for foreign invaders, and we attack ourselves. This kind of inflammation can be painful, exhausting, and debilitating. So to fight chronic pain, the first step is to look for underlying causes of inflammation.

The number one cause of the pain you are experiencing is usually the food you are eating. Yes, I am going to talk about food in every chapter of this book. Yes, I run the risk of driving you crazy. I need you to pay attention, which is why I will keep repeating it: our highly processed, additive-filled, dye-filled, GMO-compromised SAD diet triggers inflammation, creating autoimmune problems, which in turn cause our own bodies to attack themselves. To live a pain-free life without opioids, you have to remove processed foods. For many pain conditions, removing gluten and dairy will also help bring relief. For others you may need to avoid high-histamine foods. For all conditions you must avoid MSG and "natural flavors" (a code word for neurotoxins), petroleum-based food dyes, and mold inhibitors.

Adding anti-inflammatory foods to your diet helps with pain. Turmeric is a root that grows in abundance in tropical climates and is used in Indian and African cooking. Turmeric has powerful natural anti-inflammatory properties, which means it will help you reduce inflammation and pain. You can add it to a stir-fry, roast it with other root vegetables, use it as a spice, add it as a healthy extra to everything from applesauce to pancake batter, or juice it. Oily fish (like salmon and sardines) is a standard component of both Japanese and Mediterranean diets, considered among the healthiest in the world. Like turmeric, oily fish is anti-inflammatory. You need to give it a little bit of time, but if you start adding turmeric to your daily diet and eating fish once or twice a week, along with other dietary improvements and lifestyle changes, you will noticeably reduce your body's aches and pains. Other anti-inflammatory foods include broccoli, olives, chia seeds, blueberries and other fresh fruits, green tea, and dark chocolate.

Food Solutions to Help with Pain

1. **Always eat real food.** Strive for a diet of fresh organic fruits and vegetables; high-quality proteins including eggs, chicken, fish, and free-range grass-fed, grass-finished red meat; high-quality healthy fats like avocados, coconuts, olives, extra virgin olive oil, and nuts; healthy starches like sweet potatoes, yams, and rice; and probiotic foods like fermented vegetables and plain yogurt. Stock your freezer with frozen organic vegetables like green beans, kale, and peas (often on sale!) and add them to your morning scrambled eggs, your afternoon salad, and whatever you're having for dinner.

2. **Avoid refined sugar.** Sugar causes inflammation, blood sugar dips and spikes, and a host of other problems, including acne. Some researchers believe that sugar feeds disease[22] and that the over-consumption of sugar is one of the reasons so many Americans are battling cancer. Avoid candy bars, soda, cakes, and cookies. Though you shouldn't get draconian about never eating sweets, it's honestly best to avoid these foods whether you are in pain or not. For lasting good health, substitute naturally sweet foods (I recommend apples, dried mango, crushed pineapple, prunes, dates, raisins, yams, berries, overripe bananas, and shredded coconut) for refined white sugar.

3. **Take turmeric.** Just $^1/_4$ teaspoon in 8 ounces of water can cure a headache, but you may need up to 1 teaspoon. Start with $^1/_4$ teaspoon and increase the dosage until you notice results.

4. **Take purified fish oil.** Take 2,000 mg. a day, and try to eat oily fish once or twice a week.

5. **Take an enzyme before you eat.** If you've been eating badly your whole life or been taxing your digestion because of addiction, your body may not be digesting food as effectively as it should. You can be malnourished if you are not absorbing the nutrients from the healthy food you're eating. After age forty the amount of digestive enzymes your stomach secretes starts to diminish. Most people will benefit from taking a high-quality enzyme before each meal. And don't forget to chew. Aim for twenty chews per mouthful, which will help with digestion.

Exercise Helps Too

The second line of defense for inflammation is exercise. The average American office worker sits for over ten hours a day. A recent study of over 12,500 Americans, published in the *Journal of Preventative Medicine,* found that the average nineteen-year-old American is as sedentary as a sixty-year-old![23] You cannot be healthy if you are sitting for this many hours every day. Of course, I am sitting at my dining-room table looking at the red alder and Oregon white oak out the window as I write this, realizing I've been sitting now for several hours without a break. Let me get up, do some stretching, and take a walk around the block . . .

Okay, where was I?

You don't have to be an Olympic athlete. You don't even have to *like* exercise. You don't have to want to do it. Grumbling is allowed. It's not a competition, and you don't have to be "good" at sports. But to reduce your chronic pain, you do have to get up and move as much as you can throughout the day and dedicate some time daily to exercising.

Aim for 45 to 60 minutes of mild to moderate physical activity every day—walking the dog, jogging, running, weight lifting, swimming, dancing, CrossFit (my current fave), or whatever activity you enjoy. Doing daily exercise will lessen pain and improve your mood. Making love counts too. It offers an endorphin boost, reduces pain, and reminds you that pleasure is **possible** without opioids. If you have become dependent on opioids, your natural sex hormones may have become so suppressed that you have all but lost the desire and even the ability to have sex. A return of your libido is something to look forward to as you lower your opioid use.

It's also helpful to have small bursts of activity throughout the day, even just a few minutes at a time. Take the stairs instead of the elevator, jump your age in jumping jacks, convert your work space so you can stand for part of the day, park a half mile away from your destination and walk. Do your best. I know it may sound impossible, especially if you are heavier than you want to be or very out of shape, but the benefits to your health and well-being of daily exercise are immeasurable.

Integrative Solutions to Treat Back Pain

I injured my back in college lifting a huge box of books. I fell to the floor paralyzed, unable to move for hours. My doctor gave me pain pills and muscle relaxants. I used alcohol to supplement the pills, but I was in terrible pain for weeks. Over a decade later I learned I had a bulging disc. Each time I reinjured my back, I would take more pain pills and muscle relaxants. Then I began studying integrative medicine, and a colleague recommended chiropractic care. The relief was immediate after just one adjustment. I know firsthand how debilitating back pain can be.

If you are suffering from chronic back or musculoskeletal pain, there is an arsenal of Western and non-Western healing techniques to help you heal.

Acupuncture: Acupuncture is a healing technique used in Chinese medicine that stimulates specific points on the body by inserting thin needles through the skin. Several studies have shown that acupuncture is an effective way to relieve lower back pain.[24] Acupuncture is so effective that it is used in Scandinavian countries to help women in labor manage childbirth pain.[25] One of my friends has deeply benefitted from acupuncture; she finds it so relaxing she falls asleep during the sessions and then awakens refreshed and pain-free.

Chiropractic care: Your back and neck may be out of alignment, a common problem for people who are stressed, sit for long hours, lift small children, or spend too much time curving their necks to look at their smartphones. An osteopath or a chiropractor can adjust your back and neck to bring your spine back into alignment. If this is the root cause of the problem, you will most likely feel immediate relief. While you are there, talk to the chiropractor or osteopath about ways to make your lifestyle more ergonomic. This may include buying a wedge that provides proper lumbar support when you are in the car, switching from a sitting to a standing or walking desk, and incorporating more movement into your day. I recommend a 1- to 2-minute walk every 20 to 30 minutes—and less time on your smartphone.

Meditation: When neck or back pain is caused by anxiety and stress (or when the fact that you are in pain is causing you stress), stress-relieving techniques like meditation can be remarkably successful. This isn't as quick a fix as opioid pain medicine or a muscle relaxant, but it is one that will improve every aspect of your life. Sign up for a meditation class, ongoing meditation sessions, or even a retreat. Check with your local Zen center. You can also download guided meditations.

Strength training and stretching: Strengthening your core (your stomach and back muscles) as well as your legs will help cure back pain. A physical therapist can tailor a set of exercises to your specific needs, or you can start now by integrating stomach crunches (avoid sit-ups), hamstring stretches, and pelvic tilts into your daily exercise routine. Yoga, which provides strength training and stretching, is also effective in preventing and treating back pain.[26] Pay attention to your body. Find the strength training and stretching exercises that feel good, and be careful not to do any exercise that hurts your back.

Therapeutic massage: Sometimes the root cause of back pain is muscle tension and chronic stress. Therapeutic massage can be tremendously healing for both problems and works better, I believe, than prescription muscle relaxants that may have unwanted side effects (like brain fog and fatigue). The best way to find a skilled massage therapist is to ask friends who have suffered from back pain for recommendations. If money is an obstacle, most massage-therapy schools offer reduced-cost massages done by students. I recommend you get a massage once a week until the pain goes away. Ask your massage therapist to use an oil that includes camphor, lavender, or eucalyptus, which will also help with pain. You can also massage painful areas on your body with arnica lotion.

Weight loss: The backache you are experiencing might be caused by being overweight. It's very difficult to lose weight (ask me how I know), but imperative for reducing pain. Cut out junk food, processed Frankenfood, and sugar. Don't go it alone. Joining Weight Watchers or a weight-loss program at your gym or just finding a friend to lose weight with you will help you succeed. And, of course, eating a diet of real foods and getting plenty of exercise and high-quality sleep will help you lose weight too.

Integrative Solutions for Emotional Pain

There are reasons you are in emotional pain. It's not just "all in your head." When you can figure out the reasons for the loneliness, guilt, or depression you are feeling, you can actually fix your feelings by dealing with the root causes. The key is to take it one step at a time. You'll find that if you get grounded in one aspect of your life, other pieces will also start falling into place.

That's what happened for Joey. Joey is twenty-seven and thin as a beanpole. He has a two-year-old son he adores, though he and the mom are no longer together. Joey has been struggling with severe anxiety and emotional pain for two years. Today he is calm, and the wrinkle lines on his forehead are gone. He sits without squirming.

"You look great today," I remarked. "What's different?"

"I'm seeing my kid again." Joey beamed. "Work is going better. I don't have the money problems that were killing me."

The transformation in front of me was nothing short of miraculous. Joey had taken hold of his life and started to chip away at his biggest stressors. In particular he began climbing out of the financial hole his drug use had put him in. Since he had a working car, he could pick his toddler up for the much-needed father-son time. Being on time made his ex more responsive and kinder to him and helped him get better reviews at work.

Reduce stress. Identify your biggest stressors and make a plan to reduce them, one at a time.

Plug into a support system. Perhaps you prefer counseling to 12-step meetings, but if you feel uncomfortable meeting one-on-one, find an AA or NA meeting nearby (there are meeting locators online at www.na.org or download the app called Meeting Guide to help you find one). Your local hospital or church may also have an addict support group. The Substance Abuse and Mental Health Services government website also maintains a list of other ongoing meetings where you can get support: www.findtreatment.samhsa.gov/locator /link-focSelfGP.

Distance yourself from enablers. Stay away from anyone or anything that triggers your desire to use. Friends and family who use your addiction as an excuse not to get on with their own lives are best avoided for now.

Start a journal to chronicle your recovery. You can journal by speaking into your smartphone or an old-fashioned tape recorder, scrapbooking photos or drawings, writing on paper or on your computer, or sharing a blog on the internet that others can read. Set yourself the goal of making a contribution (at least one sentence) every day. Record your goals, aspirations, struggles, relapses, food choices, or anything you choose. You can carry this chronicle of yourself with you on your journey and use it to help you answer your doctor's and loved ones' questions.

Start helping others. You may feel as if your life is too big a mess for you to help anyone else, but one of the best things you can do to clean it up—even as you are in the midst of recovery—is to help someone else.

Relapse Is Expected but Not Required

Let's get real: it is hard to get off opioids and even the most motivated addicts sometimes relapse. Over 60 percent of those who have a problem with alcohol or drugs will use again within the first year after treatment.[27] Heroin addicts, especially, are at high risk for relapse, chronic mental-health problems, and even death.[28]

Addiction is a chronic, relapsing illness, and it's important for you to think about what that means. A patient whose eczema is under control thanks to diet, exercise, avoidance of toxins, and medication might have an unexpected flare-up—because of either something she ate, something she touched, or even stress. We don't think of drug relapse that way, usually, because we think addicts "should" have the willpower to keep addiction under control. But if you think of a relapse as a flare-up, something that happened and that you can get on top of—not something that shows that you are a moral failure or a bad person—you will have an easier time getting sober again.

"Relapse is expected but not required." I would actually say that to you if you were my patient, even in front of a loved one or support person (if you've given permission for the support person to be a part of the evaluation).

Why do I tell my new patients that? For many people going cold turkey is unrealistic and unfair. When you are trying to fight an addiction, you may relapse. As much as you want the problem to be over—and over *now*—life doesn't usually work that way. It took you a lot of years to get you to where you are now, and it may take as many more to move away from the severe end of the addiction spectrum. You and your support team need to know that relapse happens. When it does, you try again.

Be committed to your recovery, even as you make mistakes and even fail. Identify what situations, thoughts, and people trigger you to want to get high. When you know what your triggers are, you can learn how to avoid them. You need a new set of skills to help you get away when you find yourself triggered—like recoiling from a hot flame.

"You have two legs. They're made for walking or running," I tell Amanda, a thirty-year-old recovering heroin addict who's been coming to me for just under a year.

Amanda tells me her girlfriends invited her to get high last week, and she wasn't sure what to say. Growing up in an abusive home, she had never really learned to stand up for herself.

"Just say out loud, 'I just forgot, I'm supposed to meet somebody right now,' and physically leave," I tell her. Easier said than done, I know. But I tell Amanda that it doesn't matter that she doesn't own a car and didn't have her cell phone with her. "You have two legs. You can get the hell out of there."

Have you ever watched a baby learning how to walk? He gets up, falls down, gets bruised, cries, and is comforted by loving arms; then he picks himself up and tries again. If that baby was afraid of making mistakes, he'd spend his whole life crawling!

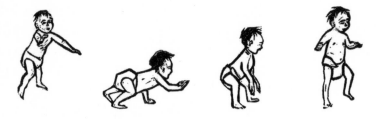

SOMETIMES, YOU HAVE TO FAIL TO SUCCEED.

It's an important life lesson for everything: sometimes we need to fail to succeed.

I don't want anyone in my clinic to fail. But I want everyone to know that I will help them try again as many times as they are willing to try, as long as they are honest with me.

I can handle relapse. What I can't handle is lies and deception, trying to game the system, or any attempts to use me as your drug dealer. I can't and won't work with anyone who comes to my clinic looking to get buprenorphine from me to sell it to somebody else in order to buy another drug of choice. But I will always be there to support you. Let's walk this long and winding road together.

A Message to Your Support Team

Support people need to know what signs of relapse to look for. Signs that a patient who's being treated with buprenorphine has relapsed include:

Excessive sleepiness

Slurred speech

Strange or intoxicated behavior

Opioids are the leading cause of drug-overdose deaths in the United States. In the time it took you to read this chapter as many as six people have died. But you do not have to be a statistic.

Remember the frogs? Be the one who jumps into the journey of recovery. Get busy getting well. Move yourself toward the mild end of the addiction spectrum before it's too late for you. Opioids might not be your only cross. It is the rare heroin or other opioid addict who doesn't use other drugs as well. So you also have to confront your other addictions. Read on.

CHAPTER 5

Braking Bad: Overcoming Your Addiction to Meth and Other Stimulants

JOSH, who's been coming to my clinic for about two years, staggers in fifteen minutes late. It's a rainy day, and he's dressed in layers—khaki pants and a gray sweatshirt with a maroon collared shirt underneath. Josh is in pretty rough shape today: dark circles under his eyes, ghostly pale skin, reeking of tobacco. He's shivering a little, though it's warm inside. He runs his hands through his brown hair, which he wears trimmed on the sides and long on top, and fidgets with both legs. He fails his urine test—again—and the time we spend together centers on how he's going to sober up enough to stay out of jail.

When Josh leaves I find myself feeling low. How did such a smart, likable, energetic kid end up making such bad choices? Why is facing life without drugs so hard for Josh and so many young people today? I think about these questions as I finish Josh's charting. As many success stories as I have in my clinic and as optimistic as I am by nature, this is really hard. I can't sugarcoat it. Addiction like this sucks. And meth. Dear God. Why is Josh doing meth?

Methamphetamine is a stimulant that can come in a bitter-tasting white powder or pill. It's sometimes bluish, and it may also look like a rock or crystal, which is why they call it "crystal" or "crystal meth." Crystal meth is the most potent form, which has been popular and cheap in the United States since the early 1980s.[1] You may also have heard meth called ice, glass, Tina, tweak, speed, crank, and a variety of other street names. It's a drug that was first synthesized from a plant used in Chinese and Ayurvedic (that is, Indian) medicine by a Japanese chemist named Nagai Nagayoshi in 1893.[2] You can crush and snort it, swallow it, smoke it in a glass pipe, and also inject it to get high.

However you use it, meth increases dopamine in your brain up to a hundred times your normal levels, which is why it gives you such a powerful high. As I mentioned in chapter 1, dopamine is an important "feel good" chemical. A neurotransmitter released in the brain during pleasurable activities like eating delicious food or making love, dopamine also helps with alertness and focus. Another of my patients described using meth as a pleasure akin to the most intense orgasm he had ever had, but one that lasted for hours. Is it any wonder, once you start using meth, it can be so hard to stop?

Yesterday's Pharma Peddling Becomes Today's Drug Scourge

In chapter 3 I talked to you about how today's pharmaceutical companies and medical doctors hawk and foster addiction, promoting your drug use to increase their bottom line. That's not a new phenomenon, unfortunately. Like cocaine (another illegal stimulant), meth was legally used by medical doctors for years. Theodor Morell, Adolf Hitler's doctor in Berlin, famously gave the Führer meth injections.[3] Soldiers fighting on both sides during World War II often took stimulants, including meth and amphetamines,[4] to stay awake and alert[5] (as do some long-distance truck drivers to this day).[6] In 1944 meth, made by Abbott Laboratories,[7] was officially approved by the FDA.[8] Back then it was used to treat everything from alcoholism to obesity to depression. During that boom time after World War II, indeed, drug companies pushed all sorts of amphetamines on consumers in the United States.[9]

One magazine advertisement targeting housewives boasted that meth is a "magic powder" to disperse unwanted fat, purify and enrich the blood, and make you feel healthier in every way.[10] Amphetamines were peddled as appetite suppressants, nasal decongestants, and energy boosters, and use skyrocketed.[11] In the decade following World War II, over half a million Americans were using amphetamines. But with the widespread use of amphetamines came reports of their harmful effects: these central-nervous-system stimulants were soon seen to have debilitating side effects, especially at higher doses. Meth was found to cause restlessness, insomnia, paranoia, convulsions, hallucinations, and even cardiac arrest.

The euphoria meth induced also turned out to be highly addictive. The 1970 Comprehensive Drug Abuse Prevention and Control Act placed meth products under Schedule II, which resulted in a steady decline in meth use in pill form. Cocaine became the stimulant of choice in the 1970s, followed by a new wave of meth abuse in the mid-1980s with the arrival of street "ice," "crank," or "crystal meth." The stimulant abuse that was started by the medical profession at the end of World War II, which was eclipsed by the explosion of crystal meth in the 1980s, has returned again with the skyrocketing number of prescriptions for stimulants to treat ADHD.

Worse Than Heroin?

It's hard to imagine a drug worse than heroin, but meth could be it. There was an explosion of meth-treatment admissions from 1993 to 2003, with numbers jumping from 28,000 a year in 1993 to approximately 136,000 in 2003.[12] Although the number of new meth users went down over the next decade, over a million people used meth in 2012, and there were 133,000 new users that year alone.[13] These days, *three times* as many people in Oregon are arrested because of meth (15,308 in 2016) than because of heroin (4,990), and there have been more meth-related than heroin-related deaths in our state, with meth fatalities going up 44 percent from 2014 to 2015.[14] Easy to get on the West Coast, widely available in Oregon, it is usually smuggled in by Mexican drug cartels. Worldwide meth abuse remains an intractable problem as well: the United Nations estimates there are 37 million amphetamine users globally, more than the number of cocaine and heroin users combined.[15]

Addiction specialists and emergency-room physicians are well aware of the telling signs that someone has been "tweaking" (for the uninitiated, the slang word for getting high on meth): intense energy, fever, agitation, restlessness, extreme anxiety, paranoia, and delusions or hallucinations, the last two of which can make the meth user potentially violent. If you've tried both meth and heroin, you know from firsthand experience: the extreme restlessness, pacing, and nonstop talking that happens when you've taken meth is in stark contrast to the more sedated, lethargic, depressed, underwater feeling you have after taking too much heroin or other opioid.

After the intense high and euphoria experienced from meth use comes depression and lethargy due to the severe depletion of dopamine, serotonin, and norepinephrine stores. Meth addicts, left desperate to feel anything, are shaky, apathetic, depleted of energy, and just plain miserable. Only more meth will raise their neurotransmitter levels enough so they are able to function or to relieve the anxiety, depression, and lethargy they feel without it.

What's also hard is that, unlike with opioids, we don't have any drug that can block the effects of meth. We don't have an adequate pharmacological substitute or partial agonist, like buprenorphine. We don't have a way to reverse a meth overdose, like naloxone (see chapter 10 as well as appendix 1 for more on naloxone). To say that meth addiction is hard to treat is an understatement. So if you've taken meth in the past but aren't using it anymore, give yourself a pat on the back. And never, *ever*, give yourself permission to use it again! Run from it, *literally*, if that is required.

As enticing as the high is for some, meth use can destroy your mental and physical health. If you've never tried it, but want to see for yourself how meth can age you, rot your teeth, and make your skin sallow, there are websites (one is called "Your Face on Meth") and apps where you upload a photo of yourself and the site converts it to what you'll look like if you use meth long-term.

SHORT-TERM NEGATIVE HEALTH EFFECTS FROM USING METH

Anxiety

Delusions

Disturbed sleep and insomnia

Exhaustion (when the drug wears off)

Hyperactivity

Increased aggressiveness

Irritability

Nausea

Weight loss

**LONG-TERM NEGATIVE HEALTH EFFECTS
FROM USING METH**

Arrhythmia (irregular heartbeat) that can lead to heart failure and
  organ damage

Brain damage

Confusion

Damaged blood vessels in the brain

Depression

Increased blood pressure

Increased heart rate (tachycardia)

Liver, kidney, and lung damage

Malnutrition

Severe tooth decay

Josh: Gifted, Then Addicted

Over the time that I've been treating him, I have been talking to Josh
about how he got so entangled with drugs. Sometimes he is lucid
and articulate. Other times he talks in sentence fragments, alternat-
ing between making insightful observations and trailing off incoher-
ently, losing his train of thought. He tells me he was really outgoing
when he was little, that he had a black belt in tae kwon do by the

time he was thirteen. But, he says, he was also very oppositional, always had a problem with authority, and came from a pretty chaotic home. Though his sister never took drugs, he does have the genetic predisposition to become an addict that I talked about in chapter 1. Josh's dad is an alcoholic, and his mom, a labor and delivery nurse, is addicted to opioids.

Josh's exposure to drugs started early. He tried opioids for the first time in seventh grade when he fractured his right arm. Then in ninth grade, on the first day he used a season pass to Mount Hood, he took a jump on his snowboard at breakneck speed and fractured the growth plate in his shoulder. He needed surgery and pain medication—and the doctors gave him opioids without ever taking a family history. By then Josh already knew that he liked the effects of opioids and easily found ways to trick doctors into giving him more. His sophomore year of high school he started with weed.

Talk to him for a few minutes, and you'll quickly realize that Josh is an incredibly intelligent outside-the-box thinker who would probably have been tagged as gifted if anyone had thought to give him an IQ test in elementary school. Josh went to private Catholic school; he was constantly getting in trouble, always told to sit still, and often acted out. Gifted, high-energy kids, especially boys, are often failed by our school system. Instead of finding creative outlets for his exuberance and curiosity and trying integrative techniques to help him focus, Josh was medicated with amphetamines for his attention challenges.

Focus disorders, especially in males, have been associated with drug addiction in general and with meth addiction in particular. One study comparing over two hundred adults who were diagnosed with ADHD in childhood with adults who had no such diagnosis found that people with ADHD were twice as likely to become substance abusers and nearly four times as likely to progress from alcohol use to drug use than people who didn't have underlying attention disorders.[16] Doctors and researchers estimate that anywhere from 20[17] to 70 percent of meth addicts have struggled with lifelong ADHD.[18]

"I think I've got a genetic disposition to addiction, and giving kids speed and opiates is really dangerous," Josh says when he reflects on how he got addicted. "Most people I know who are addicted, it's all medicine related."

A Rose by Any Other Name? Methamphetamine and Other Amphetamine Drugs

Methamphetamine is an amphetamine. If you have ADD or ADHD, you are familiar with synthetic stimulants, which include Adderall (amphetamine-dextroamphetamine), Ritalin (methylphenidate), Vyvanse (lisdexamfetamine), Focalin (dexmethylphenidate hydrochloride), and a host of new preparations releasing these same compounds in different ways. Stimulants like these are commonly prescribed for focus disorders, because they increase attention and are thought to be generally helpful with performance at school or work. Amphetamines have been historically prescribed for narcolepsy, but are falling out of use.[19] All of these drugs increase the effect of dopamine by either causing the release of more or allowing it to stay in the body longer.

Although methamphetamine and ADHD stimulants are similar in structure, the effects are different, especially in their intensity. Still, amphetamines have the potential to have very serious side effects, especially at higher doses. These side effects include insomnia, poor appetite, weight loss, accelerated heart rate, irritability, hallucinations, and depression. Occasionally amphetamines will have a sedating effect, making the user look sleepy and "out of it."

I shared my concern about exposing babies to fentanyl and other opioids during labor in chapter 3. I am also concerned about exposing young children to amphetamines. Nearly *ten times* as many children are taking prescription stimulants as were taking them in the late 1980s, and prescription use among six- to twelve-year-olds is highest.[20] When I'm wearing my pediatrician's cap, I am happy to have these tools in my medical toolbox. But I also think it's important to ask the question: By putting young children and teenagers on brain-altering substances, are we perhaps priming them for much more problematic drug use in adulthood as well as for addiction?

I was hyper as a child, but never put on any medication. I always chose to sit in the back corner of every room, so that my fidgeting and restlessness would be less distracting to my teachers and peers. But I was also very lucky: I went to a one-room thatched-roof elementary school in an African village, and we had plenty of breaks to run and play outside mid-morning, at lunch, and in the early afternoon. All through grade school and high school in Africa, we had afternoon sports and activities outdoors with plenty of opportunities to let off steam. I was able to pay attention and sit somewhat still in class partly thanks to the constant movement and outdoor time that was a part of my day.

Children and adults cannot learn effectively if they are forced to sit still for hours on end. But, sadly, American educators and policymakers seem to have forgotten the importance of recess, physical education, sports, and unstructured play. In America today PE and recess are limited in favor of academic learning, even though cutting these opportunities for physical activity throughout the day actually makes it harder for children—not just kids with attention disorders—to learn.

At the same time that our kids are much more sedentary than is healthy for their bodies or their brains, the criteria for diagnosing attention deficit disorders has become much more inclusive. The American Psychiatric Association now includes "makes careless mistakes" and "has difficulty waiting his or her turn" on the list.[21] Doctors are encouraged by pharmaceutical companies and pharmaceutical-funded studies to prescribe medication for attention challenges. Educators, who may get more federal and state funding for schoolchildren with special needs, also encourage parents to have their children diagnosed.[22] The result has been a financial bonanza for drug companies, as more children in America than ever before are now being diagnosed with ADHD,[23] and children and adults are taking record amounts of amphetamine drugs.[24] Prescription stimulant sales are more than five times what they were in 2002.

At the same time, most children are being fed a nutritionally bankrupt diet, being exposed to record levels of toxins, spending too much time on screens (something I'll talk more about in chapter 8), and are vitamin D deficient. All of this harms the brain. Glyphosate, the main chemical ingredient in the weed killer Roundup, is sprayed on most corn and soybeans grown in America and is known to interfere with the precursors of the neurotransmitters, tyrosine and tryptophan.[25] Its widespread use may also be implicated in the growing numbers of children with ADD.[26]

The result of our toxic environment, the SAD way of eating I've been talking about in every chapter, and a lack of exercise, outdoor time, and free play is that ADD and ADHD in children today seem to be more severe than in previous generations. And severe ADD often does require medication if you want to keep your child in school.

Studies show many college students have started using stimulants to prepare for and take tests. Even if you have no formal diagnosis of ADD or ADHD and even if your brain already produces enough dopamine, most of us reap the benefits of alertness and focus when first taking these drugs. Which makes them very tempting to try.

Is there a risk of becoming addicted to your ADHD medications? Drug manufacturers claim that these meds are benign, and doctors often tell patients they are nonaddictive and "safer than aspirin."[27] But that's simply not true.

Doctors should not reach for the prescription pad as the first intervention when a tween or teen is having trouble focusing in school. The first line of defense must always be natural approaches, including lifestyle changes (which are admittedly very hard to implement with strong-willed teens) and an individually tailored education plan that includes extra movement and time outside. Often what is really needed is more activity and active learning throughout the day, clearer boundaries, help with organizational skills at school and outside of school, and some extra tutoring or mentoring.

In his book *The Myth of the ADHD Child*, psychologist Thomas Armstrong, executive director of the American Institute for Learning and Human Development, offers 101 different strategies to improve a child's behavior and attention span without the use of any pharmaceutical drugs, recommending everything from "wiggle-friendly furniture" (standing desks, swivel stools, exercise balls) to neurofeedback training. All of this can potentially help a child concentrate and do better in school.

If these interventions are not enough, I have found that properly treating ADD and ADHD with judicious use of the lowest doses of medication can help kids improve their self-esteem and their ability to learn in school, while also calming the agitation, depression, and anxiety that sometimes come with a severe inability to focus. Should our kids be popping amphetamines like candy? No. Might your prescription as a teen have contributed to your addiction as an adult, as Josh feels his did? Yes. At the same time, some studies have shown that *untreated* ADD or ADHD leads to *more addiction* in young adults who end up self-medicating with illegal drugs.[28] Put another way, young people who are properly treated for their ADD and ADHD seem to be less likely to become addicts.[29]

If you have diabetes and your pancreas has stopped producing enough insulin, we need to treat you with insulin. If your dopamine and norepinephrine levels are low and insufficient for focus, we may also need to treat you with pharmaceutical drugs. But it is true that stimulants can be abused, and insulin cannot. That is one of the reasons I educate endlessly. At every visit, I talk to my patients who are on prescription stimulants about the dangers of addiction and how to avoid it.

In the pediatric arm of my practice, I have had over thirteen thousand children. Of those, nearly a thousand patients have been diagnosed with ADD or ADHD. About half of them are on some low-dose amphetamine, and their families are also doing their best to follow the nutrition plan, supplement guide, and counseling advice outlined in this book. During the last ten years, only two of my pediatric patients have ended up in my addiction clinic as young adults. The success seems real, though I am not fooling myself. There is no question that those with underlying ADD or ADHD, anxiety, or depression are at higher risk for becoming addicted to mind-altering substances and that, even with the best care and attention, some young adults will succumb.

Amphetamines Should Not Be Forever Drugs

I encourage you not to think of prescription amphetamines as forever drugs. Be honest about your symptoms and any side effects you may be having from the prescription, and tell your doctor what is working and what isn't. It's important to get on just the right dose for benefit without having side effects and to only take the medicine as prescribed.

Contrary to what the drug companies and medical academies preach about the need to take these medicines every day, I prefer that you take "drug holidays" whenever possible, for example, on weekends and vacations. Take as much time off from the medication as you can without distress. Taking breaks from amphetamines helps avoid increasing tolerance and the need for higher doses.

Lessons from the Rat Park Experiments

In the late 1970s and early 1980s, Bruce Alexander, a Canadian scientist at Simon Fraser University, conducted a series of experiments with rats to try to explain the origin of drug addiction.[30] Alexander wanted to test the prevailing scientific thinking at the time that posited that certain drugs, like morphine and cocaine, were so highly addictive that anyone given unlimited access to them would succumb to addiction. Alexander had noticed that the theory was based on scientific experiments with rats in small cages in solitary confinement with nothing to do and no companions.

Like many other mammals and nearly all primates, including humans, rats are social by nature. Like humans, they are industrious and thrive on contact and communication with others. So Alexander and his team built a lush habitat two hundred times larger than a traditional rat cage. The palatial park was comfortable indeed: the rats, all housed together, were given exercise wheels, tin cans for hiding, platforms for climbing, food, and space to mate. In this environment, they were then given choices to drink from different dispensers that contained either plain water or morphine-laced water.[31]

It turned out that the Rat Park rats, after trying morphine, preferred water, even when the morphine was dissolved in a sweet liquid rats love. Happy rats with companions and plenty to keep them occupied were not interested in drugging themselves. Not only did the rats living in Rat Park not become addicted to morphine after trying it; they even preferred plain water to morphine even when it meant having physical withdrawal symptoms from previously being forced to consume morphine, which Alexander showed in subsequent experiments.[32]

Though the mainstream medical establishment, law-enforcement agencies, and public-health officials have largely ignored these experiments, they teach us what is perhaps the most important lesson about helping people addicted to meth. **It's not your drug that is destroying you. It's not your willpower or your lack of morals. It's your loneliness, boredom, and lack of true connectedness. It's your cage.** The lesson from Rat Park is one I repeat throughout this book: **change your environment to fix your life.**

Integrative Solutions for Meth Addiction, the Dr. Paul Way

Josh, like so many of my patients, was surrounded by enablers and "friends" who were either profiting by selling him drugs or using drugs themselves. His mom was supplying him with opioids, his girlfriend was giving him Adderall and using drugs with him, and his "friend" was selling him whatever other drugs he needed or wanted. Willpower will fail almost every time, if you are in the moderate or severe range of the addiction spectrum and are experiencing withdrawal symptoms every time you try to stop or are in a state of desperation that you know your drug of choice will fix.

No. This is *not* a time to rely on willpower!

You need a total change of environment. That's right. If it's your family that is keeping you sick and stuck, you have to say, "Good-bye" and "See you later" to them, as painful as that may be for a while. If your friends are using drugs with you or supplying drugs to you, you have to end those friendships or at the very least put them on absolute hold until you have a minimum of a year of sobriety under your belt.

It took me ten years. I had to avoid bars, parties, and any drinking situations for about a decade before I felt totally comfortable around people who were drinking. You must keep your environment safe for as long as it takes. But avoiding people who drink or use drugs is only half of the environment puzzle. Equally important is to surround yourself with positive people who are not using, who know how to have fun and find safe thrills, and who don't feel threatened by your sobriety.

Connectedness is key. Along with welcoming those good influences into your life, it really helps to seek out activities that motivate you and that you are passionate about. When that activity has been meth, it's hard to remember what else is out there. But there is a world of interesting people and activities waiting for you. When you start looking, you will find them. I promise. Your drug use disconnected you from allowing healthy, caring relationships into your life, along with good energy and good activities. Once you stop using, you can and will reconnect with old friends and family members and develop healthy new relationships and interests. It is time to establish healthy connections with safe people and start spending your time doing positive things.

Exercise is vital. Maybe you don't feel like doing it. Maybe you'd rather sit on the couch curled up under a blanket. Maybe you're so out of shape that you can't even imagine walking around the block. But exercise is so important to your recovery from meth. Exercise produces natural feel-good chemicals in your brain called endorphins, and you need as many endorphins as you can get right now, *sans* drugs.

I recommend doing as much exercise as you can, preferably 45 minutes to an hour a day. If you're out of shape, start by taking slow walks and build up to interspersing those walks with some jogging. But I also know that your life is busy and probably a little (or a lot) crazy, and finding time to exercise while you're also trying to make ends meet, take care of your family, and rebuild your broken relationships is not always easy. Do this: work with enough intensity to sweat for 20 minutes at least four times a week. If you find a group environment—like a dance, martial-arts, trampoline, weight-lifting, or whole-body drumming class—chances are you will start to look forward to it, replacing your meth use with a positive addiction that you miss when you don't do it.

That's what happened to Lauren who started using meth when she was nineteen because her boyfriend wanted her to get high with him. She was young and in love, and she stayed addicted for a year. To get off meth, she had to both end her relationship with him and find healthy alternatives to getting high. She started playing soccer again, twice a week, a sport she had always loved as a kid.

There is no right way to exercise. The best type of exercise is the one you will do.

I don't care if all you're doing is shuffling through the neighborhood. The trick is to make it a habit and go whether you want to or not. It will be hard to get motivated, especially in the beginning before it becomes part of your routine, but it is worth it.

Rechannel restless energy. You can channel your need for speed away from stimulants and into staying busy and finding ways to have fun, even extreme fun. Boosting your dopamine with exciting activities will give you a safe feeling of euphoria. The key here is *safe*. For me it's motorcycle riding. I push the pace just hard enough for it to be a thrill, but I never, ever, take a corner so fast that I can't hold my lane. I know recovering addicts who have taken up fire dancing, skydiving, bungee jumping, motorcycle racing, hang gliding, piloting, backcountry skiing, and ice camping. Others actually prefer to put their past of thrill seeking behind them and end up doing more relaxing activities that are just as satisfying, like fishing or yoga. The point is to replace the countless hours you spent lost in a drug fog with time doing positive activities.

Reduce stress to avoid relapse. You've heard me say it before and you'll hear me say it again: stress is one of the biggest triggers that pushes you toward the severe end of the addiction spectrum or even causes relapse. Harboring resentments is another self-inflicted stress. When we feel resentment, it's as though we're taking a poison and waiting for *the other person* to die. Usually it is you, the person holding on to that resentment, who suffers, while the person who you feel wronged you is happily going about life oblivious to your pain.

Reducing stress requires some intentional action on your part. What do you need to change in your life to feel more relaxed and less anxious? Is it an *attitude* you have about work or school or your boss or family member? If you cannot change that person or the situation, then you must change your attitude and how you respond. We only get to control our own responses. We don't get to call the shots and demand change from everyone around us, as much as we want to do that and even when we know we are right.

Do an attitude check. How do you change your attitude? You've got to practice. Pull out your phone, journal, or a piece of paper. Write down everything that stresses you out—all of it. Your list may be five miles long. That's okay. Now take each negative sentence you've written down and rephrase it into a positive one.

When my daughter was in kindergarten, one of her friends mistakenly kicked another friend, Lizzy, in the mouth as they were sliding down a corkscrew pole on the playground.

"Ow!" Lizzy cried, putting her hands to her face, tears starting in her eyes. She felt her teeth with her tongue. "Hey, you helped my loose tooth!" she exclaimed, delighted. "Awesome!"

That's what I call an attitude check.

Your stress list might include: "I feel like my boss hates me at work"; "I always fight with my mom"; "My husband never picks up his tighty-whities." And your attitude adjustments can read: "Work is giving me an opportunity to become more aware of my self-esteem issues"; "I'm glad my mom lives close enough to me that we can argue daily and that she's still alive to drive me crazy"; "My husband's really good at fixing things that break in our apartment, and I appreciate that about him." See where I'm going with this?

Use the "You may be right" technique. I teach my patients a technique to diffuse arguments that I call "You may be right." When an argument starts brewing with your significant other, your friend, your child, or your supervisor, ask yourself if winning this argument is a matter of life and death. Of course, it's not, right?! Okay, well, you've heard it's better to be happy than to be right—except that that usually doesn't sit well with us addicts and alcoholics (we like to be right!). However, here is my brilliant and simple technique to stop any argument. Put a hand on the person's shoulder, look him or her in the eye, and say, "You may be right." In your mind it's okay to *think*, "But I know you're wrong"; just don't say that out loud. End of argument. Stress reduced. Move on to something more pleasant.

Shutter your phone screen. Without your knowing it, your smartphone may be stressing you out. My phone screen, which was inadvertently set to alert me, kept lighting up each time I got an email. Well, I get hundreds of emails a day! It was a huge stress relief when I reprogrammed my phone *not* to alert me to anything other than messages from my answering service and appointment reminders. If your text messages are stressing you out, shut those off too. Don't let any apps, like Facebook or Instagram, send you alerts. We are all wired naturally to scan for danger. To your physical hormone response system all these alerts are red neon "Danger" signs—so your phone screen is unknowingly triggering the release of stress hormones in you. Turn it off. An easy way to do this is to put your phone in another room when you're not using it, or switch on airplane mode. In this age of constant phone use, I know that probably seems like old-fashioned (or impossible) advice. But getting some distance from your phone will help you with your stress levels, which will help with your recovery.

Turn off the news. Don't watch the news on TV or listen to it on the radio. I was driving to work listening to NPR and realized that everything they were talking about—North Korea, politics in the Middle East, natural disasters—were all things that I could do nothing about. The news was stressful, but I was helpless to make a difference, especially on my morning drive to the office. I switched to music, and immediately I could feel my stress level go down.

Identify other triggers. What else is causing you stress? What root causes of stress can you change? Identify them and take the necessary steps to get rid of that stress (legal ways only, of course).

Restore Your Sleep to Recover Your Body

Meth, more than any other drug, destroys your sleep. During a meth binge you may be awake for days, full of frantic energy, and doing crazy things that entire time. Then you crash, sleep fitfully, and wake up bleary-eyed and absolutely miserable. Restorative sleep is part of my protocol for everyone, regardless of where you are on the addiction spectrum, but it's even more important for those dealing with meth. Follow these basic sleep principles to help your sleep get back on track.

Say no to the Joe: No caffeine eight to ten hours before you want to fall asleep. In order to follow that rule, you may need to wean yourself off caffeinated beverages. Try a half-caf coffee; swap out that Mountain Dew for a cold-pressed organic vegetable juice with fresh ginger and parsley; go for a jog instead of a cola when you need a pick-me-up. These alternatives will give you the zing you're used to getting from caffeine without interfering with your sleep.

Go to bed at the same time every night: Establish a predictable bedtime and stick to it seven days a week. This is particularly hard if you're used to partying a lot. Which you probably are. It doesn't need to be the "correct bedtime" on anyone else's ideal schedule. I don't care if your bedtime is 7:00 p.m. or 2:00 a.m. Just try to make it consistent and at a time that will allow you at least seven or eight hours of sleep (more if you need it).

Avoid intense exercise close to bedtime: I want you to be exercising— just not two to three hours before bed, as the adrenaline rush that exercise gives you may make it harder to fall asleep.

Don't go to bed full or hungry: Avoid big meals near bedtime or going to bed hungry.

No alcohol before bed: I don't want you drinking alcohol close to bedtime. Its sedating effect may put you to sleep, but it will wear off in the night and wake you up. Alcohol is dangerous for recovering meth addicts and anyone else struggling with any addiction. Chances are you will start drinking more and start heading back toward the severe end of the addiction spectrum if you substitute alcohol for meth. Those with addictions are better off avoiding all of the mind-altering substances I discuss in this book. It's also better not to drink water before bed, so that you won't have to wake to pee in the night and then find yourself restless and awake. If you do wake needing to pee, try to ignore it and go back to sleep or practice shuffling with your eyes closed (as if you are sleepwalking) to the bathroom and not turning on any lights. That way you avoid alertness, so you can fall right back to sleep.

The darker the room, the better: Light interferes with your body's circadian rhythms. Make sure the windows have good curtains and your room is dark. If light comes in from under the door, block it with a rolled-up towel. This also means no TV or screens in your bedroom. Dock your phone, your tablet, and your laptop *outside* of the room where you're sleeping.

Be firm: A firm mattress or one that is most comfortable for you promotes restful sleep. Good pillows do too. Try a pillow filled with organic buckwheat husks. What works for you is what works. The more comfortable your bed, the more you will look forward to sleeping peacefully in it.

Go solo: If your partner is waking you up at night because of snoring, sleeplessness, or other issues (like restless leg syndrome), try sleeping separately until your partner has those sleep issues under control.

You can find the rest of my advice for restful sleep in chapter 10. This includes taking a warm bath or hot shower before bed, using melatonin, and evaluating any underlying medical issues that may be compromising the quality of your sleep.

Food Matters

You are what you eat, and you've been eating (or snorting or smoking) crystal meth. Your body has taken a beating from your drug use, and you need to get that garbage out of your system. I do want to share the good news: the cells of your body replace themselves all the time. This replacement happens at different rates: the lining of the intestines and colon replace themselves every few days, skin cells every few weeks, and white blood cells every few months. We once thought that brain cells never regenerated, and it is true that many brain cells last a lifetime, but we know now that even brain cells can be replaced.

You've been on meth, so you haven't been eating right for months, perhaps years. You eat partially hydrogenated vegetable oil that makes your cell membranes stiff. You put an artificial sweetener like aspartame in your morning beverage, which then gets converted into formaldehyde,[33] poisons every cell in your body, and disrupts your immune system. Other food you have been eating—when you've remembered to eat—is so highly processed and full of sugar that it triggers inflammation and excess insulin production, making you store fat and increasing your pain. Add to this the virtually complete lack of micronutrients in what we call food, the packaged junk that comes in boxes and bags from factories, and you have the perfect recipe for malnutrition and poorly functioning brain cells, immune cells, and energy production. Should I go on?

Yikes. Not good. But none of that matters. Your human body is an amazing and beautiful thing. It is never too late to improve your diet, and you will feel the benefits within days! I know I'm repeating myself (and yes, you will read this again in this book) but you must eat real whole food. Eat fresh vegetables, locally grown, from your own garden, the health-food store, or the perimeter of the supermarket. Try to buy organic, which I know can be hard to afford (look for sales).

Eat fruits in their whole form. (Kiwi skin is edible, as is mango skin; so are lemon and orange rinds. Don't believe me? Try them!) Don't drink packaged juice, as it breaks down in our bodies and releases some methanol, which, like aspartame, our bodies then convert to formaldehyde![34] Eat seeds, nuts or nut butters, beans, and other legumes, if you tolerate them. Unless you are vegetarian, eat a small quantity

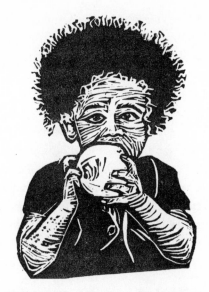

HEALTHY EATING MATTERS.

of high-quality meat and fish every week. When you can, eat free-range grass-fed, grass-finished meat in moderation as well as chicken and fish.

As much as you can, add foods that are medicinal and healing to your diet. These are foods you may have never eaten before. They include mushrooms of all kinds (including wild mushrooms), Jerusalem artichokes, bitter greens like mustard, dandelion, and nettles, as well as huckleberries, pomegranates, and kumquats.

The toxins in our world are more concentrated the higher up the food chain you go, so that larger fish and animals have the highest concentration of toxins. A vegetarian lifestyle provides a lower toxic load. If you are vegetarian, make sure you supplement with vitamin B_{12} and eat a variety of proteins such as beans, whole grains (if you tolerate them), dairy, eggs, legumes, seeds, and nuts. As much as possible, eat organic and eat local.

Be Kind to Your Biome

I don't know about you, but I like to think of myself as human. I like to think of all parts of me as "me." But it turns out that is not entirely correct. Our bodies are actually walking landscapes inhabited by colonies of microorganisms (bacteria, protozoa, viruses) and even creatures you can see with the naked eye (like the small mites that live in our eyebrows or the small symbiotic worms that may live in our colons). Your whole body and everything in it and on it is your "biome," the word scientists who geek out about this stuff like to use to describe all the organisms—macro and micro—that live on us and in us, but one you may have never heard before. What is becoming more familiar to the general public is the importance of the "microbiome." The gut microbiome refers to the microbes that inhabit your intestinal tract from the mouth to the anus.[35] Other colonies of microscopic organisms, microbiomes, can be found in the nose, the mouth, the urogenital tract, and the skin.[36] New science has been teaching us that our health is very closely tied to the health and diversity of our biome.

At birth a baby born vaginally is covered with the beneficial organisms from the mom's vagina and anus.[37] It turns out this is a good thing, especially when the mom has a healthy biome herself. These organisms help seed the symbiotic organisms that protect us for the rest of our lives, aiding in everything from fighting infectious diseases to properly digesting food. Delaying a baby's first bath for at least forty-eight hours is now known to have health benefits, largely because it allows for the proper colonization of the baby with microorganisms from the mom.

What about for babies born via C-section? What about for babies who were whisked away from their moms and vigorously scrubbed with antibiotic soap, a harmful hospital practice that deprived them of healthy bacteria and other organisms? What can we do to improve the health of our gut microbiome? Eating fermented foods, taking probiotics, and avoiding antibiotics are three crucial steps. When we have taken antibiotics, we should double and triple our efforts to eat fermented foods and take a variety of high-quality probiotics.

There has been an explosion of research on probiotics, and there are about as many strains available at health-food stores and online as there are research studies. It may be too early to tell which are the most effective and which actually survive the acidity of the stomach. As everyone's gut microbiome is different and diverse, we also don't know with real precision which strains you should be taking or how often.

My advice is to look in the refrigerated section of the health-food aisle of the grocery store and try the fermented probiotic products you see there, including fermented barley or rice water. See how you tolerate them and how they make you feel. I also recommend you rotate brands, so you potentially increase the diversity of the bacteria your body is assimilating. If you or your partner is having a baby, plan for a natural birth and be sure to get support to exclusively breast-feed for the first six months, as breast-feeding is also crucial to establishing a healthy biome.[38] Beyond that newborn and breast-feeding period, the biome becomes more difficult to change, at least in a permanent way.

There is an exciting new area of research into the use of helminths, which are very small worms, to promote a diverse gut microbiome and healthy immune system. It turns out it may be beneficial to our health to cohabitate with worms. Yes, worms. Scientists have learned that tiny worms were historically part of the human gut microbiome but have mostly disappeared from our intestinal tracts as we have modernized, become more sanitary, and sterilized our food production and distribution. Proponents of helminth therapy say that this lack of helminths in our bodies has resulted in loss of immune tolerance and is a major contributor to the autoimmune disorders we see today.[39] I suspect that they are right. The day may soon come when you can buy some form of live helminths at the health-food store, the way you can buy probiotics and nutritional supplements. Who knows?

Supplement Support to Repair the Damage Done from Using Meth

Consider taking the following supplements for two to three months after you stop using meth. Though the effects of supplements are often subtle, my recommendation is to add one supplement at a time, so you can gauge how your body responds. Wait up to a week before adding the next one.

For cravings: *Glutamine* can reduce your craving for meth as well as sugar. It stimulates production of the neurotransmitter gamma-aminobutyric acid (GABA), which can also help with sleep and anxiety. Take 1,000 mg. four times a day on an empty stomach. *Pantothenic acid* (vitamin B$_5$) can help strengthen your adrenal system, improve your serotonin levels, and also reduce sugar cravings.

For immune repair: I recommend you take between 2,000 and 5,000 IU daily of vitamin D. I have yet to find a teenager or adult who couldn't take 5,000 IU daily, but have your vitamin D levels checked to be sure. I recommend you aim for the high end of normal (50–80 ng/dL). Even if I were stuck on an island and could only have one supplement with me, it would be vitamin D. We have vitamin D receptors (VDRs) on most of our cells, including our brain and immune system cells. We make vitamin D when sunlight hits our skin, but unless you're a lifeguard with your shirt off at the equator, you likely do not have an adequate level of vitamin D, as I've said before. Very little vitamin D is available from food. You can get it by eating fish (3 ounces gives you about 300 IU) or by taking cod liver oil—yuck. Three ounces of salmon or mackerel has about 400 IU. Milk is often fortified with vitamin D, but you would have to drink a gallon a day to get optimal levels.

For neurological repair:

Tyrosine: Tyrosine is the precursor of dopamine and norepinephrine, which are extremely depleted in most meth addicts. This is the building block to enable your brain to naturally make more dopamine. It is typically taken in capsule form twice a day.

Tryptophan: Tryptophan is the precursor of serotonin. Boosting your body's ability to make serotonin will help your mood, reducing depression and anxiety.

Theanine: Theanine is a natural neurotransmitter that works to balance and calm the brain. Often this can be taken with melatonin at bedtime to help with sleep. It can also be taken twice daily.

B-complex: B vitamins are essential for many of the key metabolic pathways that support serotonin, dopamine, and norepinephrine and the detoxification pathways that enable you to rid yourself of harmful toxins. The best sources of B vitamins are nori[40] and dark green leafy vegetables, though B_{12} is found in animal products like crab, clams, liver, and egg yolks. Look for a B-complex that contains methylfolate, B_{12}, niacin, and B_6.

Do *Not* Start Using Meth Again

If you are using meth, do everything and anything you can to get away from it. If you have stopped, don't start using again. There is always hope. You can and will beat the odds. Don't let anyone tell you otherwise. Dig into this book; get yourself into an inpatient treatment program away from the drugs and drug-using friends. Do everything you can to find a new tribe of supportive sober friends. I don't care how many times you have to fall on your face. I'm here to pick you up and help you try again, but I'm fighting for your life, and I need you to fight too.

Josh's Success in Beating Meth

Six months after he came into the clinic looking so bedraggled, Josh got arrested for possession of meth. He ended up going to jail for forty-eight hours, just long enough for it "to feel really unpleasant" (his words). He told me afterward that he honestly hadn't realized how dangerously he was living and how everything he had could be snatched away in an instant.

As of this writing, Josh is on probation. If his urine tests positive for illegal drugs, he'll go back to jail for a minimum of three months. Josh's laser-focused *Why* (a concept I'll talk about more in part III) is wanting to stay out of jail and get a job as a welder. So for the first time since he was twelve, Josh has stopped smoking cigarettes and doing illegal drugs. He's even stopped taking his girlfriend's Adderall. (They're still dating but not living together anymore, a change that, he says, is good for both of them.)

It's a sunny day in June when Josh comes for an appointment, a lopsided grin on his face. He hasn't had meth or heroin in two hundred days—he's been counting—but he has started biking 150 to 200 miles a week to use up some of his restless energy and get the natural high his adrenaline-seeking self is always craving. He bikes every day. "I feel really free when I bike. I really look forward to it when I get off school."

We can all see he's got something up his sleeve. His hand shakes a little as he shows us the certificate: he's just passed his welder's exam. My office manager (herself a recovering alcoholic) lets out a loud whoop. I give Josh a hearty pat on the back and notice he seems . . . more solid. The scale confirms that he's gained 35 pounds since he stopped doing meth. I tell him he looks healthier than I've ever seen him.

"Right, Doc?" He laughs. "I don't have that angular, chiseled cheekbone thing going on anymore."

Back in the exam room he tells me he's hopeful that he's going to stay sober. "It feels permanent now. Each and every day it's gotten easier."

Although it may be inconceivable for you to think of becoming addicted to meth, maybe you've asked yourself if you drink too much. Alcohol almost became my downfall. Read the next chapter to find out how to keep it from becoming yours.

CHAPTER 6

Your Brain on Alcohol

I F YOU'D ASKED ME what I wanted to be when I grew up, I would never have said an alcoholic. No one would.

Maybe you know someone who drinks too much. Maybe you're worried you have a problem. Or maybe you know you're an alcoholic, in recovery, or trying to be. If you attend Alcoholics Anonymous meetings, you hear a lot of stories. It's easy to listen to other people's experiences with alcoholism and feel distance from them, knowing that you're certainly not as far along the addiction spectrum as they are. When I first went to AA, I would judge and compare. "I've never done that," I would think, "so maybe I'm *not* an alcoholic?" You can't medically prove to yourself or anyone else that you are or are not an alcoholic in the same way you can prove that you have cancer, diabetes, or coronary heart disease. There is no definitive blood test to diagnose alcoholism. But the more I went back to AA, the more I opened my heart, listened to the stories, and recognized my own.

Here's what everyone with a drinking problem has in common. At some point you crossed a line. You went too far. Maybe you blacked out. Maybe you drove drunk. Maybe you destroyed a relationship with alcohol-induced violence or alcohol-fueled infidelity. Regardless of the specific circumstances, you reached a point where you felt out of control. One drink triggered an irresistible, unstoppable, all-consuming craving for more. Then you started hating yourself for it. You felt despair, self-loathing, and emptiness. The alcohol you drank to feel better started making you sick and crazy, sucking the life out of you, pulling you into darkness. Ashamed, remorseful, and miserable, you inevitably drank again. As with all addictions, what may have started out as alcohol use that was sporadic, socially accepted, and even doctor-approved, on the mild end of the addiction spectrum, became an every-day occurrence, increasing in frequency and in amount.

After high school, as I told you in chapter 1, I had my first black-out. Then for nine months, from January to September 1975, before starting Kalamazoo College in Michigan, I drank beer nearly every day. I was working at a hospital as an orderly. A stout sixty-year-old named Rufus, the head orderly (these days we call them nurse's aides), took me under his wing. He introduced me to his partying friends, boasting in his booming voice, "I taught him everything I know about drinking, and he still doesn't know anything!" We would all laugh.

I wonder how much I might have drunk in college if I could have afforded to buy beer. I ate one meal a day to save money and allowed myself to drink one night a week. Those pitchers of beer at the local college bar were the highlight of my week. How I looked forward to Friday nights! I always drank to excess. I would never have just a little. If there was alcohol, I would get drunk.

After my first year in college, I noticed that most incoming fresh-men who started out premed changed majors. I wanted to be at a more science-oriented school, so I transferred to the University of the Pacific in Stockton, California. I completed my BA in biology in 1979 and became a teaching assistant while getting a master's in biology in 1981. My focus on wanting to become a doctor and the fact that I had no extra spending money kept my drinking in check. I was a weekend binge drinker.

Fifteen years later I was drinking every day. I had started breaking the self-imposed rules that I had managed to follow for the first ten years. I even drank on nights I was on call. Drinking was no longer social; it was essential. I no longer went a day without alcohol. It never ended at one or two drinks. After the first the craving for more was so intense that no amount of willpower stopped my car from heading to the liquor store.

Deep down I think I might have known I was in trouble. But I was juggling a medical career, a family with five children at that time, and my "look good." I've never admitted this outside of AA, where any-thing said at a meeting stays at the meeting, but here goes. On the way home from work I would stop at the liquor store and buy a pint of vodka. I would pour the vodka into an empty Diet Coke can and drink it on the five-mile drive home. One evening the clerk at the liquor store looked at me, astonished.

"Man, you must be desperate to put vodka in Diet Coke."

Ouch. That hurt. I avoided that liquor store for a long time. There, I showed him!

At home I prepared dinner for the family carrying my "Diet Coke" around with me. After dinner, exhausted, I went to the bedroom to finish the rest of the bottle of vodka and pass out.

I was a successful medical doctor and a devoted dad. I was well liked. I had a beautiful family and a loving wife, the love of my life. All these blessings. Yet alcohol was my master. I would wake up hung over—again—and promise myself, "That's it. No more! I'm done with drinking!" only to find the car had a mind of its own the next day after work. My head was numb every morning. The brain fog was intense. But I managed to fake-smile my way through the day. No one had any idea how miserable my body and brain felt.

But I knew. I knew the pit-in-your-stomach loneliness. I knew the profound emptiness that any problem drinker can describe for you. I knew I wanted to be able to drink the way I saw other people drinking— socially, having fun, enjoying the carefree, anxiety-free feeling alcohol gave me. But I couldn't.

So Do *You* Drink Too Much?

Have you ever said or thought any of the following things to yourself?

"I like the taste of alcohol. Why stop?"

"Of course, I can take it or leave it!"

"Sure, I drink a lot, but it's really not a problem."

"I'm in control of alcohol; it's not in control of me."

"I really should cut down my drinking."

"This _____ (person, situation, place) is really annoying me. I'd better have a drink."

"I sure wish I hadn't drunk so much yesterday."

"I know a drink this morning will help me feel better."

"I can drink most people under the table."

"I sure would have a lot more time if I didn't drink so much."

"I'm going to avoid making commitments, so I don't let anyone down if I get too drunk."

"I don't need to do _____ (activity) anymore; it's interfering with my drinking."

"How could I have done that? I put myself in danger last night with my drinking."

"My _____ (spouse, friend, mom) wants me to stop drinking. He (or she) should lighten up!"

If any of this sounds familiar, you may well have a problem. Perhaps you're not on the severe end of the spectrum, perhaps you aren't having blackouts or waking up next to strangers in bed, but I challenge you to test yourself, which is the best way to find out.

Stop drinking for two or three months. Don't drink at parties, don't drink with your family, don't drink alone. If you can be happy without alcohol and have no problem staying sober, you're probably still on the mild end of the addiction spectrum. You should still read this chapter, so you can better understand the problem drinkers in your life, but you most likely have nothing to worry about. **But if you're not able to go sixty to ninety days without a drink, you have a problem, whether you are ready to admit it to yourself or not.** Don't panic. Just holding this book in your hands, even if you're too conflicted or upset to read it, is the first step on the road toward freedom.

Why Me?

My wife's friend Joslyn was twelve years old when she had her first drink. She was at a friend's house, no parents in sight, when someone offered her a Boone's Farm strawberry daiquiri. She guzzled it down, passed out, and woke up to find herself wedged between the couch and the coffee table. Despite the headache and feeling as though she might throw up, Joslyn's first thought when she came to was: "That was fun! I want to do it again!"

When I talk to Joslyn about her alcoholism, it's easy to put the pieces into place. She grew up in a chaotic home surrounded by drinkers; alcoholism was rampant in her family. Joslyn was the youngest of six kids, her parents were exhausted, and they ignored her much of the time. The adults in her life were not good role models, and she remembers distinctly that she wasn't looking forward to growing up. "Girls Just Want to Have Fun" was the theme song of her life, she says. She spent most of her time with her peers, many of whom were as troubled as she was. As I talked about in chapter 1, early use is a big risk factor for addiction. And Joslyn got drunk for the first time when she was still a child.

But what about me? How does a firstborn missionary kid with engaged, loving, and supportive parents growing up in a teetotaling Rhodesian village become an alcoholic? I was given all the best opportunities; I was a great student and a top athlete; I attended an Ivy League medical school. My parents almost never drank when I was growing up and certainly never to excess. Yet here I was, sitting in a meeting one year sober, asking myself where things had gone wrong. That whole first year as I struggled to stay sober and listened to other alcoholics' heart-wrenching stories in meetings, I kept looking for clues as to "Why me?"

The current thinking in addiction medicine is that the pleasure-reward centers of our brains can be triggered like a switch. Once the switch goes on, it's very hard to turn it off. Repetitive addictive substance use can be activated by continually using alcohol or drugs. Everyone understands that those with family history, psychological issues, or living environments where people are drinking or using drugs are at very high risk of drinking or using and thus activating these pathways. But continually drinking or using drugs can also do the trick.

One of the hardest things about being an addict of any kind is that it damages our brains. Yet we need our brains to make healthier choices and get free from the substance or activity that is destroying us. It puts the addict in a very difficult position, as Gabor Maté explores in his book *In the Realm of Hungry Ghosts*: "If recovery is to occur, the brain, the impaired organ of decision making, needs to initiate its own healing process. An altered and dysfunctional brain must decide that it wants to overcome its own dysfunction: to revert to normal—or, perhaps, become normal for the very first time."[1]

I now understand what happened to me. I drank too much, too often, for too long. Bathing my brain in alcohol began to affect my brain and my judgment. As simplistic as that might sound, it is true. I was chemically wired to love the effect it had on me. Alcohol calmed the anxiety and restlessness I felt as a young adult, so in a sense I guess you could say I was self-medicating for stress. The more I drank, the more I wanted to drink. As much as I had protective mechanisms in place, the alcohol I drank damaged my brain. I needed good judgment—a healthy brain—to stop drinking, which is exactly what I didn't have. I progressed along the addiction spectrum and wound up on the severe end. I could no longer simply stop drinking. Willpower alone was insufficient. I needed help. If you find yourself in a similar position, it is time to put into action the suggestions in this book and get help.

Who's at Risk of Becoming an Alcoholic?

It is easier to become an alcoholic than to become addicted to illegal drugs simply because of proximity and availability. Being addicted to alcohol, like having a food or an internet addiction, which I will talk about in chapter 8, can be extraordinarily hard to kick. Alcohol, in America anyway, is ubiquitous. It is socially acceptable to drink (sometimes even more so than not to drink, as we'll see in Scot's story later in this chapter); alcohol is readily available; and the pleasures of drinking are relentlessly advertised on television and online. Most young people think it's cool. When you say "No, thank you" to an alcoholic drink, it's like saying "No, thank you" to chocolate cake or a banana split or to fun altogether. Unless you're with people who themselves have struggled with alcoholism, they don't get it. Why wouldn't you want some?!

One of the most difficult issues for drinkers young and old is the perception that drinking is normal since everyone else is doing it. Indeed, there's truth to this observation. In high school one in five Americans is binge drinking, as are one in four people ages eighteen to thirty-five.[2] If you're a drinker, chances are your friends are too. It all just seems normal.

In my clinical practice and personal experience, I've seen that there's a common thread with most addictions. Some of us are predisposed to like the effect produced by alcohol or another drug of choice. Many of these risk factors for alcoholism will look familiar to you, as they are similar to the risk factors for other addictions:

Alcoholism in the family

Chronic stress

Depression, bipolar affective disorder, schizophrenia, or other mental illness

Drinking in childhood

Early childhood trauma, including the loss of a parent, divorce, and sexual abuse

Social anxiety

Trauma in adulthood or post-traumatic stress

Violence in the home

Those Most at Risk

One of the most significant factors moving you along the addiction spectrum is how stressful your environment is. Men traditionally have been twice as likely to become alcoholics as women,[3] but recent research from Australia suggests that women are catching up.[4]

A scientific review published in October 2016 showed that men born in the early twentieth century were more than three times as likely to have a problem with alcohol as women, but for those born closer to the end of the century the gender difference has virtually disappeared. I suspect the gender gap has closed partly because women are now almost equally represented in the workforce and exposed to as much, if not more, stress as men, as they try to juggle work and family.

But there may be a more pernicious reason. Big Alcohol has been mounting aggressive advertising campaigns to get more women, especially young women, to drink more. Bud Light's new line of sweetened beer in colorful packaging with names like "Lime-A-Rita" and

"Straw-Ber-Rita" are a good case in point. Their "Meet the Ritas" campaign depicts the margarita-like beers as perfect for women of every age. There are now wine coolers targeted at stressed-out moms, and vodkas with names like "Little Black Dress," which is touted as being "designed by women, for women," because "responsible drinking is always in style."[5]

In 2018 Diageo, a British multinational and the largest producer of liquor in the world, rolled out a limited edition Jane Walker scotch, unveiled "in recognition of women who lead the way," and paired with a campaign to raise money for women's progress organizations during Women's History month, using the hashtag #MonumentalWomen.[6]

The alcohol industry also "pinkwashes" products, partnering with breast cancer awareness campaigns, to increase sales to women.[7] At the same time, we know that women are more sensitive to alcohol than men are and more prone to alcoholic hepatitis, cirrhosis of the liver, and brain damage.[8] Alcohol consumption greatly increases the risk of breast cancer. For every drink you consume a day, your risk of cancer goes up 7 percent.[9]

Any person of any ethnicity can become an alcoholic, but the prevalence of alcoholism is highest among Native Americans and whites, followed by African Americans, Hispanics, and Native Hawaiians, with the lowest rate found among Asians.[10]

People under a lot of stress, including those who are marginalized by society, often succumb to alcoholism. Transgender people have a higher rate of alcohol dependence and abuse,[11] as do war veterans. We also know that the earlier anyone begins to drink, especially if you start as a young teen, the higher the risk of moving along the addiction spectrum.

The Health Benefits of Alcohol

Health benefits. Say what? Here I am telling you how alcohol came close to destroying my life, and now I'm going to talk about health benefits? Life is messy. We want to see everything in black and white. I know I do. But it's just not that simple. Alcohol has been consumed by humans and used ceremonially since the dawn of humanity. Some anthropologists believe that beer may have appeared in human cultures before bread.[12] Analyses of the remains of simple pottery made by prehistoric peoples in the Middle East and Europe show that these early societies fermented grain. We also know that the earliest civilizations, including the Sumerians, Egyptians, and Chinese, knew how to make alcohol.[13] Alcohol served several important health functions for early humans: it was a way of preserving calories from otherwise perishable fruits and grains so you could eat them later, even without refrigeration,[14] and was an alternative to polluted water.

Indeed, before the advent of clean drinking water, alcohol may have been the drink of choice for those who could make it or afford it. Remember young David Copperfield who, in abject poverty, scrapes together just enough money to buy himself a morsel of food and a glass of beer? When Charles Dickens wrote *David Copperfield* in 1849 and 1850, the water in London was often unclean due to latrine sewage seeping into rivers and the water table. Before the twentieth century, children in Great Britain and America often drank watered-down beer or the cheap, low-alcohol beverage called small beer. In other European countries watered-down wine was the drink of choice at meals from ancient times through the twentieth century. The small amounts of alcohol in the water helped kill harmful bacteria and could make stagnant water more palatable.

Before the advent of modern anesthesia, alcohol was also used as an anesthetic in preparation for surgery or dental operations to help patients calm down and blunt their feelings of pain.[15] We no longer give alcohol to infants, but doctors just a generation ago used to recommend that parents rub whiskey on a teething baby's gums for pain relief. Today some Orthodox Jews soak a cloth in kosher wine or vodka and give it to baby boys to suck on during traditional circumcision ceremonies performed without anesthesia.

Alcohol is also a good antiseptic—putting it directly on a wound will help clean and sterilize it. Because it's so versatile, disaster-preparation classes usually recommend keeping some kind of alcohol in your emergency kit.

We know that anxiety and stress have a harmful effect on our health, one that functional medicine doctors believe is not taken seriously enough by conventional medicine. This is a subject of debate, for sure, but alcohol in moderation is also thought to be beneficial. If having a glass of wine or a beer with dinner helps you relax, that may be healthier than living in a state of high anxiety. Drinking red wine every day has also been associated with reduced risk of heart disease.[16] Drinking alcohol in moderation has been associated with longevity.[17] Numerous studies have found that when people drink a small amount of alcohol, they live longer when compared to people who don't drink at all. Mortality is highest for those who drink no alcohol and those who drink more than four to five drinks a day and lowest for those who have one or two drinks a day. What the alcohol industry–sponsored studies don't tell you is that fresh grapes or fresh-squeezed grape juice would be even better!

We can debate the reasons why, but the science seems to suggest that someone who drinks in moderation is *less likely* to die early than someone who doesn't drink at all. Also be aware that many of the studies showing the health benefits of moderate alcohol consumption were funded by the industry or by academics who have connections to Big Alcohol, which often go undisclosed. One thing I think everyone agrees on, scientists, doctors, and partygoers alike: drinking too much is never healthy.

A Matter of Life and Death

In fact, abusing alcohol can be a death sentence. I'm sure you know someone whose life was cut short from excess drinking. Alcohol abuse is dangerous for people of all ages. It is responsible for one in ten deaths in adults aged twenty to sixty-four. From 2006 to 2010 excessive alcohol use led to 88,000 deaths each year in the United States.[18]

There's more. Alcoholics are between 60 and 120 times more likely to try to commit suicide and to succeed.[19] A dear friend who had an untreated drinking problem and was struggling with depression committed suicide with a handgun while I was writing this book. He was forty-six years old. My sponsor Uncle Elliott tried to do the same. He married the love of his life and had a successful career and two children, all while his drug, alcohol, and behavioral addictions spiraled out of control. He felt so overwhelmed that he grabbed his grandfather's shotgun, put a shell in it, and put the barrel in his mouth. But, thank God, he didn't pull the trigger.

Metabolizing Alcohol

Our bodies can metabolize about one drink an hour. A woman can usually drink one drink and a man can drink two drinks without significant impairment in judgment or other physical effects like slurred speech or uneven walking. We all metabolize alcohol at a different rate, but binge drinking is considered four or more drinks for a woman and five or more drinks for a man.

A drink is:

- 12 ounces of beer (5 percent alcohol content)
- 8 ounces of malt liquor (7 percent alcohol content)
- 5 ounces of wine (12 percent alcohol content)
- 1.5 ounces of 80-proof (40 percent alcohol content) liquor (gin, rum, vodka, whiskey)[20]

Then There Are Heart Problems

A glass of red wine a day seems to be protective against heart disease, but drinking excessively can damage your heart. A heavy drinker can develop an enlarged heart (known as cardiomyopathy),[21] which can lead to compromised heart functioning, blood clots, and heart failure. Other risks are atrial fibrillation, which is a very rapid heart rate that can kill you if it goes untreated.[22] As I pointed out earlier, one drink a day actually reduces your risk of stroke and heart attack; however, for heavy drinkers, the risk of stroke[23] and heart disease (calcification and atherosclerosis)[24] is increased. Heavy drinking can also induce high blood pressure,[25] which increases all cardiovascular risks.

And Liver Problems

Perhaps you already know that chronic alcohol abuse can damage your liver. Your liver is responsible for detoxifying chemicals and metabolizing drugs. The early-stage liver dysfunction seen in mild and moderate drinkers is completely reversible if you stop drinking. Severe liver failure, common in end-stage alcoholism, is much harder to reverse. You will start turning yellow, have a bloated belly from the buildup of fluids and toxins in the body, and develop brain issues doctors call encephalopathy. No fun. You may also have swelling of the hands and feet, spider blood vessels, and broken blood vessels (petechial and ecchymoses). Liver damage from heavy alcohol use is also associated with obesity[26] and can result in alcohol-related hepatitis.[27]

And Problems with Our Gut

Heavy alcohol use can give you an uncomfortable and painful gastrointestinal disorder called GERD (gastroesophageal reflux disorder).[28] It can also cause extreme nausea and vomiting, pancreatitis (inflammation of the pancreas, which can cause abdominal pain),[29] and bloody stools.

And Increased Risk for Cancer

Heavy alcohol use has also been associated with cancer of the mouth, pharynx, larynx, esophagus, breast, colon, and liver.[30] Add smoking and you have a perfect storm, greatly increasing your cancer risk.

And Pregnancy Concerns

Every American woman has been told it's dangerous to drink during pregnancy, a health message that our government has effectively conveyed to the public. In other countries drinking during pregnancy is not as taboo, but there is no question that too much can cause problems. The most severe is having a child born with fetal alcohol syndrome. Fetal alcohol syndrome is recognized by characteristic facial features, reduced mental capacity, and learning difficulties.

Some drug addicts come to my clinic pregnant. Others get pregnant while I am treating them for opioid addiction. Many of these women struggling with addiction also drink. Babies born to moms who frequently use opioids suffer from a significant and very stressful period of neonatal withdrawal. Babies born to alcoholic moms will also suffer—getting tremors that are heartbreaking to watch and sometimes life-threatening seizures. That's the bad news. The good news is that pregnancy can be tremendously motivating. Having a baby can be a turning point in your life—a time when you examine many of your behaviors and become more open to walking a new path. If there was ever a time to stop using and drinking, it is now! Alcohol should be avoided during pregnancy, as your growing baby's brain is especially vulnerable.

And Brain Damage

I've saved the best for last. Too much alcohol is bad for your brain. The more you drink and the younger you are when you start, the worse the damage may be. If you have a drinking problem and are young enough to still be in school, your learning and memory will suffer noticeably.

Drowning yourself in drink can cause a thiamine deficiency. Thiamine (vitamin B_1) plays an important role in brain, nerve, heart, and muscle functioning. A thiamine deficiency in its most extreme form causes Wernicke-Korsakoff syndrome, which manifests as confusion. Other symptoms include poor attention, memory problems, abnormal eye movements, and unsteady gait.[31]

Your brain is made up of two kinds of tissue—gray matter and white matter. Gray matter contains neurons (brain cells), glial cells (which feed the neurons), and capillaries (which provide cells with blood and oxygen). We know from scientific studies that the more gray matter in the brain, the more intelligent a person or an animal is. One study found that alcoholics, like heroin addicts,[32] have less gray matter in their brains.[33] In another study of alcoholics, the parts of the brain that receive feelings of pleasure were found to be diminished, which in turn was associated with increased cravings for alcohol.[34]

Sound familiar? I shudder at the thought that at the height of my drinking I was often consuming a pint, roughly the equivalent of eleven drinks, in just a few hours, and twice as much on the weekends. I know I damaged my brain back then, though I have worked hard to reverse it. Research has also shown that alcoholics suffer from learning and memory problems from heavy drinking.[35]

"A Day-by-Day Decision"

Scot was a teacher before he became a prominent businessman, an accomplished journalist, and the editor in chief of an award-winning small-town newspaper. Married while still in college, he had three children in his twenties and then got divorced. When he was thirty-one, he began a relationship with a young woman who had been a student of his. They stayed together for three years and then broke up. But the age of consent in their state was eighteen, and Scot's girlfriend was just shy of her eighteenth birthday when they got together. Years later, still stung by their breakup, she pressed charges against him. Scot pleaded guilty to sexual abuse. He went to prison for four years, where he admitted to himself that he was an alcoholic for the first time:

> I drank every day for twenty years, but I never thought I had a problem. But I did. I owned a bar, and I drove home intoxicated every single night. I drank at lunch. I started hiding how much I was drinking. I was always the first one up in the morning, making breakfast, cleaning up, taking care of everyone. I was always hiding that I was hung over.
>
> The only reason I started rehab was because I wanted to get out of prison. At first they said I wasn't eligible, because I didn't have a substance abuse disorder. They asked me all these questions. Have you ever passed out from drinking? I said no. But actually I had. I just lied about it. When I went to my first AA meeting, I was like, "No fucking way. This is not me. I am not doing this. I'm not going to give up drinking for the rest of my life." But I decided I'd just do it, just get through it. I'd fake it. And then I sat in that program and realized I was totally full of shit. I was totally an alcoholic. Every therapist I'd ever been to told me I had a drinking problem. I just refused to admit it.
>
> I don't think I'm genetically wired for alcoholism. I'm the type who learned to be an alcoholic because it self-medicates. When I was drunk, I was the life of the party; it helped me with social anxiety. I don't have an addictive personality, but I definitely developed what I call addict's brain. My motto has always been: "If this works a little, then a lot is even better!" If one cup of

coffee is good, I'll have six! If I made $12,000 this month, why not $16,000 next month? I'm still like that. More is always better. Alcohol. Work. Making money. Chocolate. Sex. That's my addict's brain.

I've been sober for eight years, and I haven't smoked a cigarette in twelve. Part of the terms of my parole was that I couldn't drink. That first year out I went to AA three times a week and really worked the program. I did the 12 Steps. My sponsor was this toothless guy with scuffed shoes who looked homeless. I don't know if he was or not. I liked the equality of AA. It took away my arrogance. I worked my ass off. It was actually really hard.

I don't go anymore. My not drinking is a really small part of my life, and I don't want to be defined by something I'm not doing. For me not drinking is still a day-by-day decision. I won't say I'm never going to drink again. But if I do, I'll have to be careful of the slide. With my addict's brain I could go back into problem drinking really, really easily. My kids drink, my friends drink. People tell me I'm not an alcoholic. I can be around alcohol and not drink and still have a good time, but I won't go to functions where alcohol is the point—like wine tastings or parties where I know everyone's going to get plastered. It's hard with my family, honestly. It's almost like they want me to start drinking again.

Like Scot, a lot of recovering alcoholics and addicts don't want to be identified by what they are trying *not* to do. Many of us, myself included, avoided AA for years, feeling that going to meetings was an admission of failure. There are a lot of different paths to getting sober. Alcoholics Anonymous doesn't work for everyone. But when it does work, it works well. We realize we've found our people. We realize we are home. Most addiction specialists, like me, are aware that for lasting success most alcoholics who have reached moderate to severe levels on the addiction spectrum have greatly improved outcomes if they stay plugged into a program like AA.

In AA I rub elbows with other medical doctors, lawyers, successful businessmen, teachers, and famous authors as well as with minimum-wage workers, people getting government assistance, and those who are homeless. As Scot says, we're all equal. It is a beautiful thing.

Can't You Just Help Me Cut Back?

For about thirteen years, before I was finally able to get sober, I believed I could just cut back if I tried hard enough. Confession: I never once honestly admitted to a doctor that I had a drinking problem. If asked, I responded that I drank a couple beers once in a while. In medical school we were taught to multiply people's stated responses times three when calculating their actual alcohol, cigarette, or drug use, because patients (like me) almost always lie.

If you are an addict or alcoholic, your dream is that you can just control your drinking or using. But if a single drink triggers a craving for more, then you can never safely take a drink. You can move toward the mild end of the addiction spectrum, feeling healthy, happy, and full of energy, but you will stay there only as long as you do not drink. You have to stop using alcohol completely. At least for today.

The Sober Truth About Drinking

It is not easy to get sober. I'd like to write that sentence a hundred more times, so that you can be kind to yourself if you're struggling with your sobriety or so that you can recognize how hard it is if you have a loved one who's trying but failing in recovery. (By the way, don't get hung up on the word "alcoholism." Addiction specialists prefer to use the clunky phrase "alcohol use disorder" these days. Either way, I am referring to those who have lost the ability to control their drinking.) I am not excusing alcoholics from blame—as much as alcoholism is a debilitating condition, it is also, ultimately, a choice. However, your alcohol use may have you so far on the severe end of the addiction spectrum that you have lost your ability to choose.

If this is you, I wish for you the gift of desperation. You need to get help. And you need to do it now.

Recovering from alcoholism is about your willingness to be honest with yourself and others, to work as hard as you can to change, to understand that you may fall on your face many times, to learn to ask for and receive help, and ultimately to find a way to love yourself enough that you commit to no longer causing yourself so much harm.

Alcoholism can be a long, painful, and slow suicide punctuated, perhaps, by good times and good feelings. At some point I think most of us realize we are killing ourselves with our drinking. When you accept that you have been progressing steadily toward the severe end of the addiction spectrum as you drink more and more, please turn around before you lose the ability to choose.

Realizing the health consequences of excessive drinking is a little overwhelming. But help is at hand: integrative doctors have tools to help repair the damage you've done or are still doing to your body and your brain. The longer you abuse alcohol or any other drug, the worse the damage. I can't promise that you will be able to completely reverse the effects of your alcohol abuse, but I can tell you that there are ways to make your brain and body feel much better.

The First Step Is to Decide to Stop Drinking

You know you have a problem. You're ready to tackle it. You've made a decision to stop drinking. Now you have to detox, either on your own or with help from your team of handpicked medical professionals, an inpatient treatment center, or a detox clinic.

If you had your last drink last night and this morning you have the shakes, high anxiety, and perhaps diarrhea, it is safest to detox under the care of an addiction specialist. If you can't make it through the morning or reading this paragraph without drinking, you also need help from a competent and trustworthy medical professional. It may be safest to start the detox process in the hospital. Without treatment you may experience severe anxiety, nausea, vomiting, tremors, dehydration, agitation, sweats, disorientation, and sometimes tingling, itching, burning, numbness, or even feeling as though bugs are crawling under your skin. I'm making this sound really appealing, aren't I? I am not going to candy-coat this. It is hard now, and it may get even harder. Take it one second at a time, then one minute, then one hour, then one day. You can do this. As I said to Michael, I believe in you. Don't give up.

If you want to detox by yourself, I understand. When I say I know how you feel, I'm not feeding you lines. I went it alone, with just AA for support. Since I never drank in the morning, I was able to stop drinking without experiencing life-threatening withdrawal. But I'm also concerned about your safety, as seizures and death are possible for those who stop cold turkey without help. I shudder thinking back at my own self-detox. If you are drinking around the clock, needing to take a drink in the middle of the night or in the morning to stop your shakes, you must detox with professional help.

A doctor specializing in addiction can help you by prescribing medication for anxiety and to prevent seizures. These include chlordiazepoxide, diazepam, and lorazepam. Gabapentin may be added to prevent relapse, and you can also consider using naltrexone, which I'll talk about more below. If you have liver problems, you should not take naltrexone. You may be offered another drug, acamprosate (Campral), which is thought to help alcoholics stay away from drinking by stabilizing chemical pathways in the brain. Acamprosate should not be used by people who have kidney problems and should only be started after you have been sober for at least a month.

Aversion Therapy for Alcoholism

Another prescription medication used to treat alcoholism is disulfiram, more commonly known by its trade name, Antabuse. This drug blocks your ability to break down acetaldehyde, a toxic by-product of alcohol metabolism, which means that when you're taking disulfiram and you drink, you get really sick—with flushing, sweating, blurred vision, anxiety, vomiting, and nausea. Taking disulfiram is a form of aversion therapy. Although it works for some, it is not effective for others.

To show you the insanity of alcoholism, I have a colleague, Mark, who was so desperate to stop drinking that he took disulfiram that had been prescribed to his friend. Then Mark sat in his car outside an AA meeting drinking a six-pack of Henry Weinhard's, even as it made him sicker and sicker. Mark remembers being beet red in the face, nauseated, feeling totally humiliated. There he was, taking a medication that he knew prevented him from getting drunk but chugging one beer after another, completely desperate.

He was unable to open his car door and force his feet to walk inside that building to go to the meeting. And this was a medical doctor who knew full well what drinking was doing to his body while on that medicine!

Naltrexone

Another prescription medication your doctor may recommend is naltrexone. Naltrexone won't cure you of alcoholism, but it may lessen your desire to drink and may help you decrease the amount of alcohol you consume. Naltrexone works by binding to your opiate receptors and blocking dopamine, the neurotransmitter that helps us feel good. It removes the pleasurable effects of alcohol and may reduce the pleasure you feel from using other drugs. It is advised that you not take naltrexone until you have gone a week without drinking.

Naltrexone comes in three forms: short-acting tablets taken once or twice a day, as an injectable shot given once a month, or as an implant (a pellet placed under the skin, which lasts a few months).

CAUTION: Do not take naltrexone if you are using opioids daily along with drinking, as you will be plunged into severe withdrawal. Naltrexone should not be used during pregnancy or by anyone who has liver damage.

A single shot of naltrexone can trigger severe suicidal depression in some alcoholics. It is safer for anyone considering naltrexone to start with a week or two of oral naltrexone to make sure it doesn't compromise your mood or well-being before trying either a shot or an implant. If you can take it safely, you have two options: use it daily for an extended period of time (usually several months) or sporadically, as needed.

The Sinclair Method

The Sinclair Method, based on research done by Dr. David Sinclair, involves using naltrexone or another medicine that blocks opioid receptors on an as-needed basis when you know you are going to drink. The idea behind this is both brilliant and simple. Under the supervision of a doctor, you take a dose of an opioid antagonist like naltrexone before you plan to drink. If you know you are going to the gym after work and won't be drinking, no need to take the medicine that day. On the days you take an opioid antagonist, you will probably still drink. But the opioid antagonist blocks you from becoming drunk, though you may get a little tipsy. You will, however, still get the hangover!

You use your remorse about drinking as motivation to take a pill on days you are feeling vulnerable and likely to drink. In this way you are rewiring your brain's reward pathways. Gradually you stop associating alcohol with pleasure and relief. This method worked for actress Claudia Christian, who actively promotes it. But I have met several recovering alcoholics for whom this method failed. It's not for everyone. More information can be found at www.cthreefoundation.org.

Are you a friend of Bill W. and rolling your eyes as you read this? We are taught in AA that alcoholism is a chronic and relapsing disease for which there is no cure. I suspect there is some truth to that. I also suspect that many of us might have avoided the misery of the last years of our drinking had we had a way to dampen the opioid effect produced by alcohol. Rather than argue philosophy or get hung up on semantics, let's agree to support anything that saves lives and helps the problem drinker heal. When you understand that addiction happens on a spectrum, you can see how perhaps the use of the Sinclair Method may help a person move back toward the mild end.

A Controversial Treatment: Injectable Naltrexone

One of the newer treatments available for the alcoholic who has tried everything and just can't stop getting dangerously drunk is injectable naltrexone (Vivitrol). Injected once a month, it blocks the opiate receptors in the brain and essentially removes the beneficial effects of alcohol. You can drink while you're on naltrexone, but, as I mentioned above, all you will feel is the hangover, not the euphoria.

Addiction specialist Marvin Seppala, MD, reports that he has been using injectable naltrexone with great success. One of his patients, a twenty-year-old alcoholic on the verge of failing college, started getting monthly shots. For her it was a miracle cure, allowing her to finish school and get her life back on track.

I am not a fan of this drug, though I have seen it work in several patients. About five years ago, my son Noah was drinking excessively, missing work, driving drunk, and suffering from severe and constant hangovers. Maiya and I were terrified—it seemed a big disaster was coming any day. Within hours of a shot of Vivitrol, Noah plunged into the worst suicidal depression I have ever seen. He moved back home with us, couldn't work, and for months was on a suicide watch, needing 24/7 supervision.

During this time, he came to me and said, "Mom or the boys won't be able to stop me from taking my life." He told me in detail how he planned to kill himself. You can learn more about Noah's struggles on his YouTube channel (bignoknow). He came within inches of losing his life. We took him to the emergency room, and he was admitted for a week for his own protection. I have no doubt that this and our continuous family support saved his life. If you are feeling suicidal and have a plan to end your life, please, please tell someone or get yourself to the emergency room. No one but you knows how desperate you're feeling. You need help.

If you read the package insert and other information available on Vivitrol, you will see that it lists an up to 5 percent chance of depression or suicide.[36] A one-in-twenty chance of suicide is a chance I'm not sure I would want to take with any patient. We cannot know how much of that 5 percent is depression and not suicide; the details are not given.

Before this experience with my son, I prescribed naltrexone for a few patients. It made them feel horrible and they never stayed on it for longer than a month or two. This drug blocks your ability to experience pleasure from anything—no wonder there is an increased suicide risk when you're taking it. I choose not to use the long-acting preparations of naltrexone in my practice, though I hear other practitioners have success with it in some patients.

Ax the Access

You cannot end your love affair with alcohol if you still have it around. Get rid of every last bit of it! For most of us, if we keep going into bars or walking through the liquor aisles of the grocery store, we will eventually cave in to our cravings. Don't even look at the TV if there's an alcohol commercial on. To this day, I turn away from those ads. Not because I have any desire to drink, but because I want to be vigilant about what goes into my brain. You should too. If you've been struggling with other addictions, do not keep your problem foods or drugs anywhere in the house. Sure, perhaps you "should" be able to have access to every triggering substance and behavior and walk away. Maybe you do! But most of us need boundaries and external constraints to help us make the healthiest and safest choices. There's nothing wrong with that.

Integrative Solutions for Alcohol Abuse, the Dr. Paul Way

Whole healing involves your body, mind, and spirit. *For the body*, we order blood work to make sure you have not damaged your liver, bone marrow, kidneys, or endocrine system. *For the mind*, we use techniques to strengthen your frontal lobe pathways, so you won't be plunged back into the cycle of overuse, hangovers, withdrawal, and remorse. Anything that helps heal your body also helps your mind, and vice versa. Counseling, psychotherapy, and 12-step programs can all be part of your wellness program. Some alcoholics have also found relief using brain tapping, also called the Emotional Freedom Technique, which teaches you stress relief.[37]

For the spirit, I am not talking about organized religion, though that works well for some. I am talking about getting in touch with your spiritual side—cultivating a connection with something bigger than yourself, finding meaning in doing good deeds and kind acts, learning to sit quietly contemplating vast ideas, and understanding that your suffering is part of the larger human experience and that it is worthwhile to do inner work to seek answers to difficult questions.

An amazing amount of healing can occur if you begin to eat right, which means leaving behind the comfort foods that actually make you sick (fast food; highly processed cheeselike substances that are full of plastic and chemicals like polydimethylsiloxane;[38] bright blue slurpy

Lab Work for Alcohol Use Disorders

I encourage you to have your doctor order the following baseline blood work:

1. Blood test for B$_{12}$ and folate. These essential nutrients can be low in alcoholics.

2. Complete blood count (CBC). This test looks for anemia from bleeding, infection, or low platelets. Alcoholics can become anemic either from poor nutrition or excessive bleeding from the esophagus or the gastrointestinal tract.

3. Comprehensive metabolic panel (CMP). This test will gauge your electrolytes, liver, and kidney function. This includes liver function testing (LFT; specific liver function tests include GGT, AST/ALT, and CDT).

4. Testosterone. Excessive alcohol or drug use can suppress the pituitary in the brain, which results in low testosterone (as well as low thyroid function), among other things.

5. Thyroid function tests (TFTs). TSH, free T4, and free T3 tests are the most common and usually ordered together. The results—though they are not always accurate—will indicate to your doctor if you have a sluggish thyroid (hypothyroidism) or an overactive thyroid (hyperthyroidism).

6. Urine drug screens (UDS). Doctors order this test to find out what other drugs you may be taking. It helps you be honest and identify all the drugs you are using.

drinks; diet anything; and canned and boxed edible foodlike substances, including that staple in your cupboard, macaroni and cheese). As I've been reminding you throughout, eat lots of pesticide-free vegetables and fruits and high-quality protein (nuts, seeds, pasture-raised eggs, healthy meats) in order to heal yourself.

If you struggle with eating enough vegetables, try drinking freshly squeezed vegetable and fruit juice, adding a handful of fresh vegetables (like kale and spinach and parsley) to smoothies, and stocking your freezer with prechopped frozen organic vegetables (which you can then add to every meal). As you are transitioning to healthy, non-alcoholic eating habits, you can channel your inner hippie and walk in Birkenstocks to the food co-op or health-food store in your town. Soon you'll stop shaving and using shampoo too! (Just kidding.)

Eat foods that are:

Rich in thiamine: Vitamin B_I is low for most alcoholics. Eat beef, nuts, seeds, oats, oranges, and eggs.

Rich in B_{12}: Beef liver, clams, caviar, oysters, rabbit, Camembert, Emmental, and Gouda as well as chlorella, a blue-green algae like spirulina that is considered by many to be a superfood, are all good sources. *Note:* When purchasing chlorella, check the label, as research has found that B_{12} content in chlorella can vary widely.[39]

High in folate: Include dark green vegetables like kale, collard greens, chard, asparagus, broccoli, and Brussels sprouts as well as lentils, chickpeas, and beans.

Rich in antioxidants: Antioxidants are compounds that delay, slow, and even repair oxidative damage to the cells and tissues of our body. They're among our best food friends. My favorite antioxidant-rich foods include goji berries, blueberries, elderberries, pecans, artichokes, kidney beans, blackberries, cilantro, parsley, basil, ginger, garlic, and onions.

Repair brain damage: Remember that your body will inherently work to heal once the toxic exposure is removed. Within a week of stopping all alcohol, I was already feeling better. Within a month of being sober, I had better focus and less anxiety. By five years, I was feeling more energetic and creative than ever before. Now, fifteen years later, I feel at the top of my game.

You need to give your brain time to heal. Support that healing with 5,000 IU of vitamin D_3 daily and a high-quality B-complex or good (preferably whole foods–derived) multivitamin that includes thiamine, methylfolate, and methyl B_{12}. The brain, immune system, and detox pathways all benefit from support with glutathione. This can be done by taking liposomal glutathione or N-acetylcysteine (NAC), which the body converts into glutathione.

Repair liver damage: When you stop drinking, you stop exposing your body, especially your liver, to the ongoing toxicity of alcohol. This allows

Toss the Tylenol ASAP

Acetaminophen is the main ingredient in Tylenol and is found in over six hundred over-the-counter and prescription medications,[40] including cough syrups, pain relievers, sleep aids, and cold and flu remedies. It is also commonly combined with opioid painkillers in prescription medications. This drug is everywhere, and doctors recommend it all the time. But they should not!

Acetaminophen is dangerous for everyone, particularly alcoholics. Acetaminophen overdose is one of the main causes of liver failure in the United States,[41] and acetaminophen has also been implicated in some chronic brain and immune dysfunction.[42] Scientists know why: acetaminophen depletes the body of glutathione, a chemical that is essential for ridding the body of toxins. So if you have Tylenol in your house, toss it in the trash. If you need pain relief, try taking 2,500 mg. (about 1 level teaspoon) of organic ground turmeric in a glass of water or with plain yogurt. See chapter 4 for detailed advice about other integrative ways to manage pain.

your liver to start the process of repairing itself. Optimize your liver health with a daily dose of milk thistle, an effective detoxifying herb that has antioxidant and anti-inflammatory properties, as well as NAC and glutathione. It is imperative to avoid acetaminophen (the main ingredient in Tylenol) in all its forms, as this is a highly liver-toxic drug. If you have any in your home, toss it in the trash. In addition, drinking coffee has been shown to be beneficial to liver health,[43] as has eating foods high in antioxidants,[44] including grapefruit, blueberries, and cranberries. Grapes, beets, prickly pear, and Jerusalem artichokes will also help.

Repair gut damage: The cells lining the gut are rapidly dividing, and thus they will heal relatively quickly once you stop drinking heavily and start eating high-quality whole foods that will promote the healthy growth of beneficial bacteria. To help your gut heal, add a forkful of fermented probiotic real food to every meal (lacto-fermented sauerkraut, kimchee, or pickles; bioactive plain kefir; and probiotic plain yogurt are all good choices). Consider taking a high-quality probiotic—these come in either liquid or capsule form. Filmmakers Toni Harman and Alex Wakeford, who have been studying the gut microbiome for over five years (and who made a documentary, *Microbirth*, in which they interviewed twelve of the world's leading experts), themselves drink probiotic barley water daily. If you get capsules, break them into yogurt or a smoothie to make them more bioavailable. You must stop eating sugary foods and sweets, as unhealthy organisms in our bodies, like yeast and harmful bacteria, thrive on sugar.

Drink 2 to 4 tablespoons of aloe vera juice (which you can buy at a health-food store) once a day. It has amazing properties for your GI tract. The amino acid L-glutamine is also helpful in gut repair. Take up to 3,000 mg. a day.

If you are suffering from constipation or diarrhea, as many of us are, a healthy diet can cure you. You already know you should eat food high in fiber. High-fiber vegetables and fruits are a healthier choice than grains. Eat lots of raw veggies, especially. Pumpkin, beans of all kinds, and split peas are an excellent source of fiber as well. Here's another healthy tip: if you buy organic (which I hope you do), eat the skins. Potato skins, squash skins, carrot skins, even kiwi and mango skins are all edible and high in nutrients. Drinking lots of filtered water will also alleviate your constipation. I recommend you filter your water with a charcoal filtration system and/or by reverse osmosis.

Avoid HALT: Reducing your stress is a top priority. In the addiction world we teach recovering alcoholics and addicts to avoid the following conditions:

Hungry

Angry

Lonely

Tired

If you experience several of these stressors at the same time, your need for relief goes way up. Based on past experiences your brain tricks you into thinking it makes sense to take a drink. But it doesn't.

Hungry: If you're hungry, eat one of the healthy snacks listed on page 255. Learn to recognize the cues of low blood sugar. You can take control of hunger. Don't ever leave the house without a healthy snack in your pocket like a package of nuts. If you start feeling irritable, eat something.

Angry: If you're angry, teach yourself to rewire your brain by stopping and breathing. (Count your breaths. With each inhale say in your mind, "I breathe in calm." With each exhale, say, "I breathe out anger." I don't care if it sounds dippy; try it anyway.) Work with a sponsor or therapist (or both) to address your resentments, so you can let them go. Scream into a pillow as often as you need. Exercise is another positive outlet to express anger. Put a heavy bag in your garage and punch the heck out of it whenever you are feeling mad. Join a group fitness class and burn your anger off in weight lifting or spinning. Throughout your recovery, exercise will be an important tool to help you with stress and anger management, and if you can make new friends from a physical group activity, even better.

Lonely: If you are lonely, remember, you are not alone. We all feel lonely. It's hard, and it's awkward, and you may feel you don't want to, but get yourself connected with positive people and others who are on the same journey you are taking—to becoming sober. **Find your sober tribe.** When a herd of antelope is being hunted by lions, it is never the ones in the middle of the pack who are taken. It is those around the edges, not paying attention, doing their own thing. Perhaps they are straggling behind because they are sickly. You want to be in that safe place in the middle, surrounding yourself with and protected by addiction-free emotionally healthy friends and family.

Tired: If you're tired, you need to sleep, my friend, not drink. Rest is restorative. Alcohol is not. Only you can control whether you're getting enough sleep. You need to make sleep a priority. My best suggestions to safeguard your sleep can be found pages 124–25 and 257–61.

Help others in order to help yourself: Whenever I tell my sponsor Uncle Elliott how grateful I am for his guidance, he always answers, "Thank you for letting me be of service." When you are active in your addiction, you feel imposed upon or even angry when someone asks for your help. You likely feel too overwhelmed to even consider being of service to others. Their weaknesses do not inspire your compassion, but rather your anger and disgust.

I don't know about you, but when I was drinking, I was the opposite of Uncle Elliott: easily annoyed by anyone who was getting in the way of my ability to drink or have my well-deserved time off! Now free of the bondage of alcohol, I am grateful for opportunities to help a fellow human suffering from anything, including addiction or alcoholism. There is joy and a sense of purpose that comes with giving freely of ourselves to others.

If you have just joined AA and feel too broken to help other people fix their lives, start small by helping set up the room, making coffee, or helping clean up. Maybe you drive a friend to the airport, pick up sidewalk trash, or send an e-card to a friend. No act of kindness is too small. The idea is to seek out small ways to be of service every day.

Heal your spirit: You can find your spiritual healing in Alcoholics Anonymous, fellowship at your church, a Zen Buddhist practice, or with the Council for Secular Humanism. Practicing yoga, reading philosophy, and learning meditation are also ways to get in touch with your spiritual self. The program of AA is a program that calls for spiritual work as you go through the steps with a competent and wise sponsor. I talk more about spiritual work, as well as what AA offers, in part III.

I'm fifteen years sober. I'm the kind of sober where I put no mind-altering substance in my body, period. My life since has only gotten better. Not a "Disney movie happy ending" better, but more real, more honest, and more meaningful. Life is still messy and uncomfortable and awkward and sometimes—maybe even often—full of sadness and despair. The over half million subscribers on my YouTube channel see me upbeat and smiling, with a bounce in my step as I care for the families in my pediatric practice. I stand up straight and project confidence. Don't get me wrong, I am that person. But I also get impatient, and I snap at my loved ones, especially when I've been too busy to eat all day, but often even for no real reason. I'm quick to get defensive (though I apologize later, once I've had a chance to cool off), I'm disorganized, and I get distracted a lot, even when someone needs my undivided attention.

Ask my wife, and she'll tell you that I can also be very stubborn.

I think I know more than the GPS (and end up taking us the wrong way—every single time). I do stupid things like blaming my kids for taking my coffee cups (when I'm the one who actually lost them. Why would my kid steal a coffee cup? Duh). And, of course, I know more than the documentary Maiya and I are watching together. So what if the producers did do several years of research? They're just wrong! I could go on.

If we're willing to look at ourselves honestly, we can all make a mile-long list of our faults, even though it stings to admit them. My point is that no one is better or worse than you. You can try until they are throwing dirt over your coffin, but you will never be perfect, and you will never stop making mistakes. Being an alcoholic and trying to get sober isn't about being any worse or any better than anyone else. It is what it is.

I've had to overcome some really hard challenges in both my personal and professional life. The difference is that I now face both my personal shortcomings and these work and life challenges sober and clearheaded. I'm willing to admit my mistakes, ask forgiveness, and try again. I can laugh at myself.

Just to make a point, Maiya called our sons to ask them if they took my coffee cups. Noah was annoyed. "Say what? I'm thirty years old and married, Mom. Jessie and I have our own house and our own coffee cups." The others all said no too, some more outraged than others. I found the cups I thought they had stolen.

"The boys returned them," I joked to Maiya with a big grin.

She could've given me a hard time—I deserved it—but she didn't. We just laughed. The difference between drunkenness and sobriety is not that you figure out your personality defects or that your problems go away. It's that you're willing to be uncomfortable, make mistakes, admit when you're wrong, ask for forgiveness, and try again. I would not trade my best moments drinking for my worst moments in sobriety. I get to feel. I get to experience everything, not numb it all with alcohol.

Healing from addiction is an ongoing process for us all. Your journey is never static. You are always moving. Either you are making changes that move you toward the mild end of the addiction spectrum or you are sauntering toward the severe end, whistling in the wind as if you have not a care in the world.

Part of what helps us move toward and stay rooted at the mild end of the addiction spectrum is making sure we are not going to drink today. "Just for today, I am not going to drink." Tell yourself that the moment you get up in the morning and again at lunchtime. When evening falls and you're craving a drink, starting to feel lonely, and thinking longingly about that satisfying ritual of popping open that beer can or taking off the aluminum foil around the neck of a wine bottle, tell yourself again. "Just for today, I'm not going to drink." Don't stress about tomorrow, and certainly don't worry about forever!

Start living your life with intention. You are the master of your own destiny. You don't have to be ruled by your childhood difficulties, past failures, or self-loathing anymore. You no longer have to listen to thoughts that don't get you where you want to go. In part III I'll give you a set of tools to help you take control of every aspect of your life. But now let's take a closer look at cannabis, that green "weed" that has been gaining popularity with nearly everyone in the United States.

CHAPTER 7

The Cannabis Conundrum
Gateway Drug or Wonder Weed?

Hope was pretty sure her sleep issues were related to stress. Forty-six years old, she was working full-time, raising a daughter with severe autism, and also dealing with some worrisome health issues of her own. But even after her daughter started sleeping better, Hope was still plagued with insomnia. It would take hours to fall asleep, and she often didn't get more than two hours of sleep a night. She would jolt awake in the middle of the night. "It felt like someone put vibrating cell phones inside my body" is how she describes it.

Hope tried every recommended sleep remedy—from conventional prescription medication like Ambien to more holistic natural remedies like valerian root, meditation, and even hypnosis. Nothing worked. Sleep-deprived and increasingly anxious (partly because she was leaving a job she had had for a decade and starting a new one, but mostly because she was sick with exhaustion), she felt like a walking zombie.

Then some friends on social media suggested she try cannabis. Even though cannabis was illegal in her state at that time, she was willing to try anything. Hope managed to buy 2 grams of cannabis off the internet. She heated the sticky taffylike blob with an equal amount of coconut oil, put the tincture in a bottle, and put one drop under her tongue. Twenty minutes later she was fast asleep and, she says, she slept like a baby. "It was the first time I slept really well in years. I woke up the next day, and it was like heaven. I started to look forward to being able to sleep." These days Hope, who is fifty now, takes one or two drops of cannabis oil under her tongue every night. For Hope cannabis has been a lifeline.

Collectively called cannabinoids, marijuana and its derivatives are similar to the endocannabinoids naturally produced in our nervous and immune systems. Although "cannabis," the taxonomic term, is gaining in popularity, in this book I use the words "cannabis" and "marijuana" interchangeably. Research is emerging all the time about the importance of the body's innate endocannabinoid system,[1] which is involved in establishing and maintaining health. Our innate endo-cannabinoid system (I dare you to say that five times fast) helps us eat, sleep, and relax.[2] When you consume cannabis, the plant's cannabi-noids attach themselves to your innate cannabinoid receptors on cells throughout your body. Cannabis contains over sixty cannabinoids[3] that can affect different receptors. Using the plant for medicine seems to offer a broad range of health benefits.

Cannabis 101

Out of the more than five hundred patients I have treated at Fair Start in the last decade, over 90 percent of them started their descent into heroin or other hard-drug addiction by smoking marijuana. Does this make cannabis a gateway drug? Should you be concerned if you enjoy getting high? If your tween or teen is smoking pot? If your spouse can't function without it? Should you try medicinal marijuana for some of your health complaints or will you get addicted since you have an addictive personality? So many questions. In this chapter I do my best to provide the answers.

I have to say right up front that this isn't an easy subject. Many peo-ple believe cannabis is a miracle plant; others that it is a leafy devil. My opinion is a nuanced one that falls somewhere in between. The truth is that cannabis has legitimate medical purposes and can be used rec-reationally by many with little apparent harm, but it can also have dev-astating health and psychological effects. I'd like to explore the debate first and then offer help—nutritional, medical, and psychological heal-ing techniques—for cannabis addiction.

First some terminology, in case you're confused. *Cannabis* is the name of the genus of the plant. Marijuana (also called weed, pot, Mary Jane, ganja, 420, and many other names) is the name of the dried

Is It Legal?

Marijuana is illegal on the federal level. The American government considers it a Schedule I (or Class 1) narcotic. According to the Drug Enforcement Agency: "Schedule I drugs have a high potential for abuse and the potential to create severe psychological and/or physical dependence." As of this writing, there are only six Schedule I drugs: heroin, lysergic acid diethylamide (LSD), marijuana (cannabis), 3,4-methylene-dioxymethamphetamine (Ecstasy), methaqualone, and peyote.[4] If you think it's absurd that marijuana is on the same list with heroin and LSD, I do too. Despite the fact that it's federally illegal, twenty-nine states, the District of Columbia, Guam, and Puerto Rico allow comprehensive medical marijuana programs, and eighteen states allow medical use of cannabidiol, abbreviated CBD, which is not considered addictive or psychoactive. Twenty-two states have decriminalized its use, and eight states, including Oregon and the District of Columbia, have passed laws allowing the recreational use of marijuana.[5]

crushed flower tops and leaves of the female plant. Indeed, it is the resin-secreting flowers of the female plant that contain the highest concentration of the bioactive substance that makes you feel stoned or high, delta-9-tetrahydrocannabinol (THC). THC is one of the many cannabinoids that have now been identified, and one of several known to be psychologically active.[6]

So how and why does THC make you high? The reason is its molecular structure. As I alluded to above, the shape of THC fits into special binding receptors on cells throughout your body called cannabinoid receptors. When THC attaches itself to these cell sites, it ignites a series of chemical reactions. Everyone responds differently to these chemical reactions, which also depend on what strain you're smoking or ingesting and how much THC is in the batch you have. Some cannabis will make you sleepy and calm; other cannabis will give you crazy amounts of energy.

Your reaction to cannabis can take many forms: you may find everything hysterically funny, you may get the munchies and start eating your way through the house, you may start bouncing off the walls, have

Types of Marijuana

The cannabis plant has what taxonomist Robert C. Clarke, coauthor of *Cannabis: Evolution and Ethnobotany*, refers to as two distinct gene pools: *indica*, the original THC-containing medical cannabis from India first recognized by European physicians and a contributor to the world's supply of marijuana, and *sativa*, a low-cannabinoid gene pool used in the European hemp industry. *Afghanica*, a subspecies of *indica*, was introduced to the West from Afghanistan in the late 1970s. According to Clarke, most of today's cannabis is some hybrid of the broad-leaf Afghan varieties as well as the narrow-leaf Indian varieties and their relatives.[7]

The taxonomy of cannabis and the terms consumers and sellers employ to describe marijuana are two different things, though. For instance, when consumer sites such as Leafly.com run articles on the different uses of *indica* and *sativa*—*indica* helps anxiety and general stress, while *sativa* is generally more stimulating and gives users more energy and creativity—they aren't usually referring to *indica* and *sativa* from a taxonomic perspective. What's more, legalization has led to even more varieties on the market as growers experiment with hybridization. It's a rather confusing brew of terms and uses that warrants caution. My general advice is if you choose to use marijuana, start with very small doses to determine the effects a particular type will have on you.

the best workout of your life, get unusually horny, or be filled with a sense of peace and serenity you don't usually feel. As one friend shared: "I smoked, and it was as if I had no stress, had never had any stress, and would never have any stress again in the future. If I could guarantee that kind of high every time, I'd smoke every damn day." You may also find you're just lethargic and happy to sit and do nothing all day.

Pot's popularity is on the rise. It's hard to open the computer or turn on the television these days (at least in states where cannabis has been legalized) without seeing articles about the benefits of cannabis. We're not talking about blogs on websites like Hightimes.com about the best-tasting buds of the year, but headlines like "How Weed Helped Me Get in the Best Shape of My Life" (on Greatist) and "7 Incredible Health Benefits of Marijuana" (on AOL). With this cultural shift in our perception of pot, it seems that both recreational and medicinal marijuana use is on the rise. The number of Americans who have tried marijuana increased from 4 percent in 1969 to 43 percent in 2016.[8] Marijuana was legalized in Washington for medical purposes in 1998 and for recreational purposes in 2012.[9] Seventeen percent of Washington's tenth graders surveyed in 2016 reported using marijuana during the last thirty days. Forty-five percent of those who used it said they used it at least *six days* in the previous month.[10] That's a lot.

So how addictive is marijuana? This is a question that tends to generate heated debate. Though you may believe it's not addictive and you can stop anytime, we know that out of everyone who is using cannabis, some 6.8 million Americans (equivalent to the population of Massachusetts), about a third feel that they have difficulty controlling their use and that using is negatively impacting their lives. This has left public-health researchers at Columbia University concerned. It seems you can enjoy marijuana without getting addicted, but, as these researchers write, "The clear risk for marijuana use disorders among users (approximately 30 percent) suggests that as the number of US users grows, so will the numbers of those experiencing problems related to such use."[11]

How early you start and how often you use influence how likely you are to have problems with cannabis. I recently attended a three-day intensive review course on addiction in Dallas, Texas, sponsored by the American Society of Addiction Medicine. Carla Marienfeld, an associate professor of psychiatry from the University of California–San Diego pointed out that although only 9 percent of people who use marijuana will become addicted, 17 percent become addicts if the use starts in their teen years.[12] For anyone using it daily, there's a 25 to 50 percent chance that they are addicted,[13] meaning they will experience withdrawal symptoms if they stop.

Is What You See What You Get?

When you buy marijuana illegally from a dealer—as with other illegal drugs—you don't really know what you're getting or how strong it is. That said, it's uncommon for drug dealers to lace pot with other substances (a common practice with drugs like heroin). Still, many middle schoolers have bought and smoked what they thought was weed without realizing that it had been cut with oregano. One friend bought a joint off a guy from her high school in Louisiana without knowing that it was laced with PCP (a hallucinogen also known as "angel dust"). About twenty minutes after smoking it, she was paralyzed, with one arm and one leg hanging off her bed. She was miserable and terrified, unable to close her eyes, unable to move. She felt as if she were falling inside her head. That bad trip lasted for hours.

Whether you are buying it legally or illegally, it is hard to know the actual amount of THC in what you are smoking or ingesting. THC strengths can vary from as low as 1 percent for a product that's mostly leaves to over 20 percent for sinsemilla flower tops heavy with resin. As cannabis plants mature and flower, they produce more THC. Late harvests, after the plants have flowered, are thought to produce a more sedating mixture.

No matter what you're buying or from whom, the THC content of cannabis sold today is much higher than it was even a decade ago.[14] Marijuana smoked in the 1980s averaged a THC content lower than 10 percent.[15] One 2015 analysis of over six hundred marijuana strains sold legally in Colorado found that its THC content now averages nearly twice that (18.7 percent), and some products had as much as 30 percent,[16] making today's cannabis a *much* more potent drug.

One of the theoretical benefits of legalizing marijuana is the ability to know exactly what you're buying. However, that same Colorado study found that marijuana flowers were contaminated with high levels of fungi and that the marijuana being sold had little or no CBD.[17]

If you are using cannabis, you are also potentially exposing yourself to a slew of toxic chemicals, which are a major driver of chronic disease.[18] Marijuana can be contaminated with agricultural chemicals, metals, and microbes as well as solvents. In this highly unregulated industry agricultural chemicals found in marijuana include numerous pesticides such as bifenthrin, chlorpyrifos, diazinon, methamidophos, teflubenzuron, the fungicide tebuconazole, the growth regulator ethephon, and the mosquito repellants DEET and malathion.[19] Studies have also shown the tar from a cannabis cigarette contains higher concentrations of carcinogens such as benzanthracenes and benzopyrenes than tobacco smoke.[20]

Cannabis as Medicine

The use of cannabis as a medicine dates back thousands of years in many cultures, but it was not until the 1840s, when an Irish doctor named William Brooke O'Shaughnessy introduced it to Western medicine that it became known for its sedative and anti-inflammatory properties.[21] American production of cannabis was widely encouraged from the 1600s to the late 1800s, as the hemp plant (which is the same genus) had so many uses, including to make rope, sails, and clothing. Cannabis was added to many medicines and openly sold as a pharmaceutical in the late 1800s and early 1900s.[22]

There is no question that cannabis has medicinal benefits.[23] Here's a short list of some of them:

Eases pain

Helps calm and prevent epileptic seizures[24]

Helps with post-traumatic stress syndrome[25]

Improves irritable bowel syndrome[26]

Improves nausea

May fight some cancers

May help with Alzheimer's disease[27]

May slow progressive blindness[28]

May slow symptoms related to ALS (Lou Gehrig's disease)[29]

Reduces insomnia[30]

Relieves anxiety

Stimulates the appetite

Stops vomiting

However, its "miracle" properties are often overhyped by those that profit from its sales. We still don't know whether the medicinal benefits come mostly from CBD, THC, or a combination of both. CBD, which is the nonaddictive, nonpsychoactive part of the plant, is now believed to be anxiolytic (a fancy word for a drug that reduces anxiety), antipsychotic, and anti-inflammatory as well as antiemetic (that is, it helps with nausea and vomiting).[31] Cannabis can increase blood flow to your brain and reduce inflammation. It also boosts your immune system, so you can fight infections and reduce your risk of cancer. Studies have shown benefits in reducing cancer-related pain[32] and chemotherapy-induced nausea,[33] and cannabis has also been shown to shrink prostate and breast cancer, among others.[34] Recent animal studies have also shown a dramatic reversal of aging-related memory loss and brain function with chronic low doses of THC, restoring cognitive function in old mice.[35]

Some compelling new research shows that cannabis lotion massaged onto the skin can offer relief from the pain of arthritis[36] and that using cannabis oil on basal cell skin cancers can inhibit the growth of tumors.[37] Cannabis is also being used with both children and adults who suffer from seizures[38] as well as to treat severe autism symptoms.

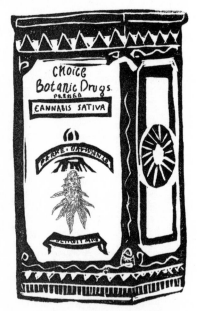

CANNABIS HAS BEEN USED IN MEDICINE FOR HUNDREDS OF YEARS.

A well-designed study of 120 children and young adults with epileptic seizures, published in May 2017 in the *New England Journal of Medicine*,[39] found that CBD oil (in the form of drops) significantly reduced the frequency of seizures compared to the number in those given a placebo. Five percent of the children and young adults taking cannabis oil became seizure-free; no children given the placebo did. (However, the rates of adverse events in the cannabis groups were also higher.) I have a patient whose parents have told me their son needed multiple pharmaceutical antiseizure medications until they used CBD, which enabled him to get off all those meds.

Donald Abrams, an oncologist and integrative medicine expert at the University of California–San Francisco, showed cannabis to be helpful in reducing pain. THC enhances the opioid effect of pain reduction, potentially reducing the need for opioid pain relief.[40] Indeed, in states where medical marijuana is legal, studies have actually found a reduction in opioid overdose deaths in marijuana users, perhaps for this reason. At Fair Start, I talk openly about the pros and cons of cannabis with my patients. Although I discourage its use because it is a potentially addictive mind-altering substance, I don't insist you stop using. **Some of my patients seem better able to wean themselves down to lower opioid doses with the help of cannabis.** This approach seems to be working: we have had no opioid overdoses over the past ten years with over five hundred opioid patients.

If you feel depressed, should you smoke pot? Hello, cannabis; goodbye, Prozac? Perhaps not. The use of cannabis for depression and anxiety has had mixed results. Some research has suggested cannabis—CBD, not THC—as a possible treatment for depression. But it appears that if you are using cannabis once a week or less, **THC actually makes symptoms of anxiety and depression worse.**[41]

Indeed, in my clinic I find that most of my opioid-dependent or -addicted patients use THC to relax, to reduce anxiety, and to help them get to sleep. For some, the short-term effect is to reduce anxiety, but as the effect of the cannabis wears off, anxiety actually increases. Thus they may be trading short-term relief for long-term worsening of their mental health.

My Middle Child's Story

Six months after Maiya and I both got sober, my African sister Tsitsi died of a massive heart attack. Tsitsi and I grew up together in Rhodesia, and she had four children—the youngest was ten and the oldest was seventeen. Tsitsi's husband had died unexpectedly just a few years earlier of pancreatic cancer. Now, living in New Hampshire, her children were orphans.

Maiya and I looked at each other after we got that early morning phone call that Tsitsi was dead. We each knew what the other was thinking—as overwhelmed as we were with juggling child care, working full-time, and trying to cope with life sober, we couldn't let Tsitsi's children get bounced around in the foster-care system or separated from each other. We brought them home to live with us.

After adding four children to the five we were already raising, the last thing we wanted in early sobriety was any drug or alcohol use in our own home. We instituted a no-drugs-or-alcohol policy. But several of our sons started smoking pot in high school anyway. When they were stoned, it was obvious to all of us. They basically checked out. The more they used, the less they were motivated to do schoolwork, participate in after-school activities, or spend quality time with the family.

That summer all nine children still living at home shared one car, a black Scion xB. With the chaos in our house at the time and our inability to keep on top of what all the kids were doing, I made the rule that to get the keys to the "kids' car" you had to pass random urine drug screens. Two of the boys chose not to drive that summer rather than be subjected to the "humiliation" of a drug screen. THC can show up in urine screens for as long as a month after your last use if you've been using regularly. In reality they knew they'd never pass. That they were both unable to stop and too ashamed to be honest about it with us was a sad indication of the hold marijuana had on their lives.

By the time the two oldest boys graduated from high school in 2005, it was clear they were into the party scene and our family's rules were meaningless to them. It was time for them to move out. They both got jobs, and I paid the first and last month's rent on their first apartment. That only lasted a year.

Desperate financially, the boys begged to be allowed back home.

"You'll live under our house rules," I said.

"Of course, we will, Dad," they reassured me.

The joke was on me. Within months they needed to be shown the door once more. By then Maiya and I had finally wised up to how we were enabling our children's addictions by not insisting that they take financial responsibility for their own lives. No first and last month's rent money was offered this time!

Their younger brother also struggled with pot. He was having such a hard time in high school that we were worried he might fail. Distracted by his girlfriend, he was smoking marijuana during the day and skipping class. Maiya and I decided to send him to San Diego to live with other family sophomore year. Grandma and Sissy were eager to take him in and watch over him. He thrived in California, away from the drug culture of his open-campus city school, earned a 3.7 GPA, and was on the honor roll. He began prioritizing schoolwork, stopped using marijuana during the day, and only smoked after he had finished all his assignments. When he came back to Portland to finish high school, he chose to attend a different school with a closed campus, Naya Early College Academy, to eliminate the distraction of going off campus during the day and to avoid senioritis.

Sometimes a change of environment,
friends, or activities is the most important step
you can take to reverse your progression
on the addiction spectrum.

My son believes his troubles with marijuana first started because of side effects from medication. In first grade we were getting exasperated reports from teachers that he couldn't sit still. By middle school he was formally diagnosed with ADHD and put on medication. He couldn't follow directions, didn't remember to write anything down, and almost never turned in even completed homework assignments. The doctor recommended first Concerta, then Focalin, and finally Adderall, trying one at a time to see if it would help. None of them did. The negative side effects from these stimulants included hallucinations, and he started secretly using marijuana to relax before bed.

At the time Maiya and I didn't realize that unhealthy eating, including food dyes[42] and too much refined sugar, can make attention disorders much worse. We didn't know that many of the over-the-counter medications (like Tylenol) and other pharmaceuticals (like antibiotics) we were routinely giving to our kids were exposing them to a toxic overload. We also didn't think about how schoolchildren are asked to sit far longer than is healthy and how creating an individualized learning plan to include extra outside time and more unstructured play would have been a better way to help him succeed. No one talked to us about alternative approaches and, honestly, we probably wouldn't have been open to them if anyone had.

The Problems with Pot

As many health benefits as cannabis may have, widespread use of this psychoactive plant brings its own set of challenges. Some of them include:

Agitation

Anxiety and panic attacks

Coordination issues

Depersonalization (a mental disorder where you feel detached or estranged from yourself)

Derealization (a mental disturbance where you experience the world as unreal)

Disinhibition (impulsivity, poor risk management, disregard for social conventions)

Dry mouth

Hallucinations

Impaired performance

Impaired reaction time

Inability to plan

Increased risk of other addictions

Increased risk of schizophrenia

Lack of motivation

Limited judgment

Lowered IQ (found in chronic users who start in adolescence)

Nausea

Poor attention

Poor memory and decreased ability to learn new things

Poor performance in school

Psychosis

Rapid heart rate

Red eyes

Sexual problems (for men), increased risk of venereal disease (for women)

Vomiting

Is Cannabis Destroying Your Brain?

When expectant mothers are smoking pot or taking THC in any form, it may disrupt a baby's brain development. Use in pregnancy has been associated with lower birth weight, hyperactivity disorders in children, and behavior problems.[43]

When young people—especially younger teens—use marijuana, it can lead to several problems. The one that worries me the most is that cannabis use can cause permanent brain changes when started in the teen years.[44] Recent research from Harvard University has revealed that when children start smoking marijuana before the age of sixteen, they damage their brains.[45] "The brain of an adolescent is still neurodevelopmentally immature," explains Staci Gruber, an associate professor of psychiatry at Harvard Medical School. When you expose the developing brain to cannabis, Gruber insists, "you can alter the developmental trajectory of the brain. This is also true for other drugs and alcohol."[46]

A high concentration of cannabinoid receptors is located in the hippocampus, the part of the brain where memories are formed and an area responsible for learning new information, which may be why using cannabis can impair your memory. Heavy use may actually diminish the volume of your hippocampus. Scientists now hypothesize that exposure to cannabis is more detrimental for adolescents' learning and memory than for adults'.[47]

We also have evidence from magnetic brain scans that chronic use of marijuana damages the brain.[48] Another study uncovered brain abnormalities and memory problems in adults in their mid-twenties even years after they had stopped.[49] This suggests heavy cannabis use can cause lasting damage to important regions of the brain. Memory-related structures of the brain appeared to shrink and collapse inward, possibly reflecting loss of brain cells. In a 2015 study published in the journal *Hippocampus*, scientists at Northwestern University's medical school propose that cannabis causes brain malformations and that cannabis-related brain changes may explain the memory loss we see in heavy users.[50]

What About Schizophrenia?

There is little doubt that marijuana users are at significantly higher risk of developing schizophrenia,[51] psychosis,[52] and other mental illnesses than nonusers. Is it that youngsters who have a genetic susceptibility to schizophrenia use cannabis to self-medicate, or is it that the cannabis itself triggers an illness that may otherwise have stayed dormant? No one really knows, though many experts argue that *early use actually causes later mental illness.*

The connection between cannabis use and schizophrenia is particularly strong if you begin use in your teen years or if you have certain genetic predispositions. This concerns me. Most people walking around with a risky genetic predisposition to mental illness don't know it. Certain single-nucleotide polymorphisms (SNPs), which I talked about in chapter 1, can put youngsters at risk for severe mental-health issues.

But that genetic potential will not be expressed if you avoid the environmental trigger that can turn it on. So cannabis becomes the environmental trigger that can catapult a young person who was doing fine, albeit at higher risk for mental-health issues, into someone who is having a full-blown mental-health crisis. Although it is true that some people with mental-health issues find cannabis helps them, for others who have a tendency toward mental illness, using cannabis may make it worse. Cannabis can also cause psychotic episodes, especially paranoia and delusional thinking. It has also been associated with depression and suicidal thoughts. Perhaps by now you are starting to understand why, for all its potential medicinal uses, cannabis is a drug I would rather you never try.

In another study published in the journal *Neuron*, schizophrenia symptoms were found to be linked to a faulty "switch" connecting two important regions of the brain (for my more technical readers, the insula and the dorsolateral prefrontal cortex).[53] Other research done by a team of scientists from Israel and the US found that there is a wide variation in the way cannabis acts in the brains of adolescent rodents, depending on their genetics. The brains of the genetically primed mice were damaged by cannabis exposure, whereas the brains of the other mice were not.[54]

It's imperative that young people and their families pay attention. As the principal investigator told *Science Daily*, "Young people with a genetic susceptibility to schizophrenia—those who have psychiatric disorders in their families—should bear in mind that they're playing with fire if they smoke pot during adolescence."[55]

Chronic Use Can Lead to Chronic Problems

I have had two chronic marijuana users develop nausea and vomiting so severe they ended up in the emergency room needing IV fluids. Jordan, twenty-five, had been a daily smoker since his early teens. His cannabis knowledge far surpassed mine, and he would patiently explain the effects of the different strains with expert understanding. Jordan had managed his inflammatory bowel disease with cannabis and told me he would never stop using it. Imagine his surprise when using cannabis began triggering severe nausea and vomiting for him.

At his appointment with me after spending more than six hours in the ER, Jordan insisted cannabis wasn't the cause. He didn't believe he had cannabinoid hyperemesis; he thought he had the flu. I pushed back. He didn't listen. But then he had several more severe episodes of vomiting and nausea, and he reluctantly decided to stop using, which fixed the problem. The second case was the same; it was only after that patient stopped being exposed to THC that his vomiting and nausea went away.

It is the largely unknown but very real risk of permanent psychosis

Is Cannabis Making You Tired?

One recent study found that 10 percent of adolescents sent to a sleep center for evaluation of excessive daytime sleepiness tested positive for THC. The scientists believed that the cannabis was making them tired, but could not rule out the possibility that some youngsters may have been self-medicating for untreated narcolepsy.[56] Another team of researchers, based in London, found that heavy long-term cannabis use leads to dopamine dysfunction,[57] essentially depleting your brain of this feel-good chemical, making you feel less motivated, less energetic, and less alive. Though cannabis may make you feel more energetic today, keep in mind that it may change your brain chemistry and actually start making you feel more tired and more lethargic tomorrow.

and debilitating schizophrenia that would scare me from pulling that Russian roulette trigger of using marijuana, hoping that I would not be one of the ones to end up with a permanent brain disorder that would forever change my personality, who I was, and my ability to function in this world. How about you? Are the benefits so great that you are willing to take that risk?

Safe Cannabis Consumption

In all honesty, I would rather you didn't consume cannabis recreationally, and if you feel you need to use it medically, I'd rather you did so only under the supervision of a smart and trustworthy doctor. But if you are going to use, here are the guidelines to follow—my tips for the best, safest, and healthiest ways to consume cannabis:

1. **Always buy organic.** We live in a toxic world, and you need to do everything you can to avoid exposures to pesticides, herbicides, and other harmful chemicals. It's worth buying certified organic cannabis or at least buying from a grower you know who is staying away from chemicals.

2. **Eat rather than smoke it.** Smoking is really bad for your health for many reasons. Sublingual drops or edibles allow your body to absorb the drug in a more natural way than by smoking it. That said, you have to be careful with edibles, as there can be a long delay from the time you eat them to the time they enter your bloodstream, and you may find yourself unexpectedly intoxicated several hours later. Never eat and drive!

3. **Vape rather than smoke it.** Vaping heats cannabis without burning it, releasing the active ingredients into a fine mist that you inhale. Vaping reduces toxic particles and carcinogens and is a healthier way to consume cannabis than by smoking it.

4. **If you must smoke, use a bong.** A bong (which is a filtered water pipe) will remove the most toxic chemical residues.

5. **Never use and drive.** You may think you can drive safely, but you can't. Drugged drivers have slower reflexes and a higher risk of accidents. If you drive under the influence of cannabis, you risk harming someone else. Police are increasingly cracking down on marijuana use and driving, which is as serious as driving under the influence of alcohol. Prison is a severe price to pay.

A Gateway Drug?

So is cannabis a gateway drug? Some can use pot recreationally and remain on the mild end of the addiction spectrum. But the more you use, the more you increase your risk of moving toward severe addiction. About 90 percent of my opioid-addicted patients started with marijuana, trying it first around age fifteen on average. Upon enrollment in my program 80 percent of them were still using THC on a regular basis (a number we extrapolated from positive urine samples), and for those in active treatment today 70 percent still use THC regularly. For those patients, cannabis often helps them with sleep and anxiety. They're worried that, without it, they would feel chronically stressed and tired. Fair enough.

But I can also say that the 10 percent of my patients who have stopped using cannabis are a testament to good health. They tell me they have more motivation in life, are more positive about their future prospects, and feel less tethered to addiction. They are more clearheaded and bright-eyed. These patients are highly motivated and moving away from the severe end of the addiction spectrum—partly, I believe, because they've cut ties with cannabis.

Does Cannabis Use Lead to Alcohol Abuse?

In one study with over twenty-seven thousand participants, people who used cannabis before they ever tried alcohol increased their risk of alcohol abuse, and people who already had an alcohol use disorder and also used marijuana were more likely to see the problem persist three years later.[58] The same study found that adults who use cannabis are five times more likely to develop a problem with alcohol compared with adults who do not use it.[59] The more teens drink or use pot, the more likely they will do both at the same time.[60]

But alcohol and marijuana, it turns out, don't go well together. A recent study of over a thousand college freshmen found that students using moderate to high levels of both alcohol and marijuana had the lowest GPAs.[61] Their grades (and presumably their motivation) improved when they reduced their substance use.

Marijuana + alcohol = a negative effect on school performance.

A Word About Nicotine and Tobacco

Cigarettes are the leading cause of preventable mortality worldwide, killing over 7 million people a year.[62] Smokers die on average nearly ten years earlier than nonsmokers.[63] Most of these deaths are from cancer or heart disease. Yet as many as 15 percent of American adults still smoke cigarettes and of the majority who do, some 68 percent say they want to quit.[64] Nicotine, the chemical in tobacco that gets you hooked on cigarettes, is a highly addictive stimulant. There is nicotine in all forms of tobacco (cigarettes, cigars, pipes, snuff, chew, and dip), nicotine gum, nicotine patches, and e-cigarettes. When you smoke cigarettes, nicotine is absorbed in seconds into your bloodstream by way of the lungs and then quickly passes into your brain. Nicotine promotes the release of dopamine in the brain, giving you a pleasurable buzz, accelerating your heartbeat, and making you feel more alert.

Although the number of smokers in the US has been steadily declining,[65] in the 1970s 34 to 37 percent of American adults smoked.[66] I'm sorry to say I was one of them. I started smoking after I graduated from high school—Camels, Marlboros, Chesterfields, all with no filter, whatever I could get my hands on and whatever would give me the biggest buzz. From age eighteen until twenty-four, I smoked at least a pack a day. Smoking increased my concentration, suppressed my appetite, and made me feel calmer. As all smokers do, I especially loved the small rituals involved in smoking—unwrapping the cellophane around a new pack, tapping one out of the pack, offering a friend a cigarette, lighting a match, blowing it out after that first inhale.

In medical school, I decided it was absolutely ridiculous to want to be a doctor and also be a smoker. By then we knew a lot more about the harmful effects of cigarettes. I saw that my professors smoked pipes. So I grew a beard, like them, and started smoking a pipe. I bought myself a beautiful hand-carved wooden pipe and justified the habit by telling myself pipe smoking was less harmful. (If you mouth-puff a pipe, it may be less toxic, but I was an inhaler, so I don't think it was actually any safer.)

Then my oldest daughter, Natalie, was born. I held her on my chest, listening to her soft breathing and feeling her warm weight. I wasn't going to smoke inside, so I had to put the baby down to walk out of the house, leaving her unattended, in order to smoke that pipe. I didn't want anything toxic near my baby. Disgusted with my own hypocrisy, I took the beautiful pipe I had bought myself and threw it in the dumpster in the alleyway. I had tried to quit several times before then, but this time it finally stuck.

Smoking is highly pleasurable and social. Having a cigarette gives you an excuse to relax. Smokers at most jobs get to leave the building and take a break to enjoy their cigarettes. Cigarette smokers also enjoy a certain camaraderie. That said, our society has become much less tolerant of smoking, especially in public places. It is much harder to light up a cigarette whenever you have a craving.

When you try to quit smoking, there are two issues. Without nicotine you experience withdrawal—anxiety and jitteriness—that can be relieved by replacing the needed nicotine through a patch, nicotine gum, or vaping. Physicians trying to help smokers quit will often recommend nicotine patches. Available in different strengths, these patches give you a continuous supply of nicotine through the skin.

The other issue is behavioral: What do you do with your hands? How do you deal with feeling awkward? You need something to replace the comfort that comes from taking breaks and socializing while you light up and also something to satisfy your hand and oral fixations. Without a cigarette, you don't know what to do with your hands and you want something in your mouth. While a nicotine patch solves the problem of nicotine withdrawal, it doesn't satisfy the need to have something in your hand or the desire to have a cigarette in your mouth.

Enter the e-cigarette, or electronic cigarette. The e-cigarette, which you hold in your hand as you would a paper one, vaporizes water that contains flavor and nicotine, which you can then inhale, meeting your need to have something in your hand that you bring to your lips. When they were first introduced a few years ago, I was excited that this might be a good solution to help people quit smoking. Sadly, I've been disappointed to notice that most smokers who try vaping as a way to quit smoking return to cigarettes when they run out of nicotine cartridges to vape. Perhaps the act of mimicking smoking a cigarette is inadvertently reinforcing the desire for cigarettes. But one advantage to e-cigarettes is that they are less carcinogenic than paper cigarettes.

Nicotine-laced chewing gum is another tool that may help to reduce your craving for nicotine. If you've tried it, you are familiar with its metallic taste. My patients don't like it—they usually find the taste so unpleasant that they go back to cigarettes.

So What Actually Helps People Quit Smoking?

It's really hard to stop smoking. Many of you manage to kick other highly addictive drug habits—heroin, cocaine—and still find yourself spending money you don't have on packs of cigarettes and dip. You need to have a true desire to quit, a supportive environment, and workable strategies to redirect your need to have something in your hands and in your mouth.

It's a fact that a doctor's recommendation to quit, individual counseling, phone counseling, and group therapy will increase your success to kick the tobacco habit. Experiment with other ways to keep your hands busy—try a puzzle pen, a fidget spinner, a Rubik's cube, or knitting. Try natural gum, toothpicks, or unshelled peanuts or sunflower seeds (that you have to dehusk) to have something in your mouth.

It won't be easy—you may experience anxiety, agitation, and some weight gain. After you quit, stay on guard and be vigilant for triggers that prompt you to buy cigarettes. Just as most alcoholics cannot safely take a drink, tobacco smokers cannot safely have just one cigarette.

Your doctor may recommend bupropion, an antidepressant thought to help people stop smoking by increasing dopamine, norepinephrine, and serotonin and decreasing nicotine withdrawal. Bupropion should be avoided if you have a history of seizures. Doctors also sometimes prescribe varenicline, a medication that binds to your nicotine receptors to block you from feeling the pleasurable effects of smoking. Varenicline should be avoided if you have a risk of depression or suicide. Some of my patients have been successful quitting cigarettes with the help of bupropion. I don't use varenicline in my practice, because I am wary of medication that carries a suicide risk.

Cannabis: When Use Turns into Abuse

Although for some, cannabis can be used regularly without any apparent harm or negative side effects, for others, it becomes a real problem. The classic features of cannabis withdrawal include lack of motivation, tiredness, irritability, anxiety, restlessness, trouble sleeping, depression, poor appetite, headaches, mood swings, lethargy, and sometimes muscle spasms.[67] When your next use takes priority over everything else, is affecting your relationships, or is causing you psychological angst or physical problems (like lung infections or cannabis hyperemesis), you clearly need help tapering down or stopping your use.

As with other addictions, it is often hard to break free on your own. Get help if you need it. I am here for you, as are other empathetic, smart, and caring health-care professionals. An addiction specialist or treatment center may be required—you can read more about those options in part III. You also need a detox protocol to help you with your cannabis-induced health issues as well as the depression, anxiety, and sleep problems. Read on.

Cannabis and Smoking Detox Support, the Dr. Paul Way

Take the following supplements to support detox:

A high-quality B-complex: B vitamins play an important role in giving you energy, converting your food into fuel, and staving off depression and anxiety. If you're suffering from high anxiety, talk to your integrative physician about trying B_{12} injections. In the meantime, take a high-quality B-complex vitamin once a day or as directed.

Vitamin C: Ascorbic acid is well known and well loved for its immune-supporting properties. It also helps the body absorb iron (which is why it's beneficial to eat leafy greens or red meat with citrus) and plays a crucial role in repairing and maintaining healthy bones and teeth. Vitamin C is water soluble. Some doctors recommend a one-day vitamin-C flush, that is, taking vitamin C every hour until you have diarrhea. I prefer you take 1,000 mg. two or three times a day.

Vitamin D_3: Vitamin D_3 is vital to a healthy-functioning immune system and protective against cancer. Many smokers and cannabis users, like the rest of American adults, are deficient in vitamin D_3. Have your doctor test your D_3 levels, so you can individualize a protocol. I usually recommend 5,000 IU daily.

N-acetylcysteine (NAC): The amino acid cysteine, when taken internally, can help restore your cells' ability to respond to oxidative stress.[68] NAC is also used by pulmonary specialists to repair and heal the lungs. Among other things, NAC restores the body's glutathione,[69] the enzyme we need to rid ourselves of toxic chemicals, making it a lifesaving intervention in the case of acetaminophen overdose[70] or other toxin-induced liver failure. Take 600 to 1,200 mg. twice a day or as directed.[71]

Support your brain:

Ditch the Doritos: It's time to embrace that nutritious, delicious, and life-enhancing real-food diet that I have been telling you about in, yep, every chapter of this book. Real food will fix your brain and improve your memory. It's hard at first—you'll be craving both the crud food and the cannabis—but your better habits will so quickly lift the brain fog, reverse your memory loss, and improve your mood that you won't look back. Ditch the Doritos and instead eat your food as it comes from the earth (vegetables, fruit, nuts, seeds, meat, fish, beans, whole grains) as much as possible. Avoid Frankenfood that is in a box, bag, or can. Anything made in a factory? Put it back on the supermarket shelf where it belongs. Remember there is no such thing as junk food. It is either food, or it is junk.

Find the forgotten brain cure: Exercise is the forgotten medicine that feeds and repairs your brain. Get yourself moving and sweating at least four to five times a week for 45 minutes to an hour. You can do this. You will be surprised at how those natural endorphins boost your mood and how much better you feel physically. Your clothes will start to fit better, and you'll also get the reward of looking in the mirror and seeing a more vibrant version of yourself.

Master mindfulness: For those of you battling anxiety, I highly recommend adopting a meditation or mindfulness practice. This has been scientifically proven to reduce stress, lower blood pressure, and increase well-being. If Buddhism and yoga just aren't for you, find activities that get you out of your worrying mind and set you free. For me, my most relaxing time is riding a motorcycle on a warm day down a winding road. My mind is so occupied with being vigilant for hazards, the wind on my face so refreshing, that my worries scatter like fall leaves in the breeze.

What activity will do that for you? Where's your happy place? For my friend Mary it's at the yoga studio. For Wendy it's in her garden. For Emma it's curling up with a good book. For Brian it's walking in the woods with his tail-wagging puppy who streaks ahead and then leaps back to be by his side. For Rodney it's running the trails on the hills above his home, shooting bows and arrows in the backyard, and taking his daughter shooting at the gun club. Find that sweet spot and visit it often. The best activity to bring relief from anxiety is the one you will do.

Support your lungs:

It's damaging to your lungs to smoke cannabis every day. Even just one joint a day can lead to pulmonary infections, bronchitis, and eventually lung cancer. Even if you don't stop smoking cannabis or nicotine, you need to do everything you can to boost your lung health.

Start an indoor garden: You should have living plants in every room of your home or apartment. Choose ones that are easy to keep alive like philodendrons, jade plants, and rubber trees. These plants will keep your indoor air cleaner by absorbing carbon dioxide and releasing oxygen.

Get an air purifier: Since your lungs are working overtime due to your cannabis use, you want the air in your home to be clean. In addition to indoor houseplants, put a HEPA-approved air purifier in your bedroom.

Eat pineapple: Pineapple contains high amounts of vitamin C and manganese, but, more important, it is a good source of bromelain, an enzyme that aids digestion and is thought to support lung health by reducing inflammation. Eat fresh or frozen pineapple as often as possible. If you don't like pineapple, take a high-quality bromelain supplement for two to three months.

Exercise, exercise, exercise: In addition to the brain healing I talked about above, you increase lung capacity, reduce inflammation, and jump-start detoxification by exercising. Anything that gets your heart rate up and has you breathing hard will improve your lung health.

Practice deep breathing: If you're anything like me, you rarely take a nice deep breath. Take a moment right now, and take as deep a breath as you can. Do this a few times throughout the day, as deep-breathing exercises jump-start healing your lungs. The American Lung Association has videos of deep breathing techniques on its website.

Support your sleep:

Life feels rotten when you're sleep-deprived. Here's a quick rundown of tips to help you get the ZZZs you need. If you've been using cannabis to help you sleep, you'll have to change your sleep habits, and you may want to try other natural sleep aids. More sleep suggestions can be found on pages 124–25 and 257–61.

Cut the caffeine: A lot of us take great pleasure in a morning coffee or tea. We also drink caffeinated beverages throughout the day, eat chocolate, and use pain medication that contains caffeine. While the energy you get from caffeine helps you stay awake, caffeine can also really interfere with your ability to fall asleep. If you are a slow metabolizer and it takes your body a long time to break down the caffeine in your system, it may actually be the coffee you drank twelve hours ago that is causing your insomnia. Caffeine affects everyone differently, of course, but no one should be drinking coffee or other caffeinated beverages in the afternoon. My general rule is no caffeine after 2:00 p.m. Why? Because most of us need between eight and twelve hours to clear the caffeine from our bodies. You may feel like your sleep problems are intractable. But try extending the time between your last caffeine intake and bedtime and watch what happens.

Avoid intense exercise right before bed: I'm all about exercising as much as possible throughout the day, but if you exercise right before bed you're telling your body, "Wake up! Be alert! Pound your heart!" Instead of exercise, you want to do calming things in the evening. An after-dinner walk or some lovemaking is fine (and encouraged), but don't hit the heavy bag right before bed.

Don't go to bed hungry or right after a big meal: Too much food in your belly will make it uncomfortable to lie down. Too little food in your belly will leave you too hungry to sleep.

Turn off the screens an hour before bed: Blue light emitted from electronics wakes up your brain, when your goal is for it to power down. Keep your electronics in a separate room, and use blackout shades in your bedroom, so it is nice and dark. More on that in the next chapter.

Tell yourself you're going to have a restful night: Your mind can be your most powerful ally in the fight to get better sleep, but not if it's spinning with anxiety. In your mind, crumple your worries and throw them in the trash or pack them into a rocket ship and blast them into space. It is easy to panic about not sleeping, especially if you were left to cry as a child or scolded before bed. Try listening to a guided meditation before bed. Or make up your own serenity script that you say quietly to yourself each night. Affirm to yourself that you are ready to let go of the day, you're not afraid of missing anything, and you welcome restful sleep. Feel gratitude for your comfortable bed and cozy blankets. Pay attention to your breathing. With every inhale say, "I inhale peace and calm." With every exhale, "I exhale anxiety." With practice, that quiet moment before you fully settle into sleep will become so pleasant and relaxing that you will find your brain looking forward to it.

Find your new tribe:

As with alcohol or opioids or any drug you might abuse, when everyone in your social circle is using cannabis, it can be especially difficult to stop. If you are serious about stopping—or even just cutting back—you will need to seek out sober, emotionally healthy new friends.

These days you can't go for a walk in Ashland, a town that is only six and a half square miles, without passing one of the five cannabis dispensaries. Growers are experiencing a boom market, barely able to keep up with demand. As cannabis is legalized across the country, we will undoubtedly learn more about its benefits and harmful effects. Some states are very happy with the tax revenue generated by the pot industry. I hope they will save some for drug-treatment programs. It still remains to be seen what effect legalization will have on total use and early use by teenagers, which is known to be harmful to their developing brains. As a pediatrician and an addiction-medicine specialist, I worry.

In 2014 WebMD did a physician survey of 1,544 medical doctors from 12 specialties in 48 states. Sixty-seven percent of those surveyed believed cannabis should be a medical option for patients, and 82 percent of oncologists agreed.[72] No doubt it was pediatricians and addiction specialists who were not as keen on the idea of using cannabis, as we are the ones who see the abuse potential and negative consequences more often than other doctors.

If you feel marijuana is entirely harmless, you are wrong. As I mentioned earlier, most of my patients who are addicted to heroin, opioids, or meth began with cannabis and alcohol and then moved on. By the time they come to me, their brains are already damaged. When you start using in your teens, marijuana has damaging effects on your brain functioning, motivation, school performance, and mental health. Early use can cause permanent changes to the brain, pushing you to a place of anxiety, depersonalization, depression, and even psychosis and schizophrenia. Marijuana may be one of the triggers without which you could have avoided untold suffering.

"If I had known what was going to happen to me, I would have never taken that first hit." How many times have I heard someone in recovery admit as much, in a voice filled with remorse? Exposure to cannabis carries the very real risk of moving a young person toward the severe end of the addiction spectrum. Parents, do everything you can to keep marijuana from being introduced into your child's life. Teachers, if you know your students are smoking pot, they need your help.

For some of my patients, using cannabis helps with anxiety, sleep, and pain. It allows them to taper down the opioid dose more easily. There is a place for cannabis, particularly CBD, as a medical treatment for a host of conditions. I have a friend who's a successful lawyer who has smoked marijuana his whole life. He has a healthy relationship with the drug, much as many social drinkers have with alcohol, and has stayed on the mild end of the addiction spectrum. As cannabis becomes more accepted in the United States, we all will have to learn to find the right balance.

Moderation is something we are also seeking in our use of screens, the internet, and other addictive activities, which is the subject of the next chapter.

CHAPTER 8

Screens, Dopamine, and Recovering from Digital and Other Addictions

IT WAS FATHER'S DAY 2010. I had five young adult children sitting with me in the living room. I had just finished preparing a huge brunch of scrambled eggs, bacon, sausage, pancakes, French toast, and fruit. I pulled the lever to the La-Z-Boy to put up my feet, looking forward to having a meaningful conversation with the kids. A happy family. Except that every one of them had their smartphone in their hand, their gazes locked on those small rectangular screens. They were paying no attention to me. Or each other.

I put my coffee on the side table and folded my arms across my chest, deciding to see just how long it would take for just one of the kids to look up. At first I smiled wryly. This was an amusing experiment. After all, I was the reason we were all together. How long would it take for them to notice me? Anyone? Anyone? I waited and observed. I waited, waited, and waited. Their attention remained riveted on their devices. I wish I had been able to keep waiting until one of the kids actually bothered to look up of their own volition, but I was too impatient (one of my character defects).

No longer amused, I told them to put their *&$%)#@ phones away. Not a happy memory.

There are a million reasons to celebrate smartphones and the digital revolution we have been going through in the past twenty years. We were an urban family, and my wife and I both worked outside the home. Our kids had to navigate public transport and were often home alone after school. We would have felt as though we were neglecting our children if we hadn't given them smartphones. I'm sure many parents feel the same way.

There's so much good that comes of having technology at our fingertips—easy access to friends, instant walking or driving directions, a weather report no farther away than your back pocket, to say nothing of the ability to dictate or jot down notes the minute you think of something important, take and post photographs, set alerts, and check in with the family. For those of us who are easily distracted and don't do well sitting quietly for more than a minute or two—as addicts tend to be—a smartphone is a lifesaver. It gives us so much to do, with just a few thumb scrolls.

Maybe you feel that way too. To have so much information, so many opportunities, movies, games, and activities available to you at the touch of a button is exciting. An iPad makes the perfect babysitter for busy parents. And surfing the internet, checking Facebook—or a little online shopping—is a satisfying way to unwind at the end of a stressful day.

The digital world is an integral part of modern-day life for the vast majority of Americans: 95 percent of us own some kind of cell phone, 77 percent own smartphones, and nearly three-quarters of adults have a laptop computer.[1] Americans spend a lot of time on devices both creating and consuming (but mostly consuming) digital media. But for all the opportunities created, using this much digital media has repercussions for both your mental and your physical health. As I mentioned in chapter 4, research reveals that today's nineteen-year-olds are as sedentary as sixty-year-olds.[2] Although the researchers don't explain *why*, consider how many times you've been inside watching TV or on your phone on the couch instead of going for a walk, bike ride, or hike; doing physically active chores like mowing the grass or gardening; or heading to the park to play ball. Even on a beautiful sunny day, it's very enticing to while away the hours on our derrières playing video games or instant-messaging.

The numbers say it all. The average teen in the United States spends as much as *nine hours* a day on a screen.[3] But it's even worse for adults—a survey of media consumer habits done by the Nielsen Company found that in the first quarter of 2017 the average baby boomer spent *thirteen hours and fifteen minutes a day*—more time than they spent sleeping—consuming media.[4] And they were not writing the great American novel, inventing a clever new app, or devising the next generation of a role-playing game.

So what *are* we all doing on screens for so many hours a day? This is a question marketing firms are keen to answer. The media that most capture our attention also capture our pocketbooks. So the Nielsen Company gives a detailed breakdown by age group of where we lend our consciousness: watching TV, listening to the radio, or on our smartphones, computers, tablets, and TV devices.

Our Digital Lives: Hours of Daily Use

	Age 18–34	Age 35–49	Age 50+
TV	3	4.5	6.75
Smartphone	2	2	1
Radio	1.5	2	2
PC (computer)	1.5	1.25	1
TV connected device	1	0.5	0.25
Tablet	0.5	0.75	0.25
TOTAL	9.5	11	11.25

Adapted from the Nielsen report, rounding to nearest quarter hour.[5]

Do your eyes hurt thinking about this? Or do they hurt because even as you've been reading this book, you've hopped on your smartphone to check email, taken a short break to play your favorite video game, decided on a lark to buy another book, or paused to look up an article? Or maybe tweeted a quote you like?

Even if your mind doesn't tend to spin in several directions at once, as mine does, this endless access to information and digital technology is probably fragmenting your attention too. You may suspect you are spending too much time on screens. If you have struggled with digital gaming or any other behavior addiction, you probably already know you have a problem. But if you are moving toward the moderate or severe range of the spectrum for digital addiction or any other nonsubstance use, you may not have realized it.

I'll talk more about behavioral addictions below, but first let's find out where you currently fall on the addiction spectrum for digital use with a self-test.

Where Do You Fall on the Addiction Spectrum for Screen Time?

I. How many electronic devices do you own?

Smartphones _____

Tablets (iPad, Kindle, etc.) _____

Computers (desktop, laptop) _____

Game consoles (Xbox, Wii, PlayStation) _____

Televisions _____

Give yourself 1 point for each device. **Total points:** _____

II. Smartphone: If you own a smartphone, circle True or False for each statement. If you don't own a smartphone, skip to III.

I use my phone for games, social media, and/or internet surfing more than as a phone (to call or text).   TRUE / FALSE

I check my phone before I get out of bed every morning.   TRUE / FALSE

I've skipped the bathroom, a meal, or sleep because I was on my phone.   TRUE / FALSE

I use my phone when I'm in the bathroom, even just to pee.
TRUE / FALSE

I can't watch a movie all the way through without also being on my phone.   TRUE / FALSE

I'm anxious when I have to turn off my phone or be without it.
TRUE / FALSE

If my phone is running out of power, I panic.   TRUE / FALSE

I check social media or play video games on my smartphone for more than an hour a day.   TRUE / FALSE

When I feel awkward in social situations, I get on my phone.   TRUE / FALSE

When I feel bored, anxious, or depressed, I get on my phone.
TRUE / FALSE

I'm more comfortable with my social media than my real-life friends.
TRUE / FALSE

My phone use interferes with my ability to get things done.
TRUE / FALSE

A friend or loved one has complained to me about my phone use.
TRUE / FALSE

I'm concerned I use my phone too much.   TRUE / FALSE

Give yourself 1 point for each time you circled True. **Total points:** _____

III. Gaming: If you play video games, circle True or False for each statement below. If you don't, skip to IV.

I've skipped the bathroom, a meal, or sleep because of gaming.
TRUE / FALSE

It feels hard to control how many hours I spend gaming.   TRUE / FALSE

Sometimes I feel my gaming controls me more than I control it.
TRUE / FALSE

A friend or loved one has complained to me about my gaming.
TRUE / FALSE

I'm concerned about my gaming; I think I have a problem.   TRUE / FALSE

Give yourself 1 point for each time you circled True. **Total points:** _____

IV. Television

The TV is always on in my house.   TRUE / FALSE

I watch more than four hours of TV a day on average.   TRUE / FALSE

I don't really care what I watch on TV, as long as I'm watching it.
TRUE / FALSE

I'm irritable or upset if I can't watch TV for a day.   TRUE / FALSE

My TV watching interferes with getting things done.   TRUE / FALSE

I watch TV when I feel stressed or upset to help me cope.   TRUE / FALSE

When I watch TV, I always want to watch more.   TRUE / FALSE

A friend or loved one has complained about how much I watch TV.
TRUE / FALSE

I'm not truthful about how much TV I watch.   TRUE / FALSE

I watch TV more than I think I should.   TRUE / FALSE

Give yourself 1 point for each time you circled True. **Total points:** _____

Scoring

0–10 points: Good news. You are in control of your digital use and it's not controlling you. Be sure to continue to practice good digital hygiene and to pay attention to any red flags that might suggest you're overdoing it.

11–20 points: Not such good news. You may be spending too much time on your device, which may be starting to interfere with your quality of life. You may be progressing toward the moderate or severe range of the addiction spectrum. It's important to put the brakes on now, so you don't end up on the severe end of the spectrum, where your digital addiction starts to negatively affect your life and the lives of your loved ones.

21–35 points: Cause for concern. You're scoring in the severe range for digital disorders, and your happy media time has become digital dope. You need help to overcome something that is now compromising your quality of life, your relationships, and your productivity. Use the techniques in this chapter and throughout this book to return to the mild end of the spectrum and regain control of your digital life.

Why Would Feeling Good Be Bad?

You love binge-watching your favorite Netflix series with your best friend. You spend four or five hours a day playing video games. You enjoy the back and forth on Twitter and regularly chime in on political debates. So what? After all, a marathon session of *American Vandal* on the weekend is a fun and harmless way to disconnect from the stress of the work week. Feeling good is not bad, is it? It certainly doesn't make you an "addict."

Though I could tell you that it's not healthy to watch more than a couple of hours of TV at a time, the problem is not the Saturday binge. The problem comes when you start disconnecting from your life, lying to yourself and to others about your behavior, and choosing to pursue that behavior—whether it's compulsive buying, gaming, or eating—to the exclusion of all other activities.

Throughout this book I've been discussing addiction to drugs and alcohol, which are chemical addictions. These chemical addictions affect the reward center of the brain, increasing dopamine levels and creating intense but fleeting feelings of pleasure. When you come down from the "high" produced by alcohol or your drug of choice, the dopamine levels in your brain are depleted, and you start to feel poorly, craving the next hit or the next drink. You might be surprised to know that nonsubstance addictions—to video games,[6] the internet,[7] shopping,[8] food,[9] sex,[10] pornography,[11] gambling,[12] exercise,[13] anger,[14] codependent relationships,[15] you name it—can actually create a similar vicious reward cycle of increased and then depleted dopamine.[16]

Every time you get a new email message, text, or alert on your phone—ding!—your brain feels a rush of pleasure, a hit of dopamine. Dopamine, as I talked about earlier, is a chemical messenger that is released in your brain when you anticipate or receive something positive or pleasurable. This dopamine signals the brain to pay attention. Its message is that whatever is about to be experienced—a delicious scent, eye contact with an attractive potential mate, a glass of wine—is worthwhile. Screens are so enticing to the brain that Peter C. Whybrow, director of UCLA's Semel Institute for Neuroscience and Human Behavior, calls them "electronic cocaine."[17]

We are creatures of the animal kingdom, wired to scan for danger. The problem in our connected world is that the triggers for possible danger are almost constant. Each time you get an alert or a text message on your phone or you watch the news, you also may have a release of epinephrine, the hormone that increases your alertness and prepares you to gear up for a fight or to get ready to run, the "fight or flight" response. Our hormones do not distinguish between the true danger of a wild animal attack from the "danger" of alert or text message. This stress signal overload is exciting and captivating to our minds, but it also sets us up for hormone depletion, fatigue, anxiety, and depression, which is partly what has been happening with my patient Shandra.

I've been seeing Shandra monthly to treat her digital addiction. She used to be a talkative straight-A student, but has become withdrawn from her family and friends and at risk of failing school. Shandra's excessive screen time has also been compromising her sleep and has resulted in a severe clinical depression.

All addictions are not created equal. Some are obviously more harmful than others. You will hurt your body more by smoking crystal meth

Normal Behavior or Unhealthy Obsession?

Most activities that can turn into behavioral addictions are normal—and even healthy—in moderation. So when do these pleasurable activities slide into destructive addictive behavior? You move farther along the addiction spectrum when you become obsessed. You look for more and more opportunities to engage in the behavior. You do it despite negative consequences. Your family and friends express concern. You experience withdrawal, profound frustration, and other negative emotions when you can't do it. The activities that once brought you joy—spending time with loved ones, hobbies, creative endeavors—no longer hold your interest. Day-to-day living becomes a struggle.

Clues Your Behavior Is Becoming an Addiction

- You think about it all the time.
- You spend inordinate amounts of time doing it.
- You use it to cope with negative emotions.
- You keep doing it even when it starts to cause you physical or mental harm.
- You start neglecting your work, school, or family.
- You try to cut back but can't.
- You feel irritable or depressed when you try to stop.
- You actively hide the extent of the problem from family and friends.
- You feel isolated and totally alone because of your behavior.

than you will by overworking. But the common thread with any addiction is that you engage in it in total excess—in a way that starts to cause you physical or emotional harm (like an $80,000 credit-card bill, a severe weight gain, or a web of lies). In moderation most of the behaviors that become addictive for some people are normal and perfectly acceptable, even essential. No one can survive without food. Most jobs require daily use of the computer and phone. Exercise is both essential and one of life's great pleasures. But taken to excess, any of these activities can potentially derail your life.

It has taken the medical establishment a long time to recognize nonsubstance addictions, including relentless and uncontrollable use of digital media, as "addiction." But in a watershed moment that happened just as this book was going to the printer—in June 2018—the World Health Organization released a new international classification identifying compulsive gaming as a mental-health condition and, essentially, recognizing it as an addiction. This announcement came five years after the *Diagnostic and Statistical Manual of Mental Disorders* also recognized a different behavior—gambling—as an addiction. The 991-page fifth edition moved compulsive gambling into a section called "Substance-Related and Addictive Disorders." Though these may not sound like major breakthroughs if you are not a mental-health professional, the 2018 WHO announcement as well as the 2013 change in the *DSM-5* mark a gradual shift in thinking among addiction and mental-health experts that many of us believe has been long overdue.

The 2013 classification came about partly because scientists had been finding, over the course of nearly twenty years of research and with the help of imaging technology, changes in the physiology of the brains of compulsive gamblers. Several studies showed that the brains of pathological gamblers actually looked similar to the brains of hardcore drug addicts,[18] although these results have not been entirely consistent.

The WHO's recognition of video gaming as a mental-health condition acknowledges something that loved ones of those addicted to nonsubstance behaviors—including gambling, pornography, video games, shopping, and food—have long known to be true: these behavior addictions can be just as devastating as substance abuse. My patient Armando is a good case in point. With the help of buprenorphine and

A Word of Caution About the *DSM*

The *DSM*, the *Diagnostic and Statistical Manual of Mental Disorders*, is the definitive publication of the American Psychiatric Association and the book that health-care professionals, including psychiatrists, psychologists, and general practitioners, usually refer to in order to define and understand mental illnesses. But I'll be honest, the *DSM* is my least favorite medical book (no apologies to my psychiatrist friends). Cited as an authoritative reference, it is actually just a book of labels for doctors to place on patients based on what is often an arbitrary list of symptoms.

Unlike for cancer or diabetes, there is no definitive physical testing that will prove you have ADHD, bipolar affective disorder, or schizophrenia. Yet because your symptoms and behaviors fit the group of symptoms defined by this manual (which changes every time it is revised), you are given a "definitive" diagnosis. This diagnosis allows your doctor to prescribe a host of pharmaceutical medications to treat your symptoms. Making matters worse, as I've mentioned earlier in this book, if that pharmaceutical treatment results in other symptoms, your doctor will put you on more medication!

Doctors love to hand out labels and give patients "forever" diagnoses, hinting or telling them outright that they have an incurable or nonreversible disease that can *only* be treated with pharmaceutical intervention. But what you need is a functional or integrative physician who will take the time to figure out root causes of your mental disturbances and address them. You will be delighted to find out that as you implement the mind-body suggestions in this book, many of your symptoms, and hence your "*DSM*-approved" diagnosis, will disappear. You are not your diagnosis. You are not Ritalin-deficient or Prozac-deficient. You may not even need that pharmaceutical your doctor prescribed.

counseling Armando had been able to get his opioid addiction under control. He also stopped using meth, alcohol, and marijuana. But Armando's craving for gambling was still making him suicidal. At this point Armando was more severely affected by his compulsive desire to gamble than by his heroin addiction.

Kerry, an addiction specialist and recovering heroin addict and alcoholic, struggled more with her food addiction than anything else. Both Kerry's parents were alcoholics, and she grew up in a house full of rage. There often wasn't food in the refrigerator, but there was always beer. When the family ate meals together, if Kerry or her brothers stumbled over a word while saying grace, her father would smack them in the face. Kerry began eating compulsively when she was a child. "I felt so empty," she explains. "I wanted to be full." But though food—especially macaroni and cheese, mashed potatoes, and anything sugary or fatty—comforted her, Kerry had no off switch. Once she started eating, she couldn't stop. "You're putting your hand in the food bag, and in your mind you are screaming, 'Don't do it!'" Kerry says. Kerry shot heroin for the first time when she was fourteen years old and describes the feeling it gave her as "total nirvana." But she says it has been her food addiction that has been the hardest to overcome. Even after she had kicked the heroin habit and been sober for years, she still couldn't stop compulsively eating.

Like addiction to opioids, meth, and alcohol, these nonsubstance addictions can compromise your health, alienate you from your friends and family, and destroy your life.

Dr. Paul's Screen Struggles

Last year I was talking to my personal doctor about my health. She had run labs, and the results were of some concern. My thyroid was suppressed, my testosterone was low, and my blood sugar was borderline high, indicating that I was at risk for diabetes. She asked me when my last day off was.

"Last weekend," I said. "Two days off."

She raised her eyebrows. "And you didn't check emails, write blogs, spend more than an hour on social media, or work on your book or any other project?"

I think I guffawed. It's not an exaggeration to say that I'm working on something virtually every waking hour of every day!

My doctor wasn't done. "Are you taking a lunch break where you're off screens and off-line?" she asked.

No again. During my ten- to thirty-minute lunch break I always do my charting (slang for entering patient information into our computer's electronic filing system). You'll often find me wolfing down lunch between patients and rushing back to an exam room. My doctor told me what I already knew: my body was essentially in a constant state of fight or flight. This explained why my blood sugar was higher than it should be, why I was collecting fat around my waistline, and why I was suffering from chronic fatigue and sinus infections. She patiently explained that it is vital for our brains to get off-line and off screens, and that multitasking all day every day harms us.

Problem? Who me? I was just being productive! I *was* being productive. I didn't feel I had a problem. And certainly not an addiction. But after talking to my doctor, I forced myself to examine my screen time, and I realized what I was doing *was* a problem. I literally felt like my body was falling apart. I was too obsessed with all the tasks I felt were vital. There's no question I'm a workaholic and I was spending too much time on screens. I now have rules: no computer or phone use after supper during the week and I disconnect for at least one half day on the weekends. I'm working up to longer stretches. I now make sure I'm exercising vigorously at least four times a week and I insist on getting adequate sleep for myself, even when I feel like I have a thousand things to do. Like many things in my life, limiting my time on the computer and my smartphone is a work in progress.

The ABCDEFGs of Screen Overuse

"People really totally lose control, and they cannot stop themselves from engaging," says Hilarie Cash, cofounder of a digital addiction residential program near Seattle. There is so much demand for her residential program for younger adolescents needing to detox that she cannot hire employees fast enough to staff it. "There are all kinds of negative consequences—like being seriously underweight or overweight, being sleep-deprived. Some have serious strains on their tendons and back. And then there are social and academic consequences. That's what digital addiction is."[19]

Even if you are on the mild end of the addiction spectrum, too much time on screens can lead to:

Anxiety: You hop on Facebook only to see that a friend from college just had her fourth baby, on a moonlit night, in the comfort of her home. The photos, backlit with candles, are gorgeous. In the meantime, you've been unsuccessfully trying to get pregnant for the last year, or you had a hospital birth that was beyond stressful, and you're finding it very hard to adjust to being a mom. Reading your friend's update makes you feel like crap. Being constantly on social media, like Facebook, Snapchat, and Instagram, can make you feel both anxious and jealous. And it can lead to depression and anxiety too. A 2017 study found that people ages nineteen to thirty-two who used seven or more online platforms were more than three times as likely to experience anxiety and depression than those who used two or fewer.[20]

Back and neck problems: My medical colleagues, including chiropractors and osteopaths, tell me they have been seeing a remarkable increase in back and neck pain, mostly from too much screen time. There's even a name for it: text neck. Whether you have a full-blown addiction or just an overuse disorder, bending your neck to look at your phone for hours at a time can compromise your posture and lead to headaches and other pain. If you go to a conventional doctor with back or neck pain, they may prescribe you opioid pain relief, the beginning of a vicious circle that encourages addiction.

Compromised sleep: One of my daughters was fourteen years old when she got her first cell phone. Cell phones were new back then and she and her friends became a little obsessed. She started staying up half the night texting her friends, which became her main way of socializing. Certainly it was a habit that was safer than drugs, drinking, or nightly partying. But she would come to breakfast with dark circles under her eyes, exhausted, and even grouchier than is normal for a teenager. Maiya and I were worried. We came up with a solution together—our daughter agreed to turn in her phone when we went to bed, so she wouldn't be tempted to use it at night. But we were never good at policing the kids, and we learned years later that she struck a deal with her older brothers—she would clean their rooms during the day in exchange for access to their cell phones at night.

Disrupted sleep is often the first sign of a mental-health problem like depression or bipolar affective disorder. It is also a side effect of screen addiction. If there is one thing you do to increase your happiness, it is getting an hour more of sleep each night.[21] But though you know you should be sleeping, it's easy to get sucked into the vortex of the internet or video gaming at night. There is little controversy about the fact that overuse of screens harms our sleep.[22]

Deficiency of vitamin D: As I have been telling you in every chapter, vitamin D is essential for your immune function, bone growth, and even mood. Ninety-nine percent of patients whom I've tested—both adults and children—have had insufficient levels of vitamin D, which dovetails with research that has shown that up to three-quarters of Americans may be vitamin D deficient.[23] The more time you spend in the digital world and the less time in the sunshine, the less vitamin D and the less robust immunity you will have.

I recommend supplementation, though the preferred way to get vitamin D may be to spend more time outside. Dr. Paul's prescription: turn off your computer and try some nude sunbathing on your back porch. Full disclosure: my integrative colleagues and coauthor recommend this, but *I* don't actually tell patients in my practice to do that and you won't find *me* outside in the buff. A funny story: When we first moved back to Oregon from California, I took my young family for a picnic along the Columbia River, at Rooster Rock State Park. As I was setting up our food, I saw an elderly man standing fifty yards away—buck naked. I was a little concerned he was a flasher. I walked over to find him standing next to a sign stating, "Nude Beach Starts Here."

Excessive weight gain or loss: Digital addicts can become dangerously underweight, a phenomenon I see with meth and heroin addiction as well. When you get obsessed, you forget to take care of your basic needs: eating, sleeping, hygiene. Gaming can also lead to mindless overeating and excessive weight gain. Poor quality sleep can play a role in weight gain.[24] Researchers have found that money spent on technology is a significant factor in the rise of global obesity.[25]

Feelings of low self-esteem: A large Norwegian national survey found that addictive social-media consumption is linked to poor self-esteem.[26] Screen time taken to the extreme causes you to feel isolated and depressed.

Growing vision problems: Too much time on computers, tablets, and smartphones can cause eye strain, other vision problems (like seeing double or trouble focusing), and the headaches I mentioned above. Doctors have a name for this: computer vision syndrome (CVS). CVS seems to be worse for adults over forty than children, but doctors are also seeing unique vision problems in youngsters who have unlimited use of handheld devices. Constantly looking at screens can compromise your ability to recognize people's faces. It turns out your eyes—and your brain—need to look at the horizon in order for vision to develop normally, for your eyes to track properly and focus.[27]

Electromagnetic, Say What?

An electromagnetic field (EMF) is a force field produced by any object that is conducting electricity. The appliances and electronics in your house—your refrigerator, computer, wireless router, electric stove—are all generating EMFs. Because EMFs are invisible, you are most likely blissfully unaware of them. If you could see them, though, you would see lines of energy streaming through the windows, ceilings, and walls. We know EMFs can penetrate living tissue, creating charges in our bodies that have been linked to cancer,[28] heart issues,[29] and brain damage.[30]

Remember high-school science when you learned that the earth itself has its own magnetic field, which makes a compass point north and is used by birds and fish for navigation? EMFs naturally occur in nature, of course. So a lot of people raise their eyebrows at the question: Can EMFs really be dangerous? Unfortunately, the answer seems to be yes.

Remember that the cells in your brain continuously convert chemical signals to electrical signals in order to communicate with other

Addiction and Self-Esteem

Do you think positively about yourself? Know deep down that you are worthy and lovable? Feel you are living to your full potential?

When you have good self-esteem, you are at peace with yourself and with the people around you. You treat yourself with compassion and give yourself the benefit of the doubt. You don't gravitate toward drama and abuse, and you seek out healthy activities.

My addiction patients struggle with self-esteem, as do many of my pediatric patients. Perhaps we all do? We all have parts of ourselves that we would like to change and times when we feel great remorse. As a parent, pediatrician, and addiction specialist, I try to promote positive self-esteem in my own children and my patients. But addiction makes it difficult to have good self-esteem. You may have moved toward the severe end of the addiction spectrum because of low self-esteem to begin with, or it may be that being addicted is destroying your confidence.

Either way, your self-esteem is suffering. As you get more obsessed with your addiction, you feel that you are being self-indulgent. You are aware that you are neglecting your responsibilities, avoiding people you love, and imposing on others. Your sense of well-being and self-confidence, even if you are "high-functioning," disappears. Anxiety or depression often takes hold with an ever-tightening grip. Self-loathing sets in.

How do you fix your broken self-esteem? As soon as you can, find a volunteer opportunity or a meaningful way to give back. In helping others we help our self-esteem. As impossible as that might feel right now, try it anyway.

In an 1899 magazine article, the American philosopher William James (who also trained as a medical doctor) wrote: "Action seems to follow feeling, but really action and feeling go together; and by regulating the action, which is under the more direct control of the will, we can indirectly regulate the feeling, which is not."[31] In other words, act the way you want to feel, and the good feelings with follow. James called this "mental hygiene."

You can practice good mental hygiene by cultivating positivity and a sense of purpose in every aspect of your life. You can tell yourself positive affirmations throughout the day, over and over, so that you start to believe them. Even if you dislike your work, be the most positive person there. Work the hardest. Be kind to everyone you meet. Smile when you greet each person. When you feel yourself slip into negativity, remind yourself you are worthy, lovable, and loving. Because you are. And making small changes like this will help move you toward the mild end of the addiction spectrum, which builds your self-esteem, helping you realize you are going to be okay.

Following all the guidelines I outline in this book, especially in chapter 10, will help you improve your self-esteem and propel you toward finding what we call in the addiction world . . . serenity.

cells and that your heart is using electrical signaling all the time. The concern is that electrical signaling from human-made devices may interfere with our body's signaling and alter and harm our brains.[32] Scientific studies have linked EMF exposure and the risk of leukemia[33] and some researchers, including Harvard neurologist Martha Herbert, argue that even weak signals may have physiological consequences.[34] We know, for example, that the long-term use of mobile phones greatly increases your risk of brain tumors and brain cancer.[35] This risk is highest among those who start using cell phones before age twenty.[36]

So as an integrative physician I believe it is very important—and not that difficult—to take steps to limit your EMF exposure in the digital age. Follow these tips:

No laps for laptops: Laptops are a high-energy source of EMFs, so it's best to avoid putting yours directly on your lap. Keep your computer on a tabletop. Pregnant women, especially, should avoid having laptops on their laps. If you must use your laptop on your lap, buy a highly rated heat and radiation shield to put between the device and your legs.

Don't be a phone head: As much as you can, avoid holding your phone up to your head or wearing your electronics like jewelry. Talk on speakerphone or use headphones. No matter what you do, do not sleep with your phone plugged in by your head. In general, as I've mentioned, it's best to keep your phones and computers *out* of the bedroom. You don't want electronics that generate EMFs—alarm clocks, lamps, computers—plugged in nearby while you're sleeping.

Unplug your devices while you're using them: You reduce EMF exposure if your computer, tablets, and cell phones are unplugged and running on battery power.

Choose cable: Connecting electronics (including printers) via cables instead of WiFi greatly reduces your EMF exposure.

Say "No, thank you" to smart meters: Smart meters, which automatically tally and transmit utility use, are one of the worst sources of EMFs. Most communities have opt-out options. Call the power company or city hall to find out.

Shield thyself: Make sure all electrical wires in your living and work space are properly shielded with conduits or armored cable, which will prevent unnecessary exposure to EMFs.

Kerry's Story

Kerry, whom I talked about earlier in this chapter, is celebrating thirty-five years of sobriety from heroin and alcohol this month. But she has only been free of her food addiction for three years.

Kerry was such an angry person that when her oldest was born, she felt no love, just fury. "I'm going to teach you how to get them before they get you," she whispered to her baby.

Kerry, who is only 5 feet 3 inches, used to weigh over 300 pounds. But she didn't mind being so big. She didn't want people pushing her around, and she didn't want to be pathetic. "Being fat really protects a person," she explains. "People don't want to get close to you."

In 2015 Kerry had to get surgery for a hernia that was bleeding into her abdominal cavity. After the surgery she felt exhausted and weak; she had a fifteen-inch incision, and her iron and ferritin levels were dangerously low. The doctors told her she could have nothing by mouth. But instead of resting in bed, Kerry hauled herself up, shuffling along with the help of a walker and pushing the IV pole, and went in search of food. The compulsion to eat was so overwhelming that she could not heed the doctors' orders, even though she knew it could kill her. She ate the food feeling so ashamed and so alone, tears streaming down her cheeks.

> *"It's all about secrets—that's what a food addiction is. Secrets from yourself and everybody else. You are living in your addiction instead of living your life."*
> —KERRY, 67, RECOVERING FOOD ADDICT

For Kerry to get her food addiction under control she realized she could not make independent food choices. Instead, she needed a food plan from which she would never deviate. She also needed accountability—she has a sponsor she checks in with daily and an overeaters group she attends weekly. She realized the ritual of weighing food and eating in a similar way each day could give her the same comfort she was getting from obsessing about food and overeating. She cut all fattening and unhealthy foods out of her diet and no longer eats anything processed, starchy, or sugar-laden. She weighs every meal, allows herself only a prescribed amount of protein, vegetables and fruits, carbohydrates, and healthy fats, and does not snack between meals.

In her job as an addiction specialist, Kerry works best with "hopeless" cases. The people who come to her raging and anxious and the ones who have devastating histories of abuse, neglect, and self-harm are her favorite clients.

"I was that person," she tells me. "If you had read my case history, you would have said to yourself, 'She doesn't have a fucking chance!'"

But Kerry is not just alive. She's thriving. She is one of the most poised, well-spoken, generous, no-nonsense people I know.

"I'm nothing special," Kerry insists. "If I can do it, anyone can."

So how do you get yourself to stop compulsive shopping, compulsive eating, or compulsive gaming? Here are some solutions to get you started today. I outline the rest of my 13-Point Addiction Recovery Plan in chapter 10.

Integrative Solutions for Digital and Other Nonsubstance Addictions, the Dr. Paul Way

Fix your physical health: Your brain and body must be healthy in order to overcome any addiction. This means daily exercise to bathe your brain in endorphins and oxygenate your blood; a diet of nutritious foods, which will improve every aspect of your health; a diversified biome; adequate vitamin D to support your immune system; and enough sleep so you can rejuvenate your brain and your body, as I've been talking about throughout this book. For more on exercise, see pages 261–62. For more on sleep, see pages 124–25 and 257–61.

Track your time and/or amounts: As with any addiction, it's important to honestly assess the scope of the problem. Keep a record. That sounds simple, but this is often one of the hardest steps. Start by keeping a journal of exactly how much food you're eating, doing an audit of your credit cards and other finances to see how much you are spending, or clocking time spent online to figure out how much of your life is actually being lived in cyberspace.

There are a variety of—you guessed it—electronic apps that track how many times a day you check your phone, allowing you to see how your score compares to other people's. There are dozens of food tracking apps out there as well, designed mostly for people who want to lose weight. Is it making your palms sweat just to think about being honest about how much you are overdoing it? I know this is hard. It's not going to be easy, my friend, but do it anyway. If you're not an app-y person, you can print a tracking sheet off the internet, buy a blank book, or keep a record in your phone's notes.

Send an S.O.S.: You need help. You can't do this alone. For Kerry, though she wanted to go it alone, the only way she could overcome her food addiction was by being accountable to a sponsor every single day. Find a good therapist, life coach, or addiction specialist who understands the pitfalls of nonsubstance addiction and can guide you in behavior modification techniques, mindfulness, and accountability. If your addiction seems impossible to stop with weekly outpatient counseling, there are now inpatient options for behavioral addictions. It may be time to check into a residential program. A good residential program—one that includes individual therapy, group work, meditation training, exercise, and time in nature—can revolutionize your life. More on how to decide if residential treatment is right for you in chapter 9.

Control your access: Alcoholics should not have alcohol in their homes. Drug addicts must get away from the drug scene. It may be even harder, though, with behavioral addictions. A food addict cannot avoid all food. But you can control your access to *problem* foods by not keeping any, ever, in your home. If you are a digital addict, you will most likely need computers for work or school, but you can take steps to control your access. If you cannot follow self-imposed limits for non-substance addictions of any kind, an addiction counselor or personal coach can help.

For digital addiction: Start by going consecutive hours without your phone, the internet, or gaming. Once you are comfortably able to get off screens for two or three hours in a row, try going half a day without them. Actually scheduling a walk or run or trip to the gym, where you leave the phone behind, is a good way to start.

Until very recently, we all lived just fine without 24/7 access to phones, texts, the internet, and Instagram. At least once a week leave your smartphone at home when you go out for the day, or at least silence it or turn it off, and use it only for true emergencies.

Although complete abstinence from screens would be as unrealistic as complete abstinence from food, you can place your screen use into proper perspective by remembering what matters most to you and filling your life with activities that free you from your screens.

> **Block problem programs:** If certain games or programs are sucking the life out of you and you cannot stop once you get started, remove these from your device completely. You may find yourself sucked into Facebook for hours at a time and feeling worse, the longer you stay online.[37] If this is you, suspend your social-media account for one to three months to allow yourself to detox. Or use an app or website designed to electronically control your access.

> **Commit to "screen-free Sundays" and try "Tech Talk Tuesdays":** The best-case scenario is that you commit to having one day when your smartphone, computer, Wii, and other electronics simply stay *off*. If you are observant, this can coincide with

your day of worship. A screen-free Sunday helps you reset, reconnect, and remember all the things not in the digital world that are important to you and your loved ones: time in nature, a motorcycle drive up the coast, going roller skating, cooking a feast, pickup basketball, a free concert in the park, board-game night, contra dancing. Tech Talk Tuesdays are a guided activity that was started by medical doctor and *Screenagers* filmmaker Delaney Ruston to encourage open conversations about screen time. Download conversation starters online or make up your own. Taking time with friends and family to talk about how digital technology can be both a creative and a consumptive activity is a good idea for everyone.

Connect in real life: No matter how "connected" you feel compulsively gaming, gambling, or engaging in other nonsubstance addiction, remember that these activities ultimately make you feel lonely and disconnected.[38] There is no substitute for being face-to-face with other people. The times when you want to isolate yourself by staying in bed gaming or bingeing are actually the times you need real-life connection the most. The good news is that there are dozens of nonsubstance addiction recovery groups out there, whatever issue you are battling (see the resources section at the end of the book).

Turn off the social media and turn to real-life interactions. This can take a thousand different forms. I have patients who have found connection and community going fishing, taking community college classes, joining a knitting club, becoming politically active, and studying photography, among other things. The key is to get your mind, eyeballs, and consciousness away from screens, shopping, gambling, or food.

Shandra, my patient struggling with screen addiction and depression, was moving toward the severe end of the addiction spectrum, but by implementing the integrative approaches I outline in this book, and with a lot of support from her family and community, she was able to free herself from digital addiction. She is now seeing a digital addiction counselor once a week for as long as insurance will cover the sessions. With her therapist's help, Shandra and her parents came up with an agreement about appropriate amounts of screen time that they all felt they could implement. I also helped them remember the family

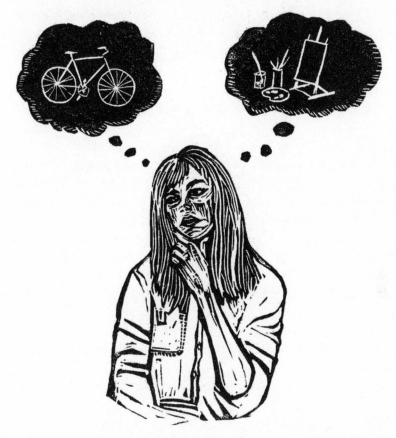

SCREEN - FREE SUNDAY? WHAT WILL I DO?

activities they loved to do, and they committed to spending at least a half a day together every weekend off screens. They signed Shandra up for stress-relieving extracurriculars—a local art class, a jewelry-making workshop, and a monthly nature walk—and also reached out to her guidance counselor at school to get more help and support in improving her grades and managing her time online. Shandra also started eating a diet of real whole foods, taking vitamin D, avoiding stressful friends and online bullies, getting to bed earlier (which is easier now that she docks her smartphone outside her room instead of sleeping with it by her bed), and walking the dog daily to guarantee she gets some exercise.

Shandra came into my office last week. She feels she's doing much better now, she said with a smile, though she still has bad days. Her smartphone use is down, and her grades are climbing back up.

"I'm glad to hear it," I said, offering a high five.

She laughed and whacked my hand.

"Hey, how 'bout a selfie, Dr. Paul?" Shandra asked, whipping her phone out of the pocket of her jeans.

So now that you are taking the steps you need to recover your health and well-being, how do you get a medical system predicated on illness to work *with you* instead of against you?

Glad you asked. Turn to part III to find out.

PART III

The Addiction Solution

CHAPTER 9

Navigating the Medical Maze

N AVIGATING THE MEDICAL MAZE while you're recovering from addiction is extremely challenging. As you've undoubtedly experienced yourself, conventionally trained medical doctors aren't really known for their patience. Yet treating addiction takes patience, persistence, a willingness to fail and try again, and an ongoing commitment to the patient and the process.

As I mentioned in chapter 2, exceptionally smart people are disproportionately represented among addicts. In all honesty, one of the frustrations for some addicts is that we often feel *smarter* than the doctors who are supposed to treat us (and able to outsmart them when it comes to getting drugs)—but over and over again we are treated as inferiors.

So how do you find a good doctor who can really help and support you? If you're already working with a doctor, how do you get him or her to try a different approach? How do you talk so your doctors will listen and listen so your doctors will talk?

THE BEST DOCTORS . . .

Aren't afraid to admit what they don't know.

Are willing to learn about any safe treatment that might help, even if it's outside their scope of experience.

Ask insightful questions.

Help you figure out what you *really* need, not just what you think you need.

Listen closely.

Pay attention.

Are smart enough not to let you take advantage of them.

Understand that sometimes they and their patients have to fail to succeed.

Finding a Program That Works *for You*

Addiction is big business. Nearly anything you google about the subject on the internet is search engine–optimized to lead you to a for-profit program that will happily lighten your wallet, sometimes to the tune of hundreds of thousands of dollars. Some of these programs are wonderful and worth the price (if you can afford it); others are honestly little more than the recovery version of pill mills.

Buyer beware. As with almost everything in medicine, the cost of the program does not necessarily indicate quality. If you've spent your life thinking that more expensive is better, think again. The United States spends more, by far, on health care than any country in the industrialized world,[1] yet we have the *shortest* life spans and we rank last (or near last) on a broad number of other health-care measures, including outcomes.[2] The truth when it comes to addiction is that you can often get *the most* benefit out of programs that cost *the least*. So please don't be fooled by glitzy brochures or luxury price tags. What works for one person struggling with addiction won't work for another. Getting recommendations from recovering addicts, trusted friends, family members, or your doctor is one way to find the best program for you, though your choices may also be dictated by what insurance will cover, which I talk more about below.

It's all about the right fit, which means connecting with kind, smart, no-nonsense addiction specialists who have big hearts and small egos as well as finding other conventional and alternative medical providers who will treat you with dignity and respect.

So Where Do You Start?

If you or a loved one has a medical emergency, call 911. Even if you're not in crisis, you probably have a strong sense of where you are by now and what your level of need is. But if you're not sure, I encourage you to go back to the self-test on page 21 in chapter 1 and take it again. Where you fall on the addiction spectrum at this time will determine your level of need for treatment.

Mild on the addiction spectrum: You will benefit from individual counseling once a week or once every two weeks as well as a weekly group support meeting if you find that helpful, visits to a general practitioner who understands the importance of finding root causes of illness, and, most important, the nutrition and lifestyle improvements that you can do yourself with the help of this book and a supportive network of friends and family.

Moderate on the addiction spectrum: Can you safely stop using drugs or drinking without severe withdrawal symptoms (shakes, sweats, diarrhea, paranoia, suicidal thoughts)? If withdrawal isn't acute, you can start with my 13-Point Addiction Recovery Plan in the next chapter. If you can't safely stop cold turkey or your chronic drug use or drinking is endangering your life, it's time to find an outpatient treatment center or you may need inpatient care.

Either way, moderate on the addiction spectrum requires treatment at an addiction clinic or alcohol recovery program, individual counseling one to three times a week, group support three to five times a week (or as often as every day if you are finding it helpful), and nutrition and lifestyle improvements that you can do yourself with the help of this book and a supportive network of friends and family. If this is not enough to get you to the mild end of the spectrum, you may need a longer stay at a residential treatment program.

Severe on the addiction spectrum: If you've got a suicide course charted or you're experiencing severe withdrawal, your first stop will most likely be the emergency room. The ER doctors and staff can get you hospitalized for your own safety, help you through what may prove to be a difficult withdrawal, and connect you to a residential program and community resources.

ER docs do an excellent job when there's a real medical emergency, but they won't be able to offer you a long-term solution. The sad reality is most emergency rooms are overrun with patients looking for free pain pills and other medications. That said, if you don't have insurance or your insurance won't cover a treatment center, the emergency room may be your only option, as a hospital cannot deny you care if you're in crisis.

Severe on the addiction spectrum often requires hospitalization followed by a residential treatment program. Before you leave that residential treatment program, you should have a strategy in place for implementing my 13-point Addiction Recovery Plan, which I'll walk you through in the next chapter. Until you get back to the moderate or mild range of the spectrum, you may need to go to a group meeting at least once a day (two or three times a day may not be too much), find a sponsor you can call as often as you need, especially when your cravings feel overwhelming, go to counseling two or three times a week with a trusted drug and alcohol counselor, and also have weekly check-ins with a doctor who specializes in addiction. This road is not easy. It's full of bumps and roadblocks and setbacks. But every step you take forward, no matter how small, will move you toward the mild end of the addiction spectrum and freedom from the substances keeping you in bondage. Freedom is the goal. Stay the course.

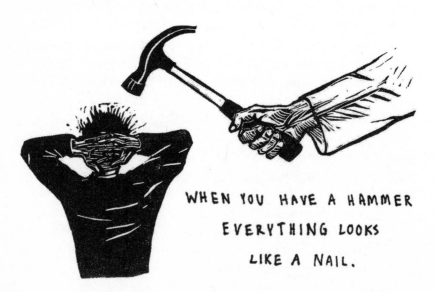

WHEN YOU HAVE A HAMMER EVERYTHING LOOKS LIKE A NAIL.

What Will My Health Insurance Cover?

Health insurance: It often costs a fortune. Many of you don't have it. And those who do find your claims denied, often for no apparent reason. It's ironic that the United States was a leader in pushing every country toward establishing human rights for their citizens. The Universal Declaration of Human Rights, adopted by the United Nations General Assembly in 1948, stipulates that every human has the right to security in the event of sickness.[3] How are we doing making sure Americans have that right? No comment.

While staying inside your insurance network may limit your treatment options, you can often find a good program, whether inpatient or outpatient, through insurance. I've found that some of the most compassionate, kindhearted, dedicated, and skilled people choose to devote their careers to addiction recovery. If you have insurance, call the mental-health number for your plan and find out what addiction treatment options are covered.

Get your doctor on board the insurance ship. It's wise to work with your primary care provider to arrange the inpatient or outpatient treatment in advance if possible. It can take days or even weeks to get preapproval, but it should save you so much hassle later on that it will be worth the wait. For two of my family members who went into treatment, their regular doctors contacted the treatment center and forwarded the relevant medical records indicating the substance-use problem and showing the urgent need for inpatient treatment. Our doctors' assistance was invaluable.

Don't let them deny you. If your insurance claim is denied after the fact, fight the denial. Many insurance companies routinely deny claims—even preauthorized claims. We have seen legitimate pre-approved claims denied multiple times. Since many—if not most—insurance holders don't realize they must fight denials, insurance companies generate millions of dollars by routinely denying legitimate claims. Get out the manual, highlight the relevant information, and then fax or email it to the clerk who's insisting your claim has been rejected. Never pay bogus insurance bills.

Is Inpatient Treatment the Best Choice for You?

One of my patients is an opioid addict whose mom is actively using meth. Another has a live-in boyfriend eager to share drugs. They have both tried to stop using as weekly outpatients, but have had a hard go of it. They are tempted all the time at home. Imagine trying to stop eating ice cream while your family brings home flavor after delicious flavor, eats them in front of you with obvious enjoyment, and suggests that you "just have one bite." You may resist for a day or two, or even a week or a month, but eventually the daily temptation for that mouth-wateringly tantalizing sweet treat becomes too great. I call this a high-risk living situation, where your cravings are constantly triggered by access to drugs or alcohol. If you're living with addicts, surrounded by drinkers or drug users, you probably need inpatient care, so you can recover in a safe and protective environment and make a plan for a new living arrangement once you're drug-free.

A good inpatient treatment program can save your life. But chances are you don't want to go. It's not easy. You have to put your life on hold; you risk losing your job, missing school, being absent when your family needs you. Plus these programs can be very expensive. If you're uninsured or have a high deductible or your insurance won't pay for inpatient treatment (expect to pay anywhere from $6,000 to $30,000

Inpatient Treatment?

You need an intensive inpatient treatment program or hospitalization if:

  You have a plan for committing suicide.

  Withdrawal makes you dangerously sick or suicidal.

  You have severe psychiatric problems that increase when you try to stop using or drinking.

  You're sick and tired of being sick and tired and are ready to stop but you can't.

a month), you may feel the price is "not worth it" and you can't afford to go. I get it. Many of my patients would benefit from inpatient treatment, which is something I often recommend to the ones who need it most. Unfortunately, most opt not to go, usually because they feel they don't have time or they're afraid of losing their livelihood if they take that time away from work.

Do You Have Time to Go into Treatment?

The number one excuse addicts use to avoid treatment is: "I have no time."

I told myself that too.

Then, when I finally got sober, I did the math. At the height of my drinking, I spent two to four hours a day drunk and as many hours hung over.

Really? I didn't have *time* to seek treatment, but I had *time* to destroy my brain and body with my beloved alcohol?

Don't let your addicted brain dupe you, folks.

Make the time!

How Long Should You Be in Treatment?

Insurance companies often only approve three to four weeks of inpatient treatment, if they approve treatment at all. But most of us who work in addiction feel that three weeks is too short. Maiya needed every one of the ninety days she was an inpatient.

For the time you're an inpatient, you are in a safe and protected environment. You are buffered from the stress of your normal life. You can focus on learning about your addiction and on the psychological challenges you've avoided until now.

At the same time, the fact that you aren't dealing with the real world and the triggers in your life that make you want to use limits how much inpatient treatment can help you. Transitioning back to real life can be like having culture shock.

A Note for Loved Ones
(and Anyone Who Needs to Go to the ER and Follow Up with Doctors)

There is nothing more heart-stopping than a 3:00 a.m. call from the police or the hospital telling you that your spouse, child, or best friend has overdosed, attempted suicide, or been in an accident. It's easy to lose your head at the exact moment when levelheaded, clear thinking is what is needed most.

Whether you're on your way to the ER or you're accompanying your addicted loved one to a follow-up appointment, there are strategies you can employ to make the medical maze less confusing.

Use these tips to improve communication with the doctors and make the best of a bad situation:

Take notes. Write down what you hear into your phone, in a notebook, or even on your hand. Turn on the voice recorder on your digital device if you need to. Or ask a friend to take notes for you. You want to write or record everything the doctors tell you, so you have a way to review it at a time when you are less stressed.

Bring support. Someone calm and reasonable, not your overly emotional BFF, should meet you at the ER if possible and accompany you to any subsequent medical appointments. It always helps to have a second set of ears and another brain in an emergency.

Ask questions. Ask all the questions you have, and don't hesitate to ask for clarification if a doctor says something you don't understand. You will most likely think of questions you wished you had asked after the ER doctor leaves. Write all your questions down. If the nurse assigned to your loved one cannot answer them, you can ask to have a doctor paged.

Pack healthy food. It's easy to live on black coffee and pastries when your loved one is in crisis, but remember, all the rules of healthy eating apply to a crisis situation too.

Cultivate an attitude of gratitude. Connect with doctors, especially those you don't know, on a personal level by paying attention to,

acknowledging, and thanking them for how hard they are working. ER doctors give a higher level of service when a patient has
loved ones beside them. I believe all doctors offer addicted patients
a higher level of care when they see family members and friends
actively involved in the recovery process.

Perfection is not the goal, recovery is. Think of it this way. We know
now that there are benefits to the brain in the process of learning a
foreign language at any age. You don't have to master that language.
You just have to try to learn. Yet a lot of adults feel as though they
shouldn't "waste their time" learning a language, because they'll never
be good at it. But the process itself will help your brain be more plastic, help you delay Alzheimer's and other cognitive decline, and make
you feel good while you're doing it. As long as your recovery is being
supported by compassionate, nurturing, nonjudgmental, emotionally
intelligent specialists and counselors, almost any addiction treatment
will be worthwhile. Any time that you're not using drugs or alcohol is
time that you are healing your brain.

The Goals of Treatment

For much of the last century, doctors believed treatment would cure
addiction. We now know that addiction and substance-use disorders
happen on a spectrum and addiction-spectrum disorders can be
chronic and relapsing. Stop right there. Addiction does not have to be
chronic. You don't have to relapse (remember that brilliant doctor who
told you relapse is expected but *not required?*), but I do believe it's more
helpful to think of addiction as we would insulin-dependent diabetes,
cancer, or depression.

You can and will get your addiction into remission if you follow
my 13-point plan described in the next chapter, which includes integrating a real-food diet, daily exercise, an effective sleep program,
judicious use of medications when necessary, ongoing social and psychological support, and daily stress relief into your life. Do all this

and you can live addiction-free—for the rest of your life.

Whether you're able to be sober in a matter of months, you relapse over several years, or you find yourself tapering down but not able to completely leave drugs behind, the real goal of treatment is to get engaged in the process and the journey of recovery, to become more self-aware, and to be in a happier, healthier, safer place.

Fighting Against Addiction Means Fighting for Good Health

Many who struggle with addiction have other health problems, which can include mental-health disorders: anxiety, schizophrenia, bipolar affective disorder, schizoaffective disorder, depression, borderline personality, post-traumatic stress disorder, social or other severe phobias, and eating disorders. Doctors call this "dual diagnosis."

Even if you feel embarrassed, try to mention all your health issues when you call to inquire about a treatment center or an addiction doctor. This is information your future health-care provider needs to know.

I'm comfortable treating teenagers and young adults with any conditions except severe psychosis or schizophrenia. Those two conditions are outside my area of expertise and best managed by a psychiatrist with addiction specialty training.

Other doctors may not be comfortable with addicts who have serious medical conditions like diabetes, heart disease, or a number of psychiatric conditions or may be inexperienced in treating younger addicts. As you navigate the medical maze for addiction, realize that you may need to select where you go based on the ability of that treatment center or doctor to manage your other health concerns.

You are not your illness. No one has the right to label you, define you, or limit you. You are a messy, complicated, interesting, multifaceted human being with health challenges that may stem from a life of poor nutrition, exposure to toxins, childhood chaos, stress, and now substance abuse. As you work to get your addiction under control, you can be proactive about your continuing recovery by surrounding yourself with people who understand the importance of nutrition, exercise, stress reduction, relapse prevention, and ongoing social support.

*You are more than your addiction or your diagnosis, and
don't let a doctor—or anyone else—tell you otherwise.*

As imperfect as our medical system is, it's the one we have to work within. For now anyway. What I want you to remember is that your real and most important recovery work happens within yourself, outside of a hospital setting or doctor's office. This is the work you do over a lifetime, and the good news is you can begin doing that important work today.

CHAPTER 10

Dr. Paul's 13-Point Addiction Recovery Plan

AS AN INTEGRATIVE MEDICINE DOCTOR, the last thing I want to do is put you on a cookie-cutter, one-size-fits-all medical program. That is exactly what we are trying to get away from with integrative medicine. My goal is to individualize treatment and care for *you*. What is best for *you*, given your family history, your medical history, your childhood exposures, your current medications, your current lifestyle, your nutritional needs, the results of your genetic and medical tests, and other factors?

In the spirit of personalization, I've crafted a plan designed for you in this chapter—a protocol to guide you—but understand that these are suggestions, not commandments. Tailor this protocol to what works and what doesn't *for you*.

How will you know what that is?

You know yourself better than anyone else. Better than your doctor, better than your mom, better than your well-meaning partner who's been trying to get you to change for all these years.

Follow the steps that make you feel better; throw out the ones that don't.

Are you ready to trust yourself and *your* approach the most? If so, read on.

Dr. Paul's 13-Point Plan for Leading Your Best Life

My 13-Point Addiction Recovery Plan is based in integrative medicine, developed from the strategies and practices I've found to be most effective at my addiction clinic and in my own recovery as well. I've tailored these points to what works to get you started immediately and also what will help keep you sober over the course of your life.

I take your sobriety very seriously, and I know you do too. Treat this chapter as your lifeline. Flag the key pages. Get out your highlighter. Tear it out of this book and keep it in your back pocket if you need to. This is your start-to-finish, A-to-Z workbook for finally getting free from whatever addictive behavior or substance that has been keeping you tethered to a life you don't love. These thirteen points are the beginning of your new life. They are your brave new path forward.

1. Start with a laser-focused *Why*.

2. Commit to honesty—*rigorous* honesty.

3. Accept and feel your pain.

4. Begin counseling.

5. Treat drug dependence as naturally as possible, with the help of pharmaceuticals as needed.

6. Seek treatment for other underlying medical conditions.

7. Devise a comprehensive nutrition and supplement plan.

8. Heal your gut microbiome to heal your brain.

9. Devise a comprehensive sleep plan.

10. Begin a consistent exercise routine.

11. Make sure you have continued social support for safe living, healthy relationships, and good stress management.

12. Distance yourself from sobriety snatchers and dream killers (aka enablers).

13. Carry naloxone.

"What if I'm not ready? What if I fail (again)?"

Are you asking yourself these questions right now? Are you sick and tired of failing to conquer your addiction?

I know what that felt like. It was horrible. But I'm here to tell you that you can break free of your own self-doubt and self-criticism. It doesn't matter how many times you may have already tried and failed. It doesn't matter what anyone else may say or think about your struggles. It doesn't even matter if you've given up on yourself a thousand times already.

You can and should draw a line in the sand and start over. You can try again. Reject bondage and embrace this journey toward freedom. Every attempt brings you one step closer to your sobriety, one step closer to your new life of glowing good health and meaningful relationships.

It's okay to fail. The only thing that's not okay is not to try.

Will it be easy?

No.

Is anything worthwhile really easy?

Probably not.

Will it be worth it?

Absolutely.

Point 1. Start with a Laser-Focused *Why*

Why did you attend that AA meeting, rehab program, or support group? Why are you reading this book? On the intake forms in my clinic we ask you to rate your willingness to change on a scale from zero to ten. Zero is none. You don't want to, you don't plan to, and you're only here because the courts or someone (your parent, spouse, child) is making you. You're in despair, lack motivation, and have no intention of kicking your habit. Ten is beyond ready: you're doing this no matter what and I couldn't stop you if I tried.

Let's see where you stand.

Circle the number that corresponds to your willingness to change and get sober:

0   1   2   3   4   5   6   7   8   9   10

Here's the best part. The number you circled actually doesn't matter. If you're sitting across from me and we're talking about how my plan can help you, I know that you can do this. I won't base your ability to succeed on your willingness in this moment. My new patients often come in raw, desperate, and hopeless, testing positive for every known drug on the planet, without any apparent support system in place and with little commitment to change. Everything seems to be working against them. And then something spectacular happens—they make it successfully into recovery. Like Michael, whose story I shared in chapter 4. Seeing this kind of transformation makes a believer and an optimist out of anyone.

Both my sponsors in AA were suicidal, looking for a jumping-off place, before they sought treatment. My first put a gun in his mouth and pulled the trigger. This was the only time in his life when a gun had misfired. "It wasn't my time," he says.

Recovery is not going to happen overnight, but when you're motivated, you can and will stop your use, even when the addiction seems insurmountable. It's not about willpower, it's about having a *Why* so big and so important that you're willing to do the work.

I'll be honest about something you know already if you've tried and failed to kick your habit. Withdrawal feels like being run over by a truck. You're peeing out the wrong hole. You have the shakes and sweats so bad you know you're going to die before the night is over. You want a drink or to use so desperately you can already taste it. You decide with certainty that suicide is a better option than sobriety. It's easy to say but hard to believe when it's happening to you, but you will get through the withdrawal. **You will get better. Every day is a new start. One day at a time.**

Modern medicine has techniques to help you survive the acute phase of drug or alcohol withdrawal and mitigate some of the symptoms. But you can have access to all of the best medicines and tools to help you recover, yet without your *Why* it's very hard to succeed. So let's find your individual *Why* right now.

It's as simple as answering this one question: **Why do you want to stop?**

Maybe it's because you love your spouse and want to stop hurting her. Maybe you've remembered the joy of calculus and you realize you want to become a math teacher to share that joy with others. Maybe your new granddaughter was born last week, and your son has made it clear that you can't be part of her life until you've been sober for a year. Maybe you're ready to face your past and make amends because you have a birthday coming up and you are ready for a life change. Or maybe it's because you'll lose everything if you don't quit now. You know that if you don't stop, you will overdose or drink yourself to death. Fear will often get you started, but realize that once you start feeling better, fear alone will not be enough. Expand your *Why* so big that it keeps pulling you toward freedom, even when the going gets tough.

Write the short version of your *Why* on an index card and put it on the mirror in your bathroom where you brush your teeth every morning and evening. Set your *Why* as an alert on your smartphone, so that you are reminded of it at the same time every day. Write it on sticky notes posted at your desk at work, in your kitchen at home, and on the dashboard of your car.

If you're a visually minded person, draw your *Why*. You can put it on a poster board, add cut-out pictures from magazines, photos of your loved ones, and inspiring quotes to imagine your future the way you wish it to be. Your vision board can be a fun project that you do over weeks or months or it can be a scrawled drawing that you whip up in an hour. You decide. Your *Why* is personal, and you get to do it your way. When it's completed, put it somewhere you can see it every day.

Every time you see your *Why*, you will remember again why you want to move toward your goal of freedom and sobriety.

Point 2. Commit to Honesty—*Rigorous* Honesty

Your secrets keep you sick. As you are moving toward the severe end of the addiction spectrum but before you get help, the last thing you want is for others to know how far gone you are. You feel it is "best" to ignore the problem. You may secretly know you're being dishonest, but you deny that you're addicted. Your addicted brain justifies itself. **It is only when you are ready to be honest—with yourself and with others—that you really start to heal.**

We are as sick as our secrets.

No one tells the truth about everything. If someone tells you he is always honest, you have caught him in a lie. You're late to a meeting and get stuck in traffic, so you tell your boss it was the traffic, not your late start. You weren't exactly lying, but you also weren't telling the truth. That's not the rigorous honesty I'm talking about. I'm talking about the big secrets that keep you in bondage.

So you must decide to be honest about your drug or alcohol use or your nonsubstance addiction, even though you may feel great shame. Find one compassionate person who you know won't judge you—your counselor, pastor, friend, parent, sponsor—and tell that person the truth. A weight will lift off your shoulders as you share. Keeping secrets sabotages your recovery physically, mentally, and spiritually. Lying is a habit that harms you. Honesty can become a habit as well, a good habit that helps you heal.

Honesty exercise: Write your deepest, darkest secrets—the ones you never want to tell anybody—on a piece of paper. It may be one sentence or it may be five pages. Write as much as you need. Then take that paper and light a match to it. (Do this in a safe place.) Collect the ashes. Go outside, perhaps somewhere in nature where you feel happy, and let the ashes go. As you watch them float away in the wind, tell yourself: "I am ready to be honest with myself. I am ready to let go of my secrets. I am ready to be loved and safe."

Josh, whom I told you about in chapter 5, had amphetamines show up intermittently in his urine drug screens, which he told me were from brief relapses. Then came the confession: he had been secretly abusing prescription amphetamines while I was treating him, grinding them into powder and snorting them up his nose, getting multiple prescriptions from other doctors and also meds from his girlfriend. He had been doing this for years, but never told anyone. And I had been considering prescribing him a stimulant for his struggles to stay focused!

Josh's honesty with me that day helped catapult his recovery into a whole new dimension. It was as if a switch had been flipped. Confidence in his life and himself replaced his fear and hesitancy.

That will happen for you too. So get honest with yourself, your doctor, and your recovery team. Honesty isn't easy, but it is necessary for lasting recovery.

Doctors ask you all kinds of personal questions and expect you to answer honestly on medical intake forms. Have you ever had a vene-real disease? How many sexual partners have you had? Has your use of drugs or alcohol led to consequences? Doctors use this information to tally data and assess the severity of your health issues, but how do we know that the information is true? Most of the time it isn't, as I mentioned earlier. It's hard enough for you to be honest with yourself, let alone on an impersonal piece of paper that a clerk behind the glass at the doctor's office handed you. Right?

If you've lied on intake forms, you're not alone. Though I'd rather you didn't, that's not the kind of honesty I'm talking about. I'm talking about being honest with yourself, honest with the people you love, and honest with the doctor who is sitting across from you, face-to-face, person to person.

There are probably some very good reasons why you're not in the habit of being honest. As a child, your innate honesty and wonder may have been met with sarcasm, ridicule, or even abuse. As an adult, you may feel shame about the things you've done. So much shame. The kind of shame that makes you want to take a pencil and erase, erase, erase. Only you know you can't.

We've all been there. I cringe remembering some of the things I wish never happened.

How do you develop a lifestyle of honesty and openness when you've had to keep yourself safe all these years with lies and deceit? Do you even want to come out as an addict in this digitally connected world where the media and the people in our lives—from family to public officials—all seem to treat honesty as optional? We see people in power lie and distort facts on a daily basis. Is it any wonder those struggling with addiction have trouble with honesty?

Who wants to admit to having a problem?

Who wants to admit to drinking or using again or too much?

Who wants to admit to stealing money for drugs, cheating on a spouse in an alcohol-infused haze, obsessing over porn, or blacking out?

Who wants to admit to lying about where we're going or who we're with?

Who wants to admit to all sorts of things we do when we are drinking or using drugs?

Just like driving a car or riding a bike, honesty is a skill that has to be learned. If you've been hit by a car while you were riding your bicycle, it's hard to get back on. It's a scary proposition—to be honest—and it takes time to cultivate.

Be honest. Be direct. Before you go in for any surgery or medical procedure, any time you meet a new medical provider, every time you start a medical file, tell your doctor you're an addict or an alcoholic. Don't hide the addict part of yourself in a misguided attempt to pretend you're someone you're not. Your ongoing sobriety is more important than anyone's opinion of you.

What if you see pity or judgment in their eyes? It doesn't matter! It doesn't matter if your doctor, neighbor, best friend, child's teacher, garbage collector, or anyone else looks down on you. It just means you are smarter and more self-aware than they are.

Know you're as good as anyone else, as capable, as compassionate, and as worthy of being loved.

Make a commitment to honesty. Remember, also, to listen to others without judgment. As we accept others, we learn to accept ourselves.

Point 3. Accept and Feel Your Pain

When my son Noah was given that shot of naltrexone to help him quit drinking, as I mentioned in chapter 6, he was catapulted into a depression that lasted over a year. Not a large man to begin with, Noah lost almost 30 pounds. That was one of the worst and most terrifying times in my life. "It was like being in a tiny sweltering room with no windows," Noah told me later. "You can't breathe, and they're slowly sucking out the oxygen." Noah's pain was unrelenting.

This is the addict's dilemma: you use a substance or behavior to self-medicate as a reprieve from pain, both physical and emotional. You turn to drugs as a relief from the depression, anxiety, or loneliness you feel when you're sober—whether you're aware that's what you're doing or not. When you try to stop, the withdrawal symptoms feel like the pain you've been trying so hard to avoid all your life. So you start again. This becomes a self-fulfilling, never-ending cycle that keeps you in bondage, no matter how hard you try to rationalize it or deny your addiction.

Getting off drugs requires a change in our mindset about pain.

It's okay to feel pain. The goal of sobriety is not to stop feeling. On the contrary, sobriety is about feeling the pain—because feeling pain is part of being human—without needing mind-altering and mind-destroying substances and behaviors to get through it. I often tell my patients, **"When you start feeling pain, you know you're doing something right."** I know it's hard, but I invite you during this point of recovery to acknowledge your pain. When you feel it, stop for a moment and breathe. Pay attention. Tell yourself that you are feeling pain and that that's okay; it's part of the recovery process.

Physical pain is information: As I talked about in chapter 4, physical bodily pain is information. It's your body's way of telling you that you are off balance and that you need to recalibrate. If my back starts to hurt, I need to change my position, lie on the floor with my knees bent, or take a walk. In my case that back pain is related to an old injury that is aggravated when I sit for hours at a time at the computer. When I listen to my body, I can heal my back and be healthier at the same time, since walking will also help me clear my head, oxygenate my blood, and lift my mood.

"That sounds easy for fleeting pain, Doc, but what about for chronic pain?" Once you start implementing the lifestyle changes in this chapter and throughout this book, you will find that you have fewer aches and pains, more energy, and a bounce to your step. If you are still in chronic pain after changing your eating habits, beginning an exercise regimen, healing your gut, and getting rid of toxic exposures, that pain is very important information—information that you need to delve into even deeper to find the root causes, so you can address them and relieve the pain. This pain is not in your head, and it does not need opioids or alcohol to remedy it. An experienced integrative or functional medical doctor will help you find and treat the underlying causes.

Emotional pain is also information: If you are struggling with emotional pain, anxiety attacks, or constant feelings of dread or panic, your psyche is telling you something. It may be that you have unresolved issues from your childhood, that you are unsafe in your current relationships or home life, that you're feeling financial insecurity, or that the problems your friends or family are having are overwhelming. It may simply be that you're having a really, really bad day. Some of your emotional pain may also be a result of nutritional deficiencies or toxic exposures. Acknowledge this pain instead of pretending it isn't there.

Put your hand on your heart (skin to skin), close your eyes, and take five long deep breaths. Pay attention to the inhale followed by the exhale. Focus entirely on your breathing—the sound of it and how it feels as the oxygen fills your lungs. Tell yourself quietly, "This breath I breathe in. This breath I breathe out." You can whisper, chant, or sing these words aloud if it helps. If your mind is spinning as you do this, acknowledge the mind spin, say hello to it, and then go back to your breath. Remember that the pain is not a sign that you need to find relief through drugs or behaviors. It is a sign that you are a human being living a full human experience. Right now is hard. Today is hard. Tomorrow will be better.

You may never be perfect, you may never be 100 percent pain-free, but you can learn to manage the pain in your body and your psyche in healthy ways. You can live in this messy, miserable, sometimes devastating and disappointing world without sleepwalking through your own life courtesy of your addiction.

"Doc, you don't understand. My pain is real," new patients say to me all the time. Whatever the cause—whether the pain is because of a serious injury, a series of complicated surgeries, or severe psychological or emotional trauma—what I say to them is this: "Yes, your pain is real! And pain sucks. But, ironically, **when we allow ourselves to feel pain, we allow ourselves to live.**"

Each and every time, as I mentioned in chapter 4, these same patients are amazed to find their pain *improves* as I help them taper off the opioids. In the case of opioids in particular, but perhaps with other addictions that stimulate various "feel good" receptors and neurotransmitters in our brains, the more we stimulate these receptors and chemicals, the more the receptors are activated. As you wean off your opioids, your pain receptors become less active and you *actually* feel less pain.

Life is not a straight line of always feeling amazing, always being happy, always doing things right. Life is not bouncing from one pleasurable experience to another. Life has peaks and valleys, ups and downs, times of great joy and times of great sorrow, good health and terrible pain. In recovery we cry a lot.

You are now in a safe place. Let yourself feel. Go ahead and cry. Cry for all the times that you could not defend yourself or protect yourself when you were a small child. Cry for all the times the people you loved the most failed you. None of this is your fault. You didn't ask to be born. You were never supposed to have to protect yourself. But you now can be the one who protects that little boy or girl who was not protected when you were small. You are safe now.

Cry because you just can't go on alone. Cry because you've been so lonely. You are surrounded and held by love. If you need to sit on the floor just to feel grounded, sit on the floor. I'm sitting right there with you. Feel the hand of someone you trust touching your shoulder and a voice gently saying, "I'm here with you. It is going to be okay. You're safe now," and keep crying if you need to. You can let that pain out. You don't have to keep it bottled up inside any longer.

In recovery we say, "You get to feel." For too long we've been numbed out. Set your sights on a realistic goal. You're not trying to be happy all the time. You're not trying to never make mistakes. Heck, you're not even trying not to relapse. You're just trying to be free from mind-altering, consciousness-sucking, two-faced, lying, physically devastating drugs for this moment, this day.

Your pain to-do list: Maybe breathing isn't enough. Maybe letting yourself cry or screaming into your pillow isn't enough either. When you're in too much pain—either physical or emotional—here is your to-do list. Before you hit the streets in search of a fix or a liquor store, promise me you'll try these things first:

1. **Take a hot shower or bath:** In the business we call this "hydrotherapy." A shower, as hot as you can stand, can work wonders for both emotional and physical pain.

2. **Stretch:** If a specific part of your body hurts, try stretching it out along with all the tight muscles surrounding it. If your psyche is bothering you, stretching your muscles will help that too. Put your hands above your head as high as they will go, stretch one and then the other to the sky, and then let them both drop. Then do this again. Repeat ten times or as many times as the number of years you've been alive. Then bend your knees softly, let your hands dangle, and try to touch your toes. Slowly roll up. Repeat this five times. Then stretch out your hips. Show off a few dance moves. While you are at it, circle your hips one way three times and then the other way three times.

3. **Breathe:** You've had a shower, you've stretched, and now it's time to sit quietly and pay attention to your breathing. Breathe in healing, breathe out hurt. The serenity verse really helps here, especially if you are having trouble quieting your mind: "Please grant me the serenity to accept the things I cannot change, the courage to change the things I can change, and the wisdom to know the difference." If you're too panicky or in too much pain to breathe and quietly say this verse, write it on a piece of paper or type it into your phone.

4. **Talk to a friend:** Always call a friend, a family member, your therapist, or even a hotline when you are in pain and craving your drug of choice. Sharing your pain in an honest way with a friend, loved one, or professional won't make it go away, but will make you feel lighter and more connected.

5. **Go outside:** In Japan there is a tradition called "forest bathing," which is a cornerstone of preventative health.[1] Spending time in nature, especially under the canopy of a living forest, can be profoundly calming and rejuvenating. If you live in a concrete jungle, this won't be something you can do every day, but try to get outside in nature at least once a week.

6. **Get a pet:** A dog will get you up and moving and help you find the time to be outside. A cat can be a cozy companion to sit with you and help you feel less alone. Pets provide us with nonjudgmental companionship that helps alleviate our pain.

7. **Rewrite your story:** Maiya has been learning to rewrite her story, and she has found it profoundly healing. Remind yourself that your thoughts are just thoughts; they're not real. Accept yourself just the way you are. Tell yourself you are beautifully imperfect, and everything is okay. Ask your loved ones to remind you that you are safe and loved, that you have everything you need.

Point 4. Begin Counseling

Being human means our brains thrive on physical and emotional connections with others. We want to be part of something, we want to be useful, we want to belong. For all of prehistory and much of early history, we connected by being part of a tribe—hunting together, gathering food and firewood, building shelters, fleeing danger, caring for each other's children. In today's world we have farmers we don't know growing our food, modern appliances doing our housework, and no immediate threats to our survival. So we have to find other ways to connect, be useful to each other, and create meaning in our lives.

Taking drugs with friends, or "partying," may seem selfish and self-indulgent from the outside, but it is actually a way that we seek purpose, togetherness, and connection. The decision to go to the party where you know there will be drinking and drugs is often far less intimidating than the loneliness and isolation you might feel staying at home. You can't stop using without filling the void that will be left in your life when you finally say, "No more," as I've been telling you in nearly every chapter of this book.

At their heart, group meetings are about helping you connect to other people. Individual counseling gives you connection too, allowing you to work on those things that may be too personal or too painful to address in a more public space. Many of you, both men and women, have suffered sexual and emotional abuse, often as children. These experiences were too painful to process, so you blotted them out with drugs and alcohol. This is where a skilled counselor will really help.

One of the advantages of going to a treatment center, whether it is day treatment or inpatient, is that there are intensive counseling, group therapy sessions, and meetings on-site. You get all these vital services provided as part of your program.

Once you reenter the "real" world after treatment, you need to continue self-care. The most important aspect of this self-care beyond good nutrition, adequate sleep, and not drinking or using drugs is your **continued program of counseling and meetings**. There are dozens of groups (including Alcoholics Anonymous, Narcotics Anonymous, Overeaters Anonymous, Sex Addicts Anonymous, Gamblers Anonymous, Cocaine Anonymous, and Crystal Meth Anonymous) and self-help programs (like SMART Recovery, Women for Sobriety, Secular Organizations for Sobriety, LifeRing Secular Recovery, and more). Most of us who manage not to relapse continue seeing a therapist for years or even decades. Many of us also go to 12-step or other group meetings to support our ongoing recovery. If you feel triggered or stressed—or start to crave drugs—your first response should be to call your counselor, sponsor, or friend or get to a meeting.

A good counselor is someone who can also help guide you toward healthy, productive, satisfying activities to replace your self-destructive ways of "having fun." Try to go to both individual therapy and an emotional support group.

A note about AA: There are a lot of different paths to getting sober. Alcoholics Anonymous doesn't work for everyone. But when it does work, it works well. Regardless of what the meeting is called or what organization is hosting it, if it feels safe, if you can identify with the stories being shared, if you leave feeling better than when you came (and you don't head instantly for the bar or a drug dealer), you have found your tribe.

Remember to always listen for the similarities when someone shares, instead of focusing on the differences. Everyone experiences despair, loneliness, isolation, and self-loathing, though we may experience them in different ways. Everyone is battling their cravings and trying to accomplish the seemingly impossible task of not just stopping abusing drugs or alcohol but staying sober.

Instant AA

Perhaps you live in a place where Alcoholics Anonymous meetings are difficult to find or you aren't sure going to AA or another 12-step program is right for you at this time. Or perhaps you've gone to meetings before and it didn't work. You're an atheist and you can't stomach the God talk, or you feel you just don't have time. There are a million reasons why addicts don't attend meetings.

It is no exaggeration for me to say that AA saved my life. I hope you'll find the courage and energy to get to a meeting. These days there are even meetings available online. Shut this book, find the nearest meeting, and attend it right now. Here's a sense of what those meetings will offer you, adapted from AA's 12 Steps. This is the distilled version, and I present it to you with as little religious talk as possible, as I know that aspect of AA can be difficult for some recovering addicts and alcoholics to relate to.

1. **We've all been where you are now.** The first step in AA is to learn to acknowledge that we indulged until we had lost the option of

choice. This is a *we* thing. We are unable to stop, and our lives have become unmanageable.

2. **You are not alone.** This step teaches you to envision a power greater than yourself.

3. **There is a higher purpose in your life.** Even though you may not be in touch with the higher purpose yet, you make a decision to be open to its being revealed to you. One of the real blessings of the 12-step programs is the concept of giving our will over to a Maker as you understand that word (it can be God, the universe, the Buddha, Mother Nature—whatever you choose). That Higher Power loves you unconditionally and helps give you the power to stay sober.

4. **Now is the time to do self-searching.** Where did I go wrong? When was I selfish and self-centered? When have I been resentful or fearful, self-seeking, dishonest, or unkind? Like a business taking inventory, you list your assets and your liabilities. This process requires the rigorous honesty I was talking about earlier. Put to paper your fears, resentments, mistakes, and all those things that you feel are preventing you from moving forward in your life.

5. **Share the results of your self-searching.** It's only when we actually admit to ourselves and to someone else the exact nature of our wrongs that we can release them. You share your self-inventory, which includes your moral failings, with your sponsor, counselor, or cleric. Some of us may be sharing stories of crimes or other situations that would be self-incriminating. This is why this process should only happen with someone sworn to maintain confidentiality.

6. **Get ready to have your defects of character removed.** There is no one right way. The path you are on is right where you need to be. This step helps you be emotionally prepared for change.

7. **Ask your Higher Power to remove your shortcomings.** This step is your opportunity to loosen the grip that some of your shortcomings might have on you. If you have access to a beach, go at low tide and write your shortcomings out in the sand. Wait and watch as the power of the ocean washes away each defect. Or you can write your

character defects on a piece of paper and tear it into tiny pieces. It helps to have a visual of letting go.

8. **List the people you have harmed and become willing to make amends.** Refer to your self-searching list of assets and liabilities as you think about the loved ones you may have disappointed in your struggle with addiction.

9. **Make amends.** Where possible, make amends, but not if doing so would cause anybody harm. I would advise you to consult with your mentor, sponsor, or counselor at this point of your journey. There is an amazing freedom and sense of peace that comes from apologizing to the people you have hurt. You can only control your part in this process; expect nothing in return.

10. **Continue to take inventory of yourself, admit when you are wrong, and do what you can to make it right.** Just because you're recovering doesn't mean you won't make more mistakes. Commit now to being humble and honest.

11. **Work to get out of self and self-centered living, being open to Good Orderly Direction.** Meditation, breathing, and prayer (if you are religious) can help with this step.

12. **Help others who are in the struggle, and continue this new way of honest living in everything you do.** AA teaches that when you help others, you are actually securing your own sobriety.

There is no either-or in my way of conquering addiction. Mine is a both-and approach. As you continue to read my integrative medicine 13-point recovery plan below, you'll realize that it complements and supports the process outlined above. Because we are living in a toxic and disconnected world, AA strategies may not be enough to reverse the course of addiction in this country.

I encourage you to integrate lasting lifestyle changes that will safeguard your health and protect you against relapse. I still attend 12-step meetings, and I also follow the plan I recommend for you in this book.

Point 5. Treat Drug Dependence as Naturally as Possible, with the Help of Pharmaceuticals as Needed

If you come to my addiction clinic, we work toward tapering off opioids slowly with the help of buprenorphine, personalizing the dose to your level of dependence. At the beginning I see you weekly, until you're doing well enough to start coming monthly. This means finding the right maintenance dose—so you can lead a productive, happy life. As I talked about in chapter 4, in my experience tapering down with buprenorphine is a more effective solution to opioid addiction than going cold turkey. Although cold turkey works short-term to get patients detoxed off opioids, it sometimes sets patients up for painful—even fatal—relapse. Physical cravings can last months or even years depending on how long you were using in the first place, your brain's susceptibility to drugs, and how many triggers you're exposed to as you navigate your daily life. For severe opioid dependence, a slow-taper approach can literally save your life.

At the same time, if you are addicted to opioids, it is imperative to find other nonpharmaceutical treatments to help with your underlying pain, as I also talked about in chapter 4. Alcoholics and drug addicts alike need to find *healthy* ways to have fun, feel connected, and feel excited. Get high, yes! But get high in ways that don't destroy your brain, body, and pocketbook; compromise your family life; alienate your loved ones; or disconnect you from the real world.

If you realize that your addiction started partly because of your need for adrenaline, like Josh, take up rock climbing (an activity you can do inexpensively if you join a group of enthusiasts), horseback riding, paragliding, parkour, or even skydiving. If part of your challenge was brain spin and brain fog, as it was for me, take a meditation class and start doing yoga daily to learn to quiet your brain. Go to trivia night, enroll in a community college course on the anatomy of the brain, or seek out other educational opportunities to feed your brain's curiosity. Get totally immersed in exercise by joining a CrossFit gym or some other group fitness activity to oxygenate your brain.

If you were in pain all the time partly because you were overloaded with toxic exposures that led to chronic inflammation, ridding your home and diet of unhealthy products and food will be a huge step to helping you get back on your feet. The harmful chemicals in plastics, pesticides, herbicides, and pharmaceutical products that all of us are constantly being exposed to (this long list includes parabens, flame retardants, dioxin, glyphosate, thimerosal, formaldehyde, and polysorbate-80, to name just a few) can disrupt your body and your brain. The off-gassing from new appliances, cars, furniture, and paint (yes that "new" smell that some people like so much) is also more toxic and damaging to your health than you might think.

To tame these toxins, I recommend you get a water-filtration system. I installed a reverse-osmosis charcoal-filtration system under the kitchen sink, so our drinking and cooking water would be free of harmful chemicals and residues. Attaching a charcoal filter to the faucet or even just using a pitcher with a charcoal filter is also a good, more affordable step. If indoor air quality is an issue (which it is for most of us), it is worth using a HEPA air filter, at least for your bedroom. Next time you buy a mattress, opt for an organic cotton or wool futon or at least a mattress that is flame retardant–free. Try to have furniture in your home or apartment that has been previously loved, so it is not off-gassing harmful volatile organic compounds like formaldehyde. Choose glass over plastic whenever possible.

Like everything with addiction, this is a process of awakening, understanding, and striving to do your best. Tapering off opioids, switching from harmful substance abuse to healthy activities, and swapping the toxins you're exposed to for more natural, less-toxic products allows you to find your feet and move forward.

Point 6. Seek Treatment for Other Underlying Medical Conditions

The majority of my patients have some underlying mental-health conditions in addition to addiction. Most common are anxiety and depression, ADD/ADHD, obsessive-compulsive disorders, and bipolar affective disorder.

You've probably been labeled by a psychiatrist (if you've seen one) or your general practitioner. This label guides doctors on what medications have been approved to treat the disease and gives us a way to understand your suffering. Fair enough. And yes, there are genetic and physical biochemical reasons for why you have struggled your whole life. But there is no blood test for depression, anxiety, ADD, ADHD, bipolar affective disorder, or schizophrenia. And I'm ultimately much more interested in helping you find the root cause of your psychiatric disorder than stamping you with a label.

While we pursue integrative medicine approaches to find and resolve the root causes of your anxiety, depression, or ADHD, we can also treat your symptoms. Talk to your addiction doctor about the options: SSRIs (selective serotonin reuptake inhibitors), ADHD medications, Wellbutrin, gabapentin, clonidine, and other pharmaceutical treatments for your brain struggles. My colleague psychiatrist Kelly Brogan is convinced these medications do more harm than good, an argument she convincingly makes in her book, *A Mind of Your Own*. Although I agree with her in principle and I would urge every patient to begin with natural healing, I have also seen how small doses of certain pharmaceuticals can help.

Explain to your doctor that you want to use the *lowest* dose of the fewest medications, and you want to be prescribed the safest medication that has the fewest side effects. Lithium, a simple salt, used to be used at a minimum dose of 300 mg. twice a day for the treatment of bipolar (manic-depressive) disorder. I have found that for some a dose of 10 to 30 mg. once or twice a day can be very effective. These days you can walk into any natural-food store and buy lithium pills. They may take about two to three weeks to work, so give yourself time.

If you're not sure your prescribed medication is helping, or if you notice that a medication you're taking was helping but has lost its efficacy, slowly wean yourself off it over two to three months, preferably under the supervision of a doctor.

When you start your recovery journey, an addiction doctor will probably order tests. These include HIV, hepatitis B, hepatitis C, complete blood count (CBC), comprehensive metabolic panel (CMP), thyroid-stimulating hormone (TSH), and other thyroid function tests. We also usually check for other sexually transmitted diseases, including syphilis, chlamydia, and gonorrhea. In the severely fatigued or ill patient, we might also check Epstein-Barr virus (EBV) and Lyme titers, erythrocyte sedimentation rate (ESR), C-reactive protein (CRP), and serum B_{12} and folate as well as vitamin D. There might be the need for a blood culture if you have an infection, usually indicated by a fever, and occasionally a brain scan if you've had seizures or head trauma.

Down the road we might also test for adrenal dysfunction, testosterone and other hormone levels, food sensitivities, neurotransmitters and genetic testing, and evidence of exposure to toxins. This is integrative and functional medicine at its finest. Work with an experienced clinician to personalize your plan.

Point 7. Devise a Comprehensive Nutrition and Supplement Plan

Now let's get real here. I know I've been telling you this over and over, but I also know that most of you struggling with addiction can barely find money for rent, if you even have a place to live. Your life is so disorganized that a discussion of ideal eating habits and exercise regimens seems a little pie-in-the-sky. That said, good nutrition is a goal to move toward. The further along you are in recovery, the easier it becomes. Baby steps for some. Giant steps for others. Even if you do a little, that's better than nothing. Agreed?

Nutrition matters. It really does. If you're anemic, you may be feeling extremely tired, to the point of despair. One of my patients, Elizabeth, a thirty-seven-year-old mom of two, was severely anemic but didn't know it. Elizabeth started self-medicating with stimulants just to make it through the day. After just two IV iron infusions her energy returned, and she was on the road to recovery. When another patient, Alisha, went on an iron-rich diet, it was like night and day. After being a strict vegetarian, she started eating meat again—just 2 ounces of high-quality red meat three times a week—and added lots of leafy greens and citrus (which helps your body absorb iron more effectively) to her daily diet. She also made a point of eating a lentil and bean soup, sometimes with sausage, always with kale and spinach and garlic, once a week. These nourishing foods improved her energy levels and got her recovery back online.

When you are ready, **keep a food journal for one week**. It may be quite an eye-opener to see that you have been surviving full-time on sugar, starch, and unhealthy fat. Cooking? What's that?

Supplementation, food recommendations, and dietary changes based on the results of the medical testing? This will sound very familiar if you already follow integrative medicine, but much of it will be brand new if you are used to advice from conventional mainstream doctors. The importance of a whole-food, real-food, anti-inflammatory diet cannot be overstated when it comes to healing addiction from the inside out.

Addiction-Related Nutritional Deficits

Years of poor food choices can hinder your ability to absorb nutrients, resulting in a host of nutrient deficiencies. The most common include the fat-soluble vitamins A, D, E, and K; B vitamins; vitamin C; and the micronutrients magnesium and zinc.

Chronic alcoholics are often deficient in B_1 (thiamine), which in severe cases can lead to a rare and dangerous brain condition called Wernicke's encephalopathy, which causes confusion, unsteady gait, and nystagmus (a condition where the eyes move back and forth). A B_{12} deficiency is also common in addicts, as is anemia.

Your whole-food diet to reverse these nutritional deficits must include lots of green leafy vegetables (so eat them at every meal—even for breakfast!), colored fruits and vegetables (eat the rainbow), and a variety of fish, meats, nuts, seeds, and eggs. As we've already mentioned at least five hundred times, a vitamin D deficiency is common to us indoor Americans, especially if you avoid the sun or live in areas where sun is limited. The farther from the equator you live, the less sunlight actually reaches your skin. Depending on the results of your testing, chances are you will need to take:

B-complex

Calcium-magnesium

Fish oil or other source of omega-3 fatty acids (2,000 mg.)

Probiotics (to promote healthy bacteria and gut healing)

Vitamin C

Vitamin D_3 with K_2 (which helps calcium absorption)

Zinc

Add to these a varied, interesting, delicious diet of real food, and you will be amazed at how much better you will feel.

Food sensitivities and undiagnosed food allergies may also be making you sick. I encourage you to have a BioTek IgG Antibody Assessment, or similar lab testing, to test for food sensitivities, which you can expect to cost around $159. You can also be tested for nutrient deficiencies using the SpectraCell Micronutrient Test Panel or another company's, which will cost around $300. This testing is not regarded as "valid" by mainstream medical doctors, but my integrative colleagues and I find it very helpful in guiding nutrition recommendations. You will too. How your body responds to your improved diet is the litmus test, not a skeptical medical doctor.

Food sensitivities used to be rare. But during the past decade, extensive glyphosate and other pesticide and herbicide use on commercial crops, the overuse of antibiotics, and the toxins we're exposed to from a more aggressive childhood and adult vaccination schedule than we've ever had before have resulted in some degree of leaky gut for most of us. Glyphosate is known to disrupt the gut barrier, allowing undigested foods to seep into our bloodstream and interact with our immune system in a way that forces our body to mount an immune response against food itself.[2] Our leaky gut turns food into the equivalent of an invading bacteria or virus. We are not supposed to have immunoglobulin G antibodies against food, yet we do.

In my pediatric practice and my addiction clinic over 50 percent of my patients who struggle with brain problems (depression, anxiety, ADD, ADHD, autism-spectrum disorders, fatigue, and addiction) have significant food sensitivities. The most common by far are sensitivities to gluten, dairy, eggs, and nuts (especially peanuts), in that order.

So what happens if you cut out these foods completely from your diet? Though this will not work for everyone, often you actually can feel the difference in your brain and in your body. No longer needing to fight foreign invaders, your brain becomes more focused, you have less fog and better concentration, and you feel less sluggish. I have even seen nonverbal children with autism start to speak in sentences a month or so after they changed their diets based on food-sensitivity testing.

Another confession: For years I was as skeptical about this as you may be right now and as dismissive as my mainstream colleagues that nutritional healing could have such a strong effect. But clinical evidence—brain-damaged children making what I was taught to believe were "impossible" recoveries—has convinced me that it works, although not for everyone. For some the benefits are subtler, but very real and well worth the sacrifice.

Food sensitivities are not usually permanent. When you remove the foods you are reacting to from your diet for several months and add natural fermented foods to your diet as well as a high-quality probiotic, you allow your gut lining to heal. Especially if you are able to remove other toxins from your life and start eating exclusively foods grown without toxic pesticides and herbicides, you should be able to slowly reintroduce these foods.

The exception is gluten sensitivity. Those sensitive to gluten are at risk for celiac disease and often cannot start eating gluten again without making themselves sick. You can be tested for celiac disease, but if you already know you have the tendency to be sensitive to gluten, a proactive approach is to stay away from it permanently.

Seven-Day Addiction Recovery Menu

Throughout this book I've been giving you advice about how to eat healthy and talking about the importance of eating real food. Just as we have to personalize medicine, we also have to personalize your diet. Since every one of us has different nutritional needs, beyond recommending a real-food, whole-food diet, I would rather not give you iron-clad rules about (cue deep authoritative voice here) *how you must eat.* Instead, I would like you to pay attention to what you are eating, how you are eating it, and how it is making you feel. I would rather see you enjoy eating and delight in food surrounded by family and friends than carefully measuring out only a quarter of a cup of nuts because that's what's on your protocol, eating them standing up at the kitchen sink, feeling miserable. Make sense?

What does healthy eating really look like meal by meal? Some doctors will tell you to avoid all processed grains, but the Japanese, who enjoy optimal weight and are some of the longest-lived people in the world, usually eat white rice two or even three times a day. For years doctors believed that a low-fat diet was healthier, and they pushed their patients to drink skim milk, eat low-fat yogurt, and avoid butter. Turns out they were wrong! We now have evidence that people who eat full-fat dairy tend to be thinner,[3] have a lower risk of developing adult-onset diabetes,[4] and may have fewer markers associated with heart disease.[5]

Should you avoid dairy products? If eating cheese makes you feel sluggish or drinking milk gives you a stomachache, probably yes. Or at least take a digestive enzyme or lactase before you eat dairy. But that really depends on you. What we do know, without a doubt, is the **less processed foods you eat, the healthier you will feel, the more energy you will have, and the stronger your immune system will be**. Avoiding processed sugar, eating organic (I know this is hard; it's expensive; do the best you can), and making sure your "snacks" are healthy, whole foods will benefit your brain and your body now and for the rest of your life.

When you first enter recovery, it's very hard, if not impossible, to think about what you're eating and even harder to start cooking meals for yourself. You can try this meal plan any time, now or when your addictive cravings have become less acute. You may be learning to cook for the first time, or you may be rediscovering something you once loved to do. Either way, here is an example of what seven days of healthy meals might look like when you're ready.

These are not fancy, elaborate meals that take hours to prepare, and you will find recipes for all of these meals with a quick internet search. You're in recovery. You don't have time to teach yourself to become a gourmet chef! Instead, I offer you simple, nutritious meals to support your body and your brain as you heal.

DAY 1

Breakfast: Scrambled eggs, baked sweet potato, rooibos chai tea or coffee, lemon water

Lunch: Tuna or salmon salad sandwich with or without whole-grain toast, carrot and cucumber sticks, apple slices

Snack: A handful of almonds and some water-packed olives

Dinner: Roasted basil-lemon chicken, steamed or sautéed broccoli, rice (preferably brown), forkful of sauerkraut or fermented veggies

DAY 2

Breakfast: Plain whole-fat organic yogurt (goat, cow, or coconut) with fruit and coconut flakes, green smoothie (see recipe on page 256)

Lunch: A large salad packed with your favorite raw veggies, topped with some leftover basil-lemon chicken or a hard-boiled egg

Snack: Raw organic green beans or sugar snap peas and a small handful of mixed nuts

Dinner: Fish (preferably wild-caught) with tomatoes and chickpeas, greens (collard, kale, spinach, or Swiss chard) sautéed or steamed with garlic, leftover rice or sweet potato with a dollop of whole-fat plain yogurt

DAY 3

Breakfast: Old-fashioned rolled or steel-cut oatmeal with a dollop of whole-fat plain yogurt and any healthy extras you feel like adding, like nuts or nut butter, seeds, and fresh fruit

Lunch: Grilled chicken and kale wrap with leftover chicken or fish, forkful of sauerkraut or kimchee, fresh fruit

Snack: Half an avocado sprinkled with sea salt, lemon or lime juice, or nutritional yeast

Dinner: Beans and greens, baked or sautéed grass-fed steak, baked yam, forkful of sauerkraut or fermented veggies

DAY 4

Breakfast: Eggs (scrambled, poached, fried, or however you like them), organic red bell pepper or other vegetable slices, orange quarters, forkful of sauerkraut

Lunch: Rice cakes topped with feta, tomatoes, and olives; cucumber salad; banana or other fruit

Snack: Walnuts with raisins, prunes, or dates

Dinner: Hearty lentil soup or vegetable stew, rice or mashed or baked potato, fruit salad or fresh fruit

DAY 5

Breakfast: Plain whole-fat organic yogurt with fresh mango, banana, and chia seeds, sprinkled with old-fashioned rolled oats

Lunch: A hearty salad

Snack: A handful of mixed nuts and dates

Dinner: Chicken or tofu Provençal, roasted Brussels sprouts, side salad

DAY 6

Breakfast: Scrambled eggs with vegetables and whole-grain or gluten-free toast, forkful of sauerkraut
Lunch: Leftover chicken or tofu Provençal
Snack: Carrot sticks and apple slices with lemon
Dinner: Vegetarian chili, corn bread, salad

DAY 7

Breakfast: Turkey sausages or ground turkey sautéed with garlic and vegetables, green smoothie
Lunch: Cheese melt with tomatoes, garlic, and spinach; leftover salad or a plate of sliced vegetables like cucumbers, carrots, broccoli, and red cabbage
Snack: Fresh or frozen blueberries, goji berries, and cashews
Dinner: Meat loaf (make yours packed with vegetables), roasted or steamed asparagus, forkful of sauerkraut or fermented veggies, fresh fruit

A note to new cooks: It's important to eat organic as much as you can, buy local fruits and vegetables, and have your fish be wild-caught rather than farm-raised, if possible. I know that's not always realistic, but do your best. You may have noticed there is no soda, juice, or processed foods like cookies, chips, or candy in this meal plan. If you're a vegetarian, substitute tofu or tempeh for the meat and add more beans, seeds, and nuts to get adequate protein. You can also substitute brown rice pasta, which is quite tasty, for rice. If you're having a craving for sweets, turn to fresh or frozen fruit for dessert. You may be in the habit of skipping breakfast. If you're getting adequate nutrients and prefer this way of eating, a long fast between dinner and your meal the next day can actually be helpful. Intermittent fasting has helped me lose weight and maintain optimal body fat.

Need a Snack? Reach for These

If you're hungry between meals or if you are too busy to cook, enjoy any of the foods listed below. These whole foods, unlike sugary treats and caffeinated beverages, won't spike and then lower your blood sugar, leaving you craving more sugar. Instead, they are whole foods that will give your body vital vitamins and minerals that help you have more energy and leave you feeling good all day.

Berries: bilberries, blackberries, blueberries, goji berries, raspberries, strawberries

Broccoli

Carrot sticks

Cherries

Coconut

Cucumber sticks

Dark chocolate

Dates

Green beans

Hard-boiled egg

Mango (preferably fresh)

Nori (Japanese seaweed)

Nuts: almonds, Brazil nuts, hazelnuts, macadamias, pistachios, walnuts

Olives

Oranges

Plain whole-fat yogurt

Prunes

Red cabbage

Sardines

Seeds: chia, hemp, pumpkin, sunflower, watermelon

Strawberries

Sugar snap peas

Tangerines

Green Smoothie

Makes: 2 servings
Time: Less than 10 minutes

It's great to get in the habit of drinking no-sugar-added smoothies and fresh vegetable juices. Smoothies are a quick and easy way to start your day with nutrient-dense energy-giving whole foods. All you need to make smoothies at home is a blender. *Pro tip:* As soon as you finish making the smoothie, fill the blender with water and pulse on high for quicker cleanup.

> **2 cups fresh organic mixed greens (experiment with spinach, baby kale, and arugula, whatever you like best)**
> **1 cup water**
> **1 cup coconut or other milk**
> **½ cup total frozen pineapple and/or mango chunks**
> **2 peeled frozen bananas, cut in chunks**
> **1 tablespoon honey or agave (optional)**

1. Wash the greens well so there is no grit. Add them with the liquid to your blender. Blend on high until liquefied.

2. Add frozen fruit and honey or agave, if desired, and blend until smooth. Serve immediately.

Point 8. Heal Your Gut Microbiome to Heal Your Brain

I've been talking about the importance of gut healing throughout this book. The more diversity of healthy bacteria present in your colon and intestinal tract, the less inflammation you are likely to have, both in your intestines and your brain. If you are not already eating fermented foods, it is time to start. I recommend you try eating probiotic plain yogurt, kefir, sauerkraut, fermented pickles, kimchee, or tempeh. You will also benefit from taking a probiotic supplement, generally one that contains lactobacillus and any number of bifidobacterium (bifidus) species.

Glutamine is an amino acid that helps prevent leaky gut and boosts the immune system. It will work hand in hand with your probiotics to heal your gut. Also try drinking 2 to 4 tablespoons of aloe vera juice, which you can add to your morning smoothie, once a day. The other lifestyle improvements you are making—eating real foods; removing additives, food dyes, and artificial sweeteners from your diet; reducing stress; and getting your daily exercise—will also promote lasting gut healing. Remember gut health is brain health.

Point 9. Devise a Comprehensive Sleep Plan

In Shona culture in Zimbabwe, where I grew up, our morning greeting to friends and family was *"Mangwanani. Mararahere?"* "Good morning. Did you sleep well?" It's a marvelous custom, to check in on one's sleep! The restorative power of sleep is vital for us all. Every adult has different sleep requirements, but most of us need between seven and nine hours of sleep a night. Teenagers need much more—up to twelve hours a night.

Our bodies and our brains need to sleep. Sleep is how our bodies naturally revitalize themselves. As I talked about in chapter 5, if you're addicted to certain drugs like meth, which can keep you awake for days, you experience the symptoms of your addiction tenfold because you are so sleep-deprived. But for those of us battling addiction, quality sleep is an often overlooked component of healing. Missed sleep and poor-quality sleep can compromise anyone's ability to fight disease, feel happy, and enjoy good health.

There are no two ways about it. In order to move away from the severe end of the addiction spectrum, you need to practice good sleep habits. You may be unwittingly sabotaging your sleep. A lot of my patients are compromising their sleep without knowing it.

Here are the best steps to getting a good night's sleep:

Always sleep in a darkened room. Purchase blackout curtains or shades. If you can't afford them, put black paper or dark towels over your windows to block out the light. Make sure all lights are off, unplug your watch, computer, and anything that emits light. If you're sharing space or cannot darken the room, wear an eye mask. Yes, those dorky masks can actually help. Put a pillow over your head as well, if that feels comfortable. Humans are diurnal animals—we want to be up during the day and asleep at night. If our indoor surroundings trick us into thinking it is daytime, we won't be able to sleep.

Always sleep in a quiet place. Sound insulation matters. Place rolled-up towels under the door, buy a carpet to absorb noise, and try sleeping with earplugs. Many people find they get much more restful sleep when they use an eye mask and earplugs. That said, some people find white noise to be comforting at night. If too much quiet makes you anxious, you can buy an inexpensive white-noise machine (just position it as far away from your bed as possible), or try running a small fan at night. The air purifiers I mentioned on page 186 can double as white-noise machines.

Don't drink or eat anything that contains caffeine after 2:00 p.m. I am actually amazed at how much caffeine some of my patients drink to keep themselves going during the day. And then they wonder why they can't sleep! Every person metabolizes caffeine differently, but most of us need between eight and twelve hours to get this stimulant out of our systems. So you should make a rule to not have *any* caffeinated coffee or tea, energy drinks or bars, or even chocolate after 2:00 or 3:00 p.m.

Create a sleep routine. Most of us need a wind-down time for the final hour or two before we fall asleep. This means turning off the computer, phone, and television (as I said above, these screens emit light that tricks our bodies into wakefulness) and having a bedtime ritual. Perhaps you talk to your mom, sister, or best friend for half an hour, then take a warm bath with Epsom salts and a drop of lavender oil, read a book or magazine, or write a letter. This sounds like old-fashioned advice in the age of the internet, but a nightly screen-free ritual like this will help you sleep like a baby.

Don't exercise right before bed. Yes, do exercise. At least 45 minutes, preferably an hour or more a day, as I've been recommending throughout this book. But try to have all your exercise completed an hour or two before bedtime. Call Jennifer at midnight on any

LACK OF SLEEP CAN LEAD TO...

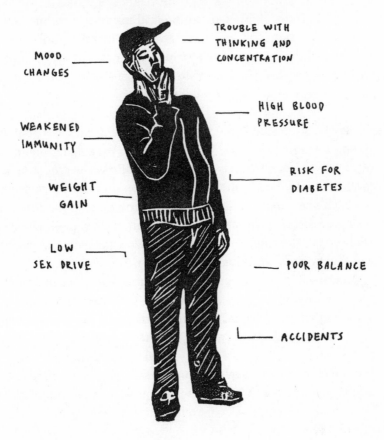

MOOD CHANGES

TROUBLE WITH THINKING AND CONCENTRATION

WEAKENED IMMUNITY

HIGH BLOOD PRESSURE

WEIGHT GAIN

RISK FOR DIABETES

LOW SEX DRIVE

POOR BALANCE

ACCIDENTS

nights her community soccer league plays 8:30 p.m. games and she'll explain more why.

Give yourself a bedtime and a wake-up time. Try to wake up at the same time each morning and go to bed the same time each night. I know our lives are hectic. Chaos is one hallmark of addiction. But the more we can create consistent routines, the better we will sleep. Once you are in that routine, do your best to stick to it. Even if you have a bad night, try to get up at your morning wake-up time. I'd rather you take a nap during the day than get off schedule.

Have a sleepy snack. Although it's not a good idea to go to bed on a full stomach (indigestion, anyone?), having the right snack an hour before bedtime can be helpful. Magnesium is a natural muscle relaxant, so try a snack high in magnesium (like almonds or a banana). Tryptophan is an amino acid used for insomnia, sleep apnea, depression, and even teeth grinding. Turkey is high in tryptophan and makes a good sleepy snack. You can also try a supplement with tryptophan along with spirulina—algae that has many health benefits—half an hour before bed.

Get tested for sleep apnea. You may be doing all this and more but still having sleep problems. Why? Because of an underlying root cause of your poor sleep that has not been identified by you or your doctor (sound familiar?). Your problem may be sleep apnea, 75 percent of which goes undiagnosed.[6] You're waking up at night dozens, if not hundreds, of times, because your breathing is being interrupted while you're sleeping. Your brain isn't getting enough oxygen, and you jolt awake, without knowing why.

A family history of sleep apnea; being male, overweight, or over forty; or having large tonsils or trouble with your sinuses all put you at higher risk for apnea. If your partner tells you you're snoring loudly or gasping in your sleep, you may have sleep apnea. Sleep apnea can be treated in a variety of ways, including with weight loss; change of sleep positions, mattress, and pillows; mouth taping; the use of a CPAP machine (you wear a mask connected to a machine); or surgery. Ask your doctor to refer you to a sleep-disorder clinic.

Try natural sleep aids, if you need them. I prefer using natural sleep aids and have had good results recommending my patients take melatonin an hour before bed. Start with 3 to 5 mg. at first and then go up to 10 mg. Don't exceed 10 mg. Other herbs that aid in sleep include valerian, skullcap, kava-kava, chamomile, and lemon balm. As part of her nightly ritual, one friend drinks lemon-balm tea, which she finds has a calming effect, and enjoys great sleep. There are also natural sleep aids you can buy at a health-food store that combine melatonin, theanine (an amino acid commonly found in tea), and 5-hydroxytryptophan (5-HTP). These herbal products work well for many of my patients, without morning drowsiness.

As I talked about in chapter 7, cannabis can also be an effective natural sleep aid for some people, though I don't recommend it. If you have a partner, mutually consensual lovemaking is a very effective, natural way to relax and get to sleep. If you don't have a partner or your partner is away, masturbating can also help you release tension and fall back asleep. You can also try essential oils, including lavender, bergamot, and ylang ylang. For more details on essential oils, see appendix 3.

Use pharmaceutical sleep aids sparingly. I will assist a new patient who is still raw, really struggling with withdrawal, and not sleeping by prescribing medication to help with sleep. Clonidine, while not a sleep medication as such, at just 0.1 mg. before bed can take the edge off. Other sleep medications that I prescribe—albeit reluctantly—include trazodone, which is an antidepressant with a side effect of drowsiness, and mirtazapine, also an antidepressant used to treat major sleep disorders. I don't love these drugs, honestly, because they can leave you feeling knocked-out in the morning; I recommend you take them only sparingly to reset your sleep cycle and not for more than a month or two.

Many doctors may also prescribe benzodiazepines, most often lorazepam (Ativan) or alprazolam (Xanax), for sleep. But benzodiazepines are highly addictive, brain-altering medications and should be used with great caution for everyone, especially those of us prone to addiction. Zolpidem tartrate (Ambien) is another popular non-benzodiazepine sleep aid. Some doctors tout its safety, but I have concerns about side effects from Ambien, especially if it is taken more than one or two nights in a row.[7] I do not prescribe benzos or Ambien for sleep.

Point 10. Begin a Consistent Exercise Routine

Everyone, whether you are addicted, in recovery, or on the mild end of the addiction spectrum, benefits a thousandfold from exercising. Even your doctor. And his coauthor. We must all add exercise into our daily routines. The best exercise is the exercise you do every day. Seriously. I don't care what exercise you do, as long as it raises your heart rate and you do it every day. Just get out and move.

I've told you this before in other chapters, but it's worth repeating again: **exercise heals the brain**. We know now that exercise can actually help your brain recover and your dopamine return to normal.[8] This is exciting and important. The science is so solid that it is even starting to be accepted in the world of conventional medicine, where doctors have long believed that the adult brain could not fix itself or regenerate!

Exercise also takes your mind off addiction. But there's another reason why those prone to addiction need to devise and follow a regular exercise routine: exercise will increase your energy and sense of well-being.

Start slowly, and give yourself goals that you can accomplish. If you haven't been exercising at all, add 20 minutes of movement into your day three times in the first week. See if you can increase the time you are exercising by 5 to 10 minutes each week. Slowly increase the intensity. If walking is your exercise of choice, add 20 to 30 seconds of jogging. In general any group activity or team sport will be more motivating, since you will be working out with others, and there's the accountability that occurs when you are in a group. Work up to 45 minutes to an hour a day, four to five days a week.

Point 11. Make Sure You Have Continued Social Support for Safe Living, Healthy Relationships, and Good Stress Management

Even if you are an introvert and need time alone, we humans are social creatures who struggle in isolation. I have found that being actively involved in a community of sober friends is one of the most important things you need to add into your life. A safe, drug-free living space is essential to breaking free.

There are shelters and sober-living homes if your living space is threatening your sobriety. Or perhaps you can find a safe relative or friend to live with short-term while you get on your feet again. Whatever you do, do *not* stay in an environment where others are drinking or using, where you're at risk for being abused, or where you are so stressed out that you know you will not be able to stay sober. Having a safe place to live helps you feel in control of your life and less stressed. When you feel in control and less stressed, you are much less likely to want to use or drink. A win-win.

Good stress management is important to keep you from going back to drugs. Back in chapter 3 I called stress the X factor in addiction. **Stress is one of the biggest triggers for our addictions and one of the most important, though often least recognized, underlying causes of sickness and disease.** I hope this doesn't sound preachy or pushy, but I'm telling you, both as doctor to patient and recovering addict to recovering addict, that you must learn to meditate, use positive affirmations, and find other effective ways to manage your stress.

I see you shaking your head. I hear you saying the word "Impossible." You're sure you'll never be able to. You're just not interested in that hooey-wooey hippie shit.

Hold on a second. *If I can do it, you can do it.*

You see, I am the world's worse candidate for meditation. Believe me. My brain never stops. I have a type A personality. Stress is my best friend. Fidgeting, restless, being five thousand places at once? That's all me.

Meditate? You might as well say "torture." Just thinking about it gave me hives.

Then my sponsor Uncle Elliott handed me Thérèse Jacobs-Stewart's book *Mindfulness and the 12 Steps: Living Recovery in the Present Moment.* I'm so ADD I probably started to read it while Uncle Elliott was in the middle of a sentence. But it worked!

How?

Jacobs-Stewart points out that all you need to do is focus on your breathing. *"Turn the mind toward noticing the breath . . . let all thoughts pass through . . . notice when the mind wanders . . . and go back to the breath."*

She explains that our "monkey brains" are hard to rein in. They're all over the place—they wander like crazy—they get into trouble—they're like pesky toddlers who draw on the walls, climb on the furniture, and refuse to behave. I thought I had to keep those wandering thoughts out of my mind to meditate and that just made it so much harder. But you don't have to stop your monkey brain from acting like a monkey. Let it do all that spinning and monkeying around; just notice it and accept it. Let the thoughts play tag in your brain and beat on the side of your skull. Then let them pass, and get back to paying attention to the breath.

Even I can do that! You can too!

Meditation classes, yoga, massage, acupuncture, mutually consensual lovemaking (if you have the appropriate outlet), and positive self-talk will all help you reduce your stress. Be selfish about self-care. And remember too that selflessness—doing kind acts for other people—will also help you de-stress and heal.

Point 12. Distance Yourself from Sobriety Snatchers and Dream Killers (aka Enablers)

There are people who feel threatened by your sobriety. There are people who would rather kill other people's dreams than pursue their own. Most enablers don't do so consciously or knowingly. But you want to surround yourself with people who love you when you're healthy, not whose greatest joy comes from picking you up out of the gutter, cleaning you up, and then gleefully watching you fall on your face again.

So what should you do if you're struggling with addiction and it's clear to you that someone or several people are sabotaging your recovery? Leave.

If you're paying the mortgage and they're freeloading, show them the door. Tell them your recovery is more important than anything, and you cannot be around them at this time. The problem is yours. You are not judging them, just following direction from your doctor (me—Dr. Paul).

What if you're married? What if you share kids? What if you will lose your job? What if? What if? What if?

Are you ready to be free? If you're ready to once and for all be done with your life of drug use or drinking, then you will have to do things you have never done before. One of the most important things you simply must do is get those who are enabling you—who are part of what is destroying your chance for a full life—out of your life. At least for a time.

Be willing to do whatever it takes.

You're probably thinking, "Dr. Paul, what could you possibly know about this? I can't leave. I can't kick him out. You don't understand."

I do understand. I know how hard it is. One of my sons was using drugs, serving as a dangerously bad role model for his siblings, and disrupting my marriage. We realized we were enabling his drug use—and that our money was going to fund his habit. Maiya and I told him if he could not follow our rules, he would have to leave. This son ended up homeless at nineteen, at the Rescue Mission in the middle of the winter to get out of the cold, and signed up for food stamps. That's right. A physician's kid, out on the streets.

I also made it clear to my wife when we finally both got into recovery fifteen years ago that relapse was not an option. I told her the house went with the kids and if either of us relapsed, that person was out! Thankfully neither of us ended up testing that ultimatum, but I was dead serious. Nothing, and I mean nothing, was going to rob me of my sobriety ever again. There's no way to say this nicely. Enablers have to be kicked to the curb.

Do not allow yourself or your loved
ones to be physically abused.

If you are in an emotionally or physically abusive relationship, you need help. Find a counselor who can help guide you in either setting up appropriate boundaries with that friend or loved one or getting out. Your sobriety is your number one goal. Put nothing above staying sober, not your parents, spouse, partner, children, work—*nothing*. Think about it. If you relapse back into a world of drinking and drugging, you will lose your loved ones and your job anyway.

A postscript: If you have an addict or alcoholic in your life who's leaning on you too much, whose actions you resent, or whose drinking or drug use is consuming all your brain space, you might have unwittingly become the enabler. Examine your role. Learn to set boundaries. It's easy for us to get addicted to our loved one's addictions and to become so immersed that we abandon our own lives. If that's you, I recommend you join Al-Anon, which holds meetings for those of us who have family and friends who are alcoholics or addicts. Please also seek weekly counseling, and use all the other tools in this book to get your *own* life back on track.

Point 13. Carry Naloxone

Opioid and heroin overdoses are now one of the biggest killers of young adults in America. Many of these deaths can be prevented if the person who finds you unconscious has naloxone to inject or squirt up your nose. Naloxone blocks and reverses the effect of what can be a lethal heroin or opioid overdose. Every heroin and opioid addict and their loved ones should carry it. It has saved thousands of lives[9] and has the potential to save millions more.

If you're struggling with opioid addiction, living with anyone abusing opioids in any form (whether prescribed for pain or from the street), or have friends who are using heroin or opioids, carry naloxone. Tell your friends and family where you keep it and show them how to use it. If you find someone unconscious from an overdose, call 911. Have the emergency team stay on the phone with you while you administer naloxone. See appendix 1 for more information about the different preparations of naloxone and how to use them.

The Gift of Addiction

Addiction is both a curse and a gift. The curse is obvious; the gift, though, is often not revealed until we are well along in our journey of recovery. In recovery we learn to do our part as best we can and let go of the results. We learn we are not in control of our kids, our partners, our employees, or anyone else. We learn we can only control and heal ourselves. As we learn truths like this, we become free.

I am responsible for my actions and my behaviors, but I am not responsible for yours. In the midst of uproar and turmoil, I can feel calm and at peace. Most of the time.

Always *believe* you can do this.

You are worthy.

Never give up.

CHAPTER 11

Embracing the Spiritual and Emotional Journey

IT'S NOT EASY to be human. For anyone. And some of us find being human excruciatingly hard. Your battle with addiction may look nothing like mine. But at our core we are the same: struggling to find our way, looking to stay safe, wanting to be connected, seeking pleasure, and hoping to feel loved.

As I mentioned in the last chapter, none of us asks to be born. You don't have a choice in that. But—even as you feel beaten down by your difficult past, shortcomings, failings, and shame—you do get to make choices about how you live your life right now.

Behavioral analysts say people struggle most when beginning new projects. If you can just manage to take that first step. Even if it's just for today. Tomorrow is a new day. You'll get there when you get there, one day at a time. Before long, those todays and tomorrows turn into weeks, then months, and then years. Suddenly you're in the driver's seat of your own life, with your hands on the steering wheel and your foot on the accelerator. Then one day you're helping others and picking *them* up when they fall down.

Maybe you feel hopeless. Maybe you feel depressed, desperate, miserable, or just bored. Life is sometimes dull and dreary. Sometimes it is unbearable. If you've ever felt that way or you feel that way right now, let me say this, and hear it well: there is always hope.

You will fail. You will get knocked down.
You will sabotage your own dreams.
That's okay. Get back up. Try again.

At first it seems as though the abstinence itself is the hardest part. It seems like an impossible task. When you think about letting go of your addiction, you probably feel you are about to lose your best friend, closest confidant, and most confidential, nonjudgmental adviser. I know that feeling. It isn't easy. Yet the really hard part is learning to enjoy life sober and being present in your own life.

You need some tools to fill that gaping hole. These are the concepts that will help you the most. They are less prescriptive than the points in my plan from the last chapter, like finding a counselor or getting proper sleep, but they are just as crucial in helping you cope with the emotional battle of sobriety and teaching you to ignore the voices in your head that will beg you to use again. In this chapter I will show you how to work toward FREEDOM:

Find your spiritual self.

Release resentment.

Expect temptation.

Embrace your flaws.

Draw on the crew sent to rescue you.

Open yourself to change.

Make progress, not perfection.

Find your spiritual self. Whether you roll your eyes at the mention of God or you used to be deeply religious but haven't been in recent years, I believe your way out of physical addiction includes becoming connected to your spiritual side. You can be an atheist, a hesitant agnostic, or a devotee of Jesus. It doesn't matter. I grew up in the United Methodist Church, where we had a traditional notion of an all-powerful Christian God. The God of your upbringing might have been angry, judgmental, or unapproachable. But your God need not be that way at all. Your God can just be a loving, gentle presence that is waiting for you, there for you, wanting to help you, always loving you.

Your God can be anything you want—anything that gives you a larger sense that there is a universe to which we all belong. You can even have no god (perhaps with a lowercase g) beyond your own breath,

The Waterfall

It was a brisk spring morning when Uncle Elliott and I drove out to the Columbia River Gorge. He gave me an assignment: without creating a dam or diverting the river, I had fifteen minutes to focus on the waterfall and stop its flow. You can try the same exercise by attempting to stop the waves at the ocean or trying to keep the sun from setting. I made a valiant and whole-soul attempt to move the waterfall, shrink the mountain, do something! I failed. No matter what I did, no matter how hard I thought or tried, I could not stop the water from falling.

Was there perhaps a *power greater than myself?*

Call it hooey-wooey, but this was one of the most powerful experiences of my life. There, in front of whoever happened to be walking past, I knelt behind the waterfall. I held hands with Uncle Elliott and gave myself over to that Higher Power.

"I offer myself to you," I said out loud. "Build me, and do with me as you will."

something that is totally undeniable and completely yours to turn to in any moment. As long as you are alive, your breath will not abandon you; and you don't have to believe in it to experience the relaxing effects of taking a deep breath. When my friend Tammy was a tormented teenager, her mother (a nurse) used to say, "Take a deep breath. It's physiologically relaxing." So even when Tammy's mind wouldn't shut off, her mother's words reassured her that there was a way to relax her body, despite herself. **Your God is any source of goodness and kindness and acceptance that works for you.**

Release resentment. Our character defects—those shortcomings, blind spots, areas of weakness—seem to crop up at the most inopportune times to sabotage our lives. We carry them with us, thinking we need them, when the real work is to let go of these burdens and false beliefs.

Perhaps you know the Zen story of the two travelers who are walking to a neighboring village in the heavy rain. They come to a river they must cross, but the bridge has been washed out by the storm. Just then, as the travelers are charting their safest course across the river, a rich woman appears at the bank of the river. Furious that the bridge is out, she's in a hurry to cross, but she does not want to soil her fancy clothing. The younger traveler's face gets hot; he's annoyed with her haughtiness, preciousness, impatience, and sense of entitlement.

The other traveler, who is slightly older, offers to help the woman across the river. He hoists her onto his back and trudges into the rushing water. The woman complains the entire way, telling him to go faster, scolding him for picking the wrong route, berating him for getting her leather shoes wet. On the other side of the river the traveler puts her down. She does not condescend to speak to him, but instead hurries away without even a thank-you.

For several hours the two travelers walk along in silence, the young man stewing about the rich woman, the older man enjoying the feeling of rain on his face, the scent of blooming flowers, and the sound of the birds.

"How could you do it? How could you bear it?" the young man finally blurts out. "That woman was so awful, so ungrateful!"

"My son," his companion replies, "I put my burden down hours ago. Why do you insist on carrying her still?"

It is easy for all of us to let anger, self-pity, selfishness, pride, jealousy, and resentment destroy our lives. When you've been fighting for your very survival, the last thing you feel like doing is being humble, grateful, or patient. But your model needs to be the strong and steady traveler who helped the woman across without expecting or even wanting thanks. It was he, after all, who enjoyed every step of his journey.

Expect temptation. Feel your temptation, and then use that feeling—that irresistible craving, that knowing that it is inevitable and that you are going to succumb to it no matter what—as information. And then, as if it were a hot flame, recoil, back up, run, get away *now*. Call your sponsor, your sober best friend, your brother, sister, mom, dad, or the other relative in your life who supports you most. Call the after-hours number for your psychologist or the National Suicide Prevention line. Call anyone who can talk you down from that irresistible desire to go back to hell.

If you stumble on a hidden bottle of alcohol or a stash of drugs, immediately destroy it! If you run into an old using friend who wants to hang out and party with you, *don't*! As I told Amanda back in chapter 4, you have two legs, use them, and get the hell out of there.

No one—not your parents, not your partner, not your kids, not your boss—gets to derail you from your sobriety. *Period!* You are not a doormat, and you cannot allow anyone to abuse or mistreat you. I know I've said it before, but I need to say it again: we need to be assertive about our recovery journey, and sometimes we must make difficult choices to maintain our integrity. We must free ourselves from the grip of people, places, and things that jeopardize our sobriety. If you have "friends" supplying you drugs, tell them you're struggling to overcome your addiction, that it's not their fault, but in order to survive you have to remove their names from your phone. Stop all contact, and ask them to honor your decision and not try to get in touch with you.

If you put sobriety above all else, you have a chance. A chance to keep that job, that awesome person you met recently, those beautiful kids who mean the world to you, that eco-friendly luxury car you purchased recently when you got an unexpected windfall, that cozy house or cool space-age apartment decorated with furniture from the second-hand store. We know that with relapse starts the downward spiral that results in losing everything.

You will be tempted. But don't give in.

Embrace your flaws. How do you move from fear, loneliness, anger, sadness, selfishness, and self-will to compassion, gratitude, joy, peace, and love? And how the heck do you find serenity? Imperfectly, with many conflicting emotions, with lots of stops and starts. There is no one right way. The path you are on now is right where you need to be. If you're veering in a direction you don't mean to go, make needed adjustments. Accept yourself, and love yourself just the way you are.

Your fears, resentments, mistakes, and all those things that you feel are preventing you from moving forward in your life don't miraculously disappear in sobriety. But as the days become weeks and the weeks become months and the months become years, you begin to understand that your flaws and shortcomings are a part of your strength.

Learning to love yourself, you also love your flaws.

Draw on the crew sent to rescue you. A man finds his home surrounded by water. Firefighters, sirens screaming, stop in front of the house and urge him to leave, offering him a lift to higher, drier ground. The floodwaters are rising, the situation is dire. It's time to go! The man declines the help. He hides inside his home. As the waters rise to the level of the windows, a motorboat with a rescue crew zooms to his house. They offer him a ride. Again he declines. He can't hide inside any longer, so he goes up onto his roof. The water continues to rise, lapping at his ankles. A helicopter chops the air overhead and drops down a ladder. The pilot screams for him to climb aboard. The man declines the help.

"God will rescue me," he shouts to the pilot. "I'll be fine." The floodwaters overwhelm him, and the stubborn man drowns. He enters the pearly gates of heaven, where St. Peter welcomes him.

"Why didn't God come to my rescue?" the man asks St. Peter, perplexed, disappointed, and indignant.

"We sent you a fire truck, a boat, and then a helicopter," St. Peter replies. "What more did you want us to do?"

On your amazing journey of recovery, you have now reached the point of action. You no longer want to stay inside and drown. You are ready to set aside everything that was destroying your life. You are moving away from the severe end of the addiction spectrum. You embrace every crew sent to rescue you. You embrace your spiritual side. You bow down before the unstoppable waterfall. You say yes to life, yes to being here where you are at this moment in all your imperfection with all your baggage, yes to the ideas of the integrative doctor wearing a Hawaiian shirt and a mischievous smile.

Open yourself to change. On this journey back to our true, authentic, messy, complicated, imperfect, *and lovable* self, we have to make the bold decision to change. We have to reexamine our core beliefs, rethink what we've been taught, consciously or unconsciously, and question how we've been raised. Are you willing to join others who have found a way to freedom? If you are, you will succeed.

We did not come into the world alone—we spent nine months growing inside another human being. We did not grow up alone—human babies cannot grow and thrive without human touch and nurturing. We also cannot kick our addiction alone—no matter how strong we tell ourselves we are. Surrender. Let go of the idea that you can do it all alone, that you don't need anyone else, that you alone in the world can fix everything that is broken. It is in partnership and in community (awkward, imperfect, sometimes annoying partnership and community) that we are finally able to heal.

It's a daily task to be open to change, surrender your self-will, and acknowledge your powerlessness over the people, places, and things that are beyond your control. You have to work to be mindful every day, so that you don't revert back to old patterns and old habits. Try to be honest about your shortcomings, open to other people's ideas, and always, always, willing to change. When we learn to surrender, we understand that what we believe with certainty today might not be what we believe tomorrow.

Make progress, not perfection. Anyone who has embarked on any spiritual or emotional journey knows that it is about progress, not perfection. I can practically hear you, after reading this book: "Well, Dr. Paul, I'm living in the real world here, and I have problems!"

You know, I agree! We all have problems. We all struggle. But when we start being kinder to ourselves, helping others, and making better, healthier, safer choices, those problems that used to keep piling up and overwhelming us start to become fewer and farther between.

We often end up getting what we're looking for. When we hate ourselves, trouble finds us. When we let go of our addiction and embrace recovery, over time we gain the tools we need to deal with the bad things. When we learn to love ourselves, good things come our way.

So now that I have convinced you to relinquish your uniqueness and separateness and now that you are willing to surrender to a force outside yourself to guide you and restore you to sanity and health, you're all done. Close this book. Stop going to therapy. All's well that ends well. Right?

Wrong. "Recover" is a verb. It's now that you're just getting started.

Remember I am with you. Every step of the way.

Epilogue

I T IS 3:00 A.M. on my second-to-last day in Maui. Waves break gently over the rocks below the balcony where I sit, tropical stars sparkle in the sky above, and a gentle breeze blows across the palm trees, their leaves flitting in the breeze like a hundred fine kite tails. I'm here with Maiya, resting, relaxing, and writing the first draft of this book. Of course, I should be sleeping. But I'm not. But I'm also not stressing about being up so early. I'm at peace—observing this outer world and my inner self, trying to find the match for the serenity of the landscape inside myself. All is well.

I've been up early every morning since we arrived, spilling my ideas onto the computer, knowing that Jennifer and I will fix them later. Maiya and I have taken long walks along the Ka'anapali Beach. Sometimes we solve the problems of the world, sometimes we fret about the children and their struggles, sometimes we argue, some-times we just walk quietly together. We walk past the Napili Bay, Kapalua Bay, Namalu Bay, across volcanic rock, bird sanctuaries, and turtle-filled coves ending at Oneloa Bay, where one morning I knelt on the sandy beach before the vast Pacific Ocean and asked my Cre-ator to take every one of my character defects from me and replace them with good qualities.

"*Mahalo*," we greet others who walk along the same trails. "Beau-tiful day," we add with the biggest of smiles. This journey we share called life has no destination. We each must find our own way. Each of us will die one day, and yet being together now makes it all easier. As you have been reading this book, my path and yours have now crossed. Whether you are my patient in the office, whether we walk past each other on forest trails, interact online, or meet each other in the pages of this book, I greet you with a smile and thank you for being in my life.

I wonder now why my motivations in the past were so self-centered and ego-driven, why I isolated myself when I needed people the most, why I tended so much toward self-sabotage when I was younger. I had an "I can do this myself attitude" that got me into addiction in the first place. When I failed at something, I thought, "I am a failure." I raged against the unfairness in the world, all the while disgusted with myself, secretly knowing I was unworthy and unlovable and on the brink of being found out. Perhaps you have felt this way too. Perhaps you feel this way right now.

I was traumatized by a thousand little failures, and I found relief in a bottle.

It took me a long time to learn to quiet my demons, stop the self-sabotage, and find ways to turn failure into success. Back then I was filled with shame. Today I am thankful I'm an alcoholic.

I couldn't say that for the first five years I was in recovery. I slunk red-faced into meetings, never wanting to be there, wanting to keep my secrets hidden in the closet instead of bringing them into the light. I thought being an alcoholic was a character defect. It was only by doing the work—with my family, with a therapist, in the rooms of AA, with my sponsor, with all the choices I made about my lifestyle and my health—that I could grow up, pay attention, and recognize the gifts my addiction has given me. I have earned a level of calm and, yes, at times serenity, that I never thought possible.

I take a break from typing furiously to watch the sunrise and listen to the enthusiastic cacophony of the sooty terns and brown boobies. Streaks of purple, yellow, and orange light fill the sky. My brain is still racing with thoughts and ideas. Whereas once I tried to suppress this energy with alcohol, I now embrace it. I am at peace with my choices, no longer driven by fear but by passion and love. I'm still a work in progress, and I still have a long way to go. To the extent that I am willing and open to new direction, it seems I am shown what that new direction will be.

When the student is ready, the teacher appears.

About the Illustrations

About the illustrations: The illustrations in this book are linocut, a multistep artistic technique that uses a sheet of linoleum as a relief surface. A design is first drawn onto the surface of the lino and then cut or carved with a razor knife or a small V-shaped gouge. The raised surface remaining after the carving is a mirror image of what is then printed. To print, the lino sheet must be covered with ink by a roller and then pressed gently onto paper by hand or rolled through a press. This printing method was first used as an artistic technique in the early 1900s by Die Brücke, a group of Expressionists in Germany (where the method had originally been used to make wallpaper), and was popularized by Pablo Picasso in the 1950s.

About the illustrator: Han Sayles is a community organizer and printmaker in Santa Fe, New Mexico, where she works as the Artist Liaison for Meow Wolf. After graduating cum laude from Colorado College with

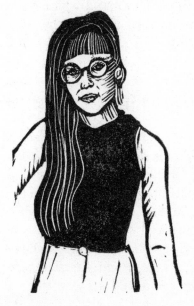

a degree in comparative literature in 2015, she became interested in the intersection between public art and political action. She taught herself to be a printmaker—an accessible art method for producing beautiful multiples to distribute a message far and wide—and uses her art to advocate for LGBTQ+ rights and social justice. In 2017 she won both the Outstanding Emerging Visual Artist Award from Pikes Peak Arts Council and an Inclusion Award from the *Colorado Springs Independent*. She continues to work primarily in silk screen and linocut prints.

Paul's Acknowledgments

I am eternally grateful to my parents, Winnie and Norman Thomas, who led by example by never drinking, smoking, or using drugs during my childhood. My mom was always there to listen and never to judge. Although she didn't understand at the time the extent of the problem that alcohol would become for me later in my life, she witnessed how I always seemed to drink to excess and at least reflected back to me what she observed. "Paul," Mom said, "I don't mind your taking a few drinks, but why do you have to drown yourself?"

In college my late aunt Carol talked to me about alcohol use and how even a drink or two, when consumed every day, could lead to problems. I wasn't ready to hear it, but I'm glad she told me anyway. I'm grateful to Dartmouth Medical School, where my psychiatry rotation required attending three AA meetings. Little did I know I would need those meetings more than a decade later. When I was ready, I knew where to go.

I'm grateful to all my children, who grew up with a dad who, while loving and nurturing, was physically and emotionally unavailable after about 8:00 p.m. until the next morning for too many years. Thank you, Natalie, my eldest daughter, for caring for your brothers all those nights when I had ceased to hear their cries. I can't take away how hard that was for you. But I can tell you that I'm forever grateful, and forever sorry.

Thanks to my nurse Jan, who, years before I won the battle and put down the bottle, gently told me she could smell alcohol on my breath. It was from the beer I drank the night before. While I never drank in the mornings or on the job, alcohol was literally seeping from my pores. We think we are holding it together, but need to be reminded when it becomes clear we are not. I'm grateful to all who in their own ways tried to help me. I recall, toward the end of my drinking career, when I felt empty inside. I recall, as vividly as if it were yesterday, making such a fake smile one morning to a nurse while rounding on babies, that the nurse mirrored my fake smile back. That stopped me in my tracks. I knew I had to do something. I knew I couldn't go on much longer with my charade.

Thank you, Brandon, my first sponsor, for your attempts to show me those parts of the Big Book that said, "The alcoholic at certain times has no defense against the first drink." I wasn't ready to hear that message yet; I just wasn't ready to accept that I could never safely take another drink, but you planted an important seed.

Thank you, Pat M., for reaching your hand out to me and saying, "I'll be your temporary sponsor," on December 22, 2002, the morning after my last drink. I didn't yet have the ability to ask for help; your presence at every meeting and gentle encouragement saved my life. Pat remained my "temporary sponsor" for a decade.

Thank you, Gary, for "working with me." You had the kind of sobriety and wisdom I wanted. I listened intently to your every word. I am grateful to so many in AA, the hurting and raw, and those with the serenity and wisdom I longed for.

Thank you to my current sponsor, "Uncle Elliott," for your deep and sincere yet gentle guidance. The exercise of trying to stop Ponytail Falls from flowing and the sun from setting was a beautiful way to drive home my powerlessness. You knew I had a challenge with that. Perhaps that is why you had me put that sign up on my bathroom mirror, so I would read it every day: "I don't need your help today. Love, God." I will never forget the experience of writing out my character defects in the sand and watching the waves wash them away.

I am grateful to Patty Van Antwerp, who forever demonstrates the joy of being in service to others and who was the patient keeper of the many, many drafts of this book. To Lisa McQuilliam, for her masterful way of keeping me organized. To all of my staff at Integrative Pediatrics and Fair Start, who have supported me throughout this entire journey. And to Michael Shaver, for all the reasons that you know so well and all the joy, compassion, and serenity you bring into my life. I could list hundreds of friends in AA who have openly shared their pain and their joy in meetings over the years and reached out in friendship to me.

Every one of my patients at Fair Start has provided me with a lesson in some aspect of the journey we call life and, specifically, in how it is, indeed, hard to be human. I've learned so much from your struggles. Thank you for trusting me to be a part of your journey. Your honesty and confidence in me is humbling. To my readers and viewers who interact with me on social media and to all who cross paths with me with openness and acceptance, thank you too.

I've learned so much from and been so blessed by the knowledge, wisdom, and willingness to share truth from the experts interviewed for the Addiction Summit: Ben Lynch, ND, James Maskell, Julie Valenti, Marv Seppala, MD, Zen Honeycutt, Joel Fuhrman, MD, David Perlmutter, MD, Mike Mutzel, Deanna Minich, PhD, Chris Meletis, ND, Niki Gratrix, Ray Lozano, Anita Devlin, Maria Watson, Jason Powell, David Jockers, DNM, Annie Grace, Mukta Khalsa, PhD, Karen Willock, Ty Bollinger, Erin Elizabeth, Sara Gottfried, MD, Peter Osborne, Sayer Ji, Kevin Griffin, Valerie Silveira, and John Dempster, ND. Thank you, also, to my son Noah Thomas, who both participated in an episode and has been my main videographer for the Addiction Summit and for YouTube. Noah's transparency with his own journey and struggles has offered me tremendous insight. My understanding of mental health and the struggle to get out of addiction has been deeply enhanced by Noah's willingness to share his battles.

Thanks to Marvin Seppala, MD, Hazelden Betty Ford Foundation CMO, for sitting by my wife's bedside holding her hand, guiding her through the difficult time of postoperative pain management while in recovery from opioid addiction. Your pioneering work at Beyond Addictions and your expertise provided the road map for outpatient detox and management and made my Fair Start addiction and detox clinic possible. I cherish our friendship and your gentle, optimistic, always smiling leadership style. Thank you, Marv, for showing us all how to embrace our past and use it to help others.

I'm grateful to all my children for loving me despite my imperfections. My life is so completely full with each and every one of you in it.

To Jennifer, my coauthor, colleague, and friend: for a "normie," you sure have grasped this topic. Thank you for always being excited about the material I gave you, even when it needed a lot of work! Your talented work on this book has made it the masterpiece that it is. We tease each other, as neither of us has seen anyone who works harder. It is always a pure joy and honor to work with you.

To my life partner and wife, Maiya: words cannot express how grateful I feel to have had you beside me these past thirty years. We struggled with family stresses that nearly tore us apart. We raised all those children, which at times was enough stress to destroy any couple. But not us. The harder it got, the closer we grew together. You battled horrible health challenges that were enough to bring anyone to their knees, but we hung in there, together. I am grateful beyond words that you have chosen to join me on this journey of sobriety and personal growth. You have always believed in me, supported me, loved me, listened to me, gently given me your input, and fearlessly challenged me when that was required. I know I am one of the lucky ones.

I'm also grateful to my Higher Power. You get me, duh. I still am fairly clueless, but I am so grateful for the ways you drop signs into my life. Point the way, and I will follow. Thank you.

Jennifer's Acknowledgments

As our editors will tell you, Paul and I tend to write long, so we need another hundred pages to express gratitude to all the people who deserve our thanks! Those editors at HarperOne, Sydney Rogers and Gideon Weil, are amazing. Not only have they done a tremendous job helping us tighten our prose and shape this book; they are also among the kindest, smartest, most patient, and most brilliant people in publishing. Stephanie Tade, our tireless champion and intrepid literary agent, has been right there with us every step of the way. Thank you, Stephanie, for *every* aspect of your support in helping us bring this book into the world. Melissa Chianta has done an incredible job fact-checking and formatting the endnotes. Thank you, Melissa. Any remaining mistakes in this manuscript are ours. Thank you also to the creative director at HarperOne, Adrian Morgan, and FaceOut Studio for the breathtaking cover design that we both love so much, Julia Kent for her patience with our IT challenges and her marketing brilliance, Suzanne Quist for her production skills, Ann Moru for outstanding line editing, and Melinda Mullin for help with publicity. We feel so lucky to be part of this team.

I was the kid who never understood schadenfreude. As a baby I would cry if I heard another baby crying. To this day I am haunted by the image of Roadrunner tricking Wile E. Coyote to fall off that steep cliff. I felt very privileged to be able to interview so many of Paul's patients and others struggling to overcome addiction, and I am very grateful for their willingness and openness in sharing their stories. At the same time, those stories wrenched my heart. There I was listening, typing notes into the computer as fast as I could, doing my best not to cry (and often failing). My grandfather was a high-functioning alcoholic, some of my closest family members have struggled with substance abuse, and my mother-in-law is also in recovery. Though I've not struggled with addiction myself, I know firsthand what it feels like to be overwhelmed by negative emotions, anxiety, and panic and to think the world would be a better place without you in it. As much as it hurts, sharing our pain, bringing our dark secrets to light, and listening without judgment really do help us all heal. Thank you to all of Paul's patients and the others struggling with addiction and substance abuse who were so honest and open with me about your pain. You helped us write this book. You help make the world a better place. We couldn't have done it without you.

At dinner last night I mentioned fretting over these acknowledgments. "I'm not sure who to thank first," I lamented.

"*Thank me!*" my daughter Athena and her friend Alex Westrick cried in unison. Athena, who just turned seventeen, is such an interesting, creative, kindhearted young woman that some days I think I deserve the Nobel Prize in parenting for bringing such a beautiful being into the world (though the truth is she was probably born that way and she inherited my husband's genes). Thank you, Athena. You had to play Mom, Dad, Santa Claus, and chauffeur and pick up a lot of slack, and I know it hasn't been easy. And thank you, Alex, for being such a good friend.

Our oldest has flown the coop and is now in college. Our house has been quieter without her. Different. As much as Hesperus was ready to start the next chapter of her life, we all miss her terribly. She likes to remind us that she was the first and the original. Though she refuses to read a word I write, she was thrilled when her roommate at Barnard said they read one of my books in her high-school critical-thinking class. Thank you, Hesperus. Your hard work, determination, sensitivity, joy, and love of life inspire me.

Etani, who's fourteen, says I may use his first name only (but not when asked to give a name for an order at the drink counter at a coffee shop). "And why would you want to thank me anyway, Mom?" Thank you, Etani, for teaching me to be the mom of a teenage son, playing soccer with me, encouraging me to get this book done, and being such a solid, engaged, and creative kid.

Baby Leone is eight now. It's been a bittersweet joy to watch her growing up so fast, trying to keep up with her three older siblings. Thank you, Leone, for being the most interesting, energetic, enthusiastic, and sometimes difficult lastborn a mom could wish for. Now, if you would stop standing on my grandmother's table and remember to floss your teeth . . .

Huge thanks to the rest of my family, including my father, Nick Margulis, my aunt Judy Margulis (who, as the honorary grandma, does so much for all of us and is so appreciated and so, so loved), my uncles Jeffrey Kessel and Michael Margulis, my aunt Laurie Olsen, and my cousins Jacob Kessel, Hannah Margulis-Kessel, Jesse Bay, Frieda Bay, and Josh Olsen. To seven-year-old Yarrow and tiny baby Altair: may the world you inherit be free from addiction. Also to my brother, Zachary Margulis-Ohnuma, who fifty years into life still has the best ideas for road trips, his wife, Mary Margulis-Ohnuma, and my nieces Miranda and Madeline and nephew Atticus. And to Dorion Sagan, Jeremy Sagan, Robin Kolnicki, Sara Fawn Sagan, Tonio Sagan, and baby Nora. I owe a debt of gratitude to all of my husband's family, especially my father-in-law, James Propis, mother-in-law, Susan Buscaglia, cousins Kristin, Paolo, and Luca Mannoni, Marya and Sarah Propis, and Great Grandma Propis, thriving at age ninety-nine. Thank you to every one of the Propis and Militello clan!

To my best friend, Sue Langston, I love you. Thank you for being there for me and the kids always in every way. To Laura Jessup, I can't imagine a better friend or more sympathetic listener. Our weekly walks helped me clear my head and follow the exercise cure recommended in this book. To Adam and Leslie Marx, thank you for always being there for us. To Michele Warrence-Schreiber, you helped launch Hesperus into the world and have been such a good friend to our family ever since. To Kimberly Ford, for those alpaca slippers, you are the best! To J. B. Hanley, a cutting-edge activist for health freedom and one of the sharpest minds I know, thank you for introducing Paul and me. Your activism and your writing are an inspiration to us. To Jake Hayes and Angie Reynick-Hayes, thank you for the amazing food (even though, dudes, you have eight kids and you have to stop bringing us dinner!). To Cammy Benton, MD, and Ilonka Michelle O'Neil for your friendship and support.

To the entire staff and community at the Siskiyou School and, especially, Catherine Dixon, Aurelia McNamara, Magda Paz, Cynthia Bower, Kristin Beers, and Katie LaCroix for holding our daughter in such a safe space. And to the entire community of parents, educators, and health practitioners in southern Oregon, especially Tangren Alexander, Valerie Arinsberg (for so many things), Mariane Ballete, Jade Bockus, Vidal Cervantes, Keith and Anne Chambers, Craig Comstock, Tony Corallo, Brigid Crowe, Pink Culver, Leslie Davis, Soshanah Dubiner, Joel Goldman, Oz Hernandez, Laurie Hicks, Linda Hopkins, Geoff Houghton, Dave Kahn, Rick Kirschner, Dannae LaQua, Paula Lynam, Jen Marsden, Rebecca Mehta, Dave Nourie, Shayna Perkinson, Sean Porter, Steve Retzlaff (Ashland Middle School's fearless leader),

Alexa and Liz Schmidt, Jim Westrick, and Jennifer and Donnie Yance.

I'm grateful to all my colleagues at Jefferson Public Radio, especially my editor (and dear friend) Abigail Kraft, our intrepid director Paul Westhelle, producer Liam Moriarty, and the ever-patient Soleil Rowan-Caneer. And to all my Thursday night soccer peeps. There are too many of you to name, but I'd be remiss without a shout-out to our captain, Nicole Rosanelli, my training buddy Jessica Allen, our bold goalie Andrea Allen Sis, and Karyssa Booth (I'm not forgiving you yet for breaking your ankle and then getting pregnant and *still* not playing, girlfriend). Go Hydra.

My husband, James, is my first reader, best editor, gourmet latte maker (from home-roasted organic green beans; come over sometime and we'll make you a cup), and closest friend. He had an unexpected and nearly catastrophic health crisis while Paul and I were finishing this book. A team of OHSU cardiologists, from electrophysiologists to heart-failure specialists, cared for James during that difficult time in the hospital, as did the best, smartest, and kindest nurses and nursing assistants (on twelve-hour shifts, and they never got grouchy). We owe a debt of gratitude to all of them, including James Mudd, MD, Babak Nazer, MD, Jonathan Davis, MD, and Luke Burchill, MD, PhD. I wish we had met you all under different circumstances, but I'm glad we found you when we did. Thank you. William Parker, PhD, Katherine Reynolds Lewis, Brian Lewis, MD, Howard Morningstar, MD, Eric Peña, MD, Robin Miller, MD, Lee Milligan, MD, Corey Kahn, MD, Dr. Paul, Leslie Cooper, MD, and the countless others who have all been part of the team lending us support, wise counsel, and expert advice. Thank you.

When James was fifteen he went to a psychologist who suggested he take up running. The fact that he has been so fit and athletic ever since is probably what kept him from flatlining after his heart went haywire. Thank you to that psychologist and to every health-care professional who has taken the time to help a young person take a health inventory and devise a healing program. That offhand suggestion that you make to a teen to implement a healthy habit may be the very thing that saves his life.

But most of all—I've saved the best for last—thank you, James, for always being there, supporting me and my work, and raising the brightest, kindest, most compassionate, most securely attached children in the world. You promised you wouldn't die. I'm holding you to your word.

Appendix i

Naloxone

Anyone on prescription pain medications or addicted to pain pills or heroin or any other opioids is at risk for an opioid overdose. Naloxone, which only works if someone has opioids in their system, is a medicine that blocks the effects of opioids and can reverse overdose. If you are with someone who is unconscious or difficult to rouse and you believe it is because of an opioid overdose, your friend or family member may need immediate naloxone. Yes, you can (and should) call an ambulance. But by the time the ambulance arrives it may be too late.

Since 2016, the availability of naloxone (also referred to by its brand name, Narcan) in a nasal spray has given first responders, family, friends, and caregivers a safe way to administer it. As of this writing, pharmacists are allowed to distribute naloxone without a patient-specific prescription in every state except Nebraska. Expect to pay between $135 and $150 for a two-dose naloxone nasal-spray kit.

The second option is injectable naloxone, which can be given by an auto-injector or in a syringe. The downside is the cost, which is typically around $400, though the price may be coming down. The Evzio auto-injector, smaller than a pack of cards, comes with voice instructions, so you can practice beforehand. You will also be guided through what to do in an actual emergency.

If you're an addict or the loved one of an addict, I recommend you carry naloxone with you and have it available at all times. It can even be used in children, should there be an accidental opioid overdose. In a life-threatening emergency naloxone can also be used on a pregnant woman as well, but her unborn baby will need to be evaluated immediately.

The safest place for someone who has overdosed is the emergency room, so even as you are delivering naloxone, call an ambulance or a friend who can drive you to the hospital. It is also a good idea for you or your doctor to call the hospital's ER and tell them you are on the way. For advice about what to do if your loved one needs to go to the emergency room, see page 224.

Emergency Treatment of Overdose: Step by Step

Is it an overdose? An overdose of opioids, including heroin, will suppress breathing. If you are unable to rouse your unconscious loved one, it may be obvious that's what's happened (a pill bottle or needle is close at hand). But you may not be sure. Snoring, gasping for breath, shallow breathing, a very slow pulse, pale skin, and small pupils are also signs of overdose. First try to wake the person by calling their name, rubbing their hands, and slapping their face.

If the person does not respond, call 911. Tell the operator it is an emergency and that your loved one is unconscious and not breathing because of a suspected overdose. Clearly state your location or street address.

Administer naloxone.

Via nasal spray: Hold the device with your thumb on the bottom of the plunger and two fingers on the nozzle. Hold the tip of the nozzle in one nostril and press the plunger to release the dose into the patient's nose.

Via auto-injector: Pull the auto-injector from its case.
Pull off the red safety guard firmly and carefully. Be very careful at this point not to inject yourself accidentally. Do not touch the auto-injector's black base, which is where the needle comes out.
Place the device against the middle of the thigh and push hard. Hold in place for five seconds. It will make a hissing and clicking sound as the needle is injecting the medicine and then retracting. Follow the voice prompt instructions, as the device will tell you what to do.

Via syringe: Either you will have prefilled syringes containing a dose of 0.4 mg. or you will draw 1 ml. (0.4 mg.) into a syringe.

Inject into the muscle of the upper thigh or upper arm. The shot can be given through clothing if necessary.

Perform CPR. If your loved one does not begin breathing right away, perform CPR. Getting oxygen to the brain may save the person's life.

1. Position the person on their back.

2. Check that the airway is not blocked. The tongue may be obstructing breathing. If that is the case, use your index finger as a hook to sweep the tongue out of the way.

3. Check for a pulse (you can feel it on the side of the neck or the wrist). If there is no pulse, give 30 chest compressions. Put your hands on top of each other on the sternum, pushing down 2 inches at a rate of 100 per minute.

4. To give rescue breaths: Pinch the nose closed with one hand. Use the other hand to keep the chin up. Blow 2 slow breaths into the mouth. Make sure your mouth is sealed around the other's mouth, so the breaths go in. Give 2 breaths every 30 compressions.

5. If someone is able to bring you an *automated external defibrillator* (AED), remove your loved one's shirt (cutting it if you have to), apply pads to the bare chest as directed, and follow the directions to stand clear so the machine can evaluate if the heart has stopped. Most have pictures or even talk you through this. The AED will read the electrical activity of the heart and deliver a shock if needed.

Be prepared to do it again. Even a person who responds to naloxone may lapse back into unconsciousness. You must be prepared to give a second dose of naloxone if the person doesn't respond in two to three minutes, or stops breathing again, or becomes or remains unconscious and an emergency team has not yet arrived.

Don't leave. Stay with your loved one until help arrives.

Best CPR practices sometimes change. I recommend you sign up for a CPR and first-aid class at the local Red Cross, YMCA, or city emergency response department to stay current.

Addictive Substances and Behaviors

ADDICTIVE SUBSTANCES

- **Alcohol**
  Beer, liquor, wine
  Cough syrups, extracts, mouthwash

- **Benzodiazepines**
  Ativan
  Halcion
  Librium
  Rohypnol
  Valium
  Xanax

- **Opiates**
  Buprenorphine
  Fentanyl
  Heroin
  Methadone
  Other pain pills

- **Stimulants**
  Amphetamine (Adderall is a combination of amphetamine and
     dextroamphetamine)
  Bath salts
  Cocaine
  Ephedrine
  Methamphetamine (meth, crystal, ice)
  Methylphenidate (Ritalin)

- **Sedatives**
  Ambien, Lunesta, Rozerem (for sleep)
  Barbiturates (amobarbital, pentobarbital, phenobarbital,
      secobarbital)
  Chloral hydrate
  GHB (gamma-hydroxybutyrate)
  Glutethimide
  Methaqualone (Quaaludes, ludes)

- **Nicotine**
  Clove cigarettes
  Tobacco

- **Marijuana**

- **Ecstasy/Molly**
  MDA (3,4-methylenedioxyamphetamine)
  MDEA (3,4-methylenedioxyethylamphetamine)
  MDMA (3,4-methylenedioxymethamphetamine)

- **Hallucinogens** (A small number of medical practitioners
      favor the use of hallucinogens in healing therapies; not all
      hallucinogens are addictive.)
  Alkaloids (belladonna, atropine, scopolamine, nightshade, etc.)
  Dextromethorphan
  Dimethyltryptamine (DMT)
  Ketamine (special K, K)
  LSD (acid, blotter, microdot, sunshine)
  Mescaline (peyote, mescal)
  Phencyclidine (PCP, angel dust)
  Psilocybin mushrooms (magic mushrooms)
  Salvia divinorum

- **Inhalants**
  Anesthesia agents (nitrous oxide, halothane, etc.)
  Nitrites (butyl- or amyl-)
  Solvents, sprays, paints, fuel (toluene, gas, glues, canned paint)

- **Herbal medication**
  Kratom

BEHAVIORAL ADDICTIONS

Codependent relationships
Digital: the internet, online gambling, social media, video gaming
Exercise
Food
Gambling
Impulse-control addictions: explosive anger, setting fires, stealing
Money
Pornography
Sex
Shopping
Work

APPENDIX 3

Essential Oils for Anxiety and Sleep

Essential oils are volatile liquids extracted from plants that can be used for medicinal purposes as well as to make homemade household and beauty products, including nontoxic laundry detergent, spray cleaner, makeup, and lotions. Some swear by them; others have no idea what they are. Although progressive medical professionals and naturopaths enthusiastically recommend essential oils in their medical practices, my more conventional medical colleagues tend to dismiss the use of essential oils as "quackery" (without ever having tried them).

Although they may be a bit overhyped by companies trying to sell them at a markup, essential oils can be helpful when you are trying to regain your health. This is not just my opinion. There are now hundreds of scientific studies that show that essential oils have medicinal benefit.[1] A study by Chinese researchers, for example, showed that myrrh can inhibit the growth of prostate cancer cells,[2] and several studies have shown that peppermint oil (the leaves of which have antispasmodic effects) can be helpful in the treatment of irritable bowel syndrome[3] and headaches.[4]

Which brand do you buy? Stay away from the aggressively marketed and expensive "name brand" essential oil lines and instead look for organic essential oils available inexpensively from health-food stores or online. With the exception of frankincense, most essential oils are very affordable. A bottle of organic lavender oil costs about $15. Since you only use a few drops at a time, it will last a long while.

How do you use essential oils? Essential oils can be inhaled via an essential oil diffuser, which disperses the oil into the air. A drop or two can be added to bathwater or to a base like coconut oil or your favorite moisturizer and then applied to the skin. You can also make a compress by soaking a washcloth in either hot or cold water that contains a few drops of oil and then applying it to your skin.

Though you will see some enthusiastic recommendations on the internet to use essential oils in cooking and take them internally, they may not be as safe to ingest, even diluted. I'd rather you be cautious. So if you want to drink lemon water, skip using essential oil and squeeze fresh lemon juice into your water instead. That said, herbal teas made from plants and herbs used to distill oils can be beneficial to your health. If you find that an essential oil is helping you sleep or relax, try an organic tea containing the same herb.

I mentioned in chapter 10 that some essential oils can help with sleep. You can find premade roll-on sleepy oil blends or balms or experiment with making your own (by combining drops of oil with fractionated coconut oil as the base). Applying a drop to the back of your neck and the soles of your feet before bed can be a calming and positive part of your nighttime sleep routine.

The effects are usually subtle, which means that the best essential oils to help with sleep can also usually help calm daytime anxiety. Try some or all of these oils and see how they make you feel:

Chamomile: A common ingredient in sleepy-time teas, chamomile has been shown to have antidepressant and anti-anxiety properties. One small placebo-controlled study done by researchers at the University of Pennsylvania found that chamomile helped with depression.[5] Don't use this oil if you are allergic to ragweed.

Bergamot: Shown to increase GABA levels and reduce the stress response in rats,[6] bergamot has a spicy, citrusy aroma that many find soothing. The oil from the peel of bergamot (which is a variety of orange) is what gives Earl Grey tea its distinct flavor. It is widely used in aromatherapy to reduce stress and anxiety.

Lavender oil: Its intoxicating scent and calming properties make lavender oil among the most popular essential oils. Some of my patients use it as perfume, as it is safe to put lavender oil directly on your skin. Put a drop in each palm, cup your palms, and inhale the scent deeply just before bed, or apply it to the back of your neck, your wrists, and the soles of your feet. This oil can also be used as a mood enhancer throughout the day.

Rose oil: Several studies have shown that rose oil increases feelings of comfort and relaxation.[7] The floral aroma is quite strong, and most rose oil is sold highly diluted already. If you like the smell of roses, you will find deep comfort in adding a drop of rose oil to your bathwater. If you have never tried rose tea, you're also in for a treat.

Ylang ylang: If you find yourself with a lot of brain spin at night, add ylang ylang to your sleep balm or Epsom-salt bath. This fragrant oil goes nicely with bergamot (see above) and can help with stress reduction[8] and lowering blood pressure.[9]

Suggestions for Further Reading

Understanding what has pushed you to the severe end of the addiction spectrum and kept you there involves understanding every aspect of your physical, emotional, and spiritual health. To truly recover from addiction, you must take back your health. Below are some of the books that have helped me both professionally and personally, as an addiction specialist and a recovering alcoholic. I don't expect you to read them all, but my hope is that you can find a book—or several—on this list that will be helpful to you right now, right where you are in your journey back toward the mild and safe end of the spectrum.

Adam Alter. *Irresistible: The Rise of Addictive Technology and the Business of Keeping Us Hooked* (Penguin, 2017). A good book to read if you're concerned that you may be addicted to your smartphone, email, gaming, television, online shopping, or binge-watching. Alter, an Associate Professor of Marketing at New York University, walks readers through how tech designers have used our understanding of human evolution to purposefully get us hooked.

Jeffrey Bland, MD. *The Disease Delusion: Conquering the Causes of Chronic Illness for a Healthier, Longer, and Happier Life* (Harper Wave, 2014). A primer on integrative medicine. Bland is a visionary medical doctor and one of the founders of functional medicine. He dispels the myth that you are destined for disease and that you need a laundry list of medications to keep you healthy. This book teaches you the keys to lasting good health.

Roy Eskapa, PhD. *The Cure for Alcoholism: The Medically Proven Way to Eliminate Alcohol Addiction* (BenBella Books, first published 2008, revised 2012). A well-done book that offers tools to help you recover from alcoholism, understand the root causes of addiction, and implement the Sinclair Method, an option that can work for some on the mild end of the addiction spectrum.

Joel Fuhrman, MD. *The End of Dieting: How to Live for Life* (HarperOne, 2015). Joel Fuhrman is a board-certified family physician best known for his *New York Times* bestseller *Eat to Live* (Little, Brown, 2011). All of his books are fantastic: he promotes a formula for health where you divide the nutrient value of your food by the calories. He promotes healthy eating, which includes maximizing vegetables and minimizing unhealthy foods. *Fast Food Genocide* (HarperOne, 2017) is his most recent book. Along with how and what to eat, this book deals with food addiction and explains how food withdrawal is akin to withdrawal from drugs and alcohol.

Annie Grace. *This Naked Mind: Control Alcohol, Find Freedom, Discover Happiness & Change Your Life* (Avery, 2015). A readable, honest, moving book that details Grace's slide from problem drinking into alcoholism and offers practical advice to help you make informed, conscious decisions about whether to drink.

Caroline Knapp. *Drinking: A Love Story* (Dial, 1996). A raw and heartbreaking literary memoir detailing twenty years living as a high-functioning closeted alcoholic. Knapp was a fearless newspaper reporter and columnist from an upper-middle-class family. She passed away from lung cancer at age forty-two.

Ben Lynch, ND. *Dirty Genes: A Breakthrough Program to Treat the Root Cause of Illness and Optimize Your Health* (HarperOne, 2018). You've heard that you have genetic risks for various health issues. Lynch is one of the leading authorities on genetic vulnerabilities. His book gives you specific simple instructions about what you can do to remove the negative effects of problem genetics. You'll be happy to learn these are mostly lifestyle changes that each and every one of us can make to have optimal health.

Gabor Maté, MD. *In the Realm of Hungry Ghosts: Close Encounters with Addiction* (North Atlantic, 2010). Maté painfully lays out the issues surrounding addiction. Working at a clinic that caters to homeless addicts in Vancouver, British Columbia, he offers a compassionate look at the lives of strung-out drug users and emphasizes the importance of human connectedness for recovery.

Deanna Minich, PhD. *Whole Detox: A 21-Day Personalized Program to Break Through Barriers in Every Area of Your Life* (HarperOne, 2016). Minich has a PhD in nutritional biochemistry and a magical way of explaining her ideas. This book teaches you how to use food to detox and heal your body.

David Perlmutter, MD. *Brain Maker: The Power of Gut Microbes to Heal and Protect Your Brain—for Life* (Little, Brown, 2015). This book explains the powerful role the gut plays in brain health and how to improve your gut microbiome to improve your health.

Joe Pizzorno, ND. *The Toxin Solution: How Hidden Poisons in the Air, Water, Food, and Products We Use Are Destroying Our Health—AND WHAT WE CAN DO TO FIX IT* (HarperOne, 2017). By eliminating toxins you can avoid you can lessen the negative effects of toxins you can't avoid. This is an excellent book filled with useful tips that will help you make lifestyle changes that will become the foundation of your health and recovery journey.

Samuel Quinones. *Dreamland: The True Tale of America's Opiate Epidemic* (Bloomsbury, 2015). A thoroughly researched and highly readable account by an investigative journalist of how the pharmaceutical industry's aggressive marketing of opioids has helped fuel the epidemic of addiction in the United States.

Julie Valenti. *Knowing How: 20 Concepts to Rewire the Brain* (Manitou Communications, 2016). If you're recovering from childhood trauma, you may not know how to process that pain without letting it overwhelm you. Valenti lays out the journey for you. She also offers remote classes that can be accessed from anywhere. I witnessed a miraculous transformation in my wife as Maiya worked through this book and attended an intensive workshop.

12-Step Recovery Books

If you go to AA or any other 12-step program, you will quickly become familiar with AA books, which are sometimes distributed for free and can usually be purchased at cost. The main book is *Alcoholics Anonymous: The Story of How Many Thousands of Men and Women Have Recovered from Alcoholism* (4th ed., 2001), often affectionately called the "Big Book." I recommend anyone dealing with any kind of addiction read the first 164 pages of the Big Book, which remain unchanged since the first printing. This is the guide alcoholics have followed for almost eighty years and remains the foundation for the AA organization, which now has over 60,000 meetings and a million members in the US and about 120,000 meetings and over 2 million members worldwide.

Al-Anon's Twelve Steps & Twelve Traditions (revised edition, 2005). Al-Anon is the organization for families of those struggling with addictions. The benefits are sometimes essential for your loved one's recovery journey and your own. You learn to focus on your journey and how to set loving but firm and appropriate boundaries.

Twelve Steps and Twelve Traditions, by Alcoholics Anonymous (2002). The second most important AA text, this book offers a more in-depth review of each of the twelve steps to guide you as you work through them.

Bill P., Todd W., and Sara S. *Drop the Rock: Removing Character Defects—Steps Six and Seven* (Hazelden, 2005). The book starts with the story of Mary swimming to catch the boat heading to an island called Serenity. She can't seem to reach it in time, can't swim fast enough to catch it, and is unable to drop the rock around her neck that is slowing her down. That rock represents the resentments, fear, dishonesty, self-pity, intolerance, and anger among other things that hold you back. This book is a masterpiece, helping you to "drop the rock."

Thérèse Jacobs-Stewart. *Mindfulness and the 12 Steps: Living Recovery in the Present Moment* (Hazelden, 2010). Meditation is something many addicts just can't quiet their minds enough to do. This book teaches you mindfulness with simple examples and practical exercises.

Resources

There are hundreds of nonprofit organizations, websites, videos, podcasts, workbooks, and articles to help you during recovery from addiction. The feel of every meeting and online chat group is different. Ask for recommendations from your doctors, counselors, friends of Bill W., and social-media connections and anyone else you know in recovery. The local library is also a great place to find community events and other helpful resources. You may find the approach that resonates with you right away, or it may take some digging. But once you are committed to recovery, you will find the help that's right for you, both online and in real life. The following is by no means an exhaustive list but provides some places to start.

Adult Children of Alcoholics: http://www.adultchildren.org; 310-534-1815. ACA, also known as ACoA, is a self-help, self-supporting program to help adults who were raised in alcoholic or other dysfunctional families. Like AA, it is a spiritual 12-step organization and it asks attendees to seek help from a Higher Power. ACA currently hosts over 1,750 meetings throughout the United States.

Al-Anon: https://al-anon.org; 757-563-1600. A self-help support group for family members of people with drinking problems, including parents, siblings, and loved ones. It welcomes anyone who has been affected by someone else's drinking. **Alateen**, which is part of Al-Anon, is the Al-Anon program for teenagers: a peer-to-peer support network for teens who are being negatively affected by someone else's drinking problem.

Alcoholics Anonymous: https://www.aa.org; 212-870-3400. An international fellowship of people battling alcoholism. AA was founded by Bill Wilson and a doctor named Bob Smith in 1935 in Akron, Ohio, and now has its worldwide headquarters in New York City. Anyone with a drinking problem is welcome, and all services are given anonymously and free of charge. AA has its members work together in groups and one-on-one with a sponsor through a 12-step program that is outlined in what they call the "Big Book," which was first written by cofounder Bill W. in 1939. They hold free meetings in the United States and nearly ninety countries worldwide.

American Society of Addiction Medicine: https://www.asam.org; 301-656-3920. The professional organization of addiction specialists, ASAM hosts an annual conference and offers patient resources, which include provider locator tools.

A Big Book Study for Compulsive Eaters: http://www.oabigbook.info/basicpage .html. A useful free website inspired by but independent of Overeaters Anonymous that has dozens of podcasts you can download to help you work a food addiction recovery program.

Celebrate Recovery: http://www.celebraterecovery.com; 949-609-8000. A Bible-centered, Christ-centered 12-step program that began in 1991 in Lake Forest, California, that applies the healing power of Jesus Christ to recovery.

Dual Recovery Anonymous: http://www.draonline.org; 913-991-2703. An independent self-help membership organization based on the 12 Steps and geared toward people who have dual diagnoses of addiction and an emotional or psychiatric illness. Based in Prairie Village, Kansas, DRA currently hosts meetings in the United States, Canada, Iceland, India, Australia, and New Zealand and has a wealth of information on their website.

FoodRelapse.com: http://www.foodrelapse.com. A free website that focuses on food addiction and relapse, through the lens of 12-step recovery.

LifeRing Secular Recovery: https://lifering.org; 1-800-811-4142. A secular recovery program that is sometimes seen as an alternative to 12-step programs, LifeRing promotes positive, practical, present-day, individualized solutions to addiction. LifeRing teaches that addicts have the power within themselves to overcome addiction and seeks to help users recover their "Sober Self." Based in Hayward, California, they host meetings in person and online in the United States, Canada, and abroad.

Local grief groups: Many hospitals and nonprofits host bereavement groups that can be a place of healing and profound support. If it was a shocking event—like divorce or a sudden death—that pushed you toward the severe end of the addiction spectrum, look for a grief support group to help you process what happened. You can find a list of grief groups in your area via https://www .psychologytoday.com/us/groups/grief.

Narcotics Anonymous: https://www.na.org; 818-773-9999. NA is a 12-step program that offers support to addicts recovering from any drug addiction. There are also other groups, such as Cocaine Anonymous (CA) and Heroin Anonymous (HA), that focus on specific drug addictions.

Rational Recovery: https://rational.org; 530-621-2667. According to RR, "recovery is not a process, but an event." This organization offers an individualized recovery approach emphasizing that addiction and recovery are personal challenges that can be resolved on your own. RR promotes recovery without groups, counselors, or rehabilitation centers. You can find a crash course on the RR approach (which is called "Addictive Voice Recognition Technique"), as well as videos and articles on their website.

SMART Recovery: https://www.smartrecovery.org; 866-951-5357. A nonprofit that supports abstinence from any type of addiction by teaching self-empowerment and self-reliance. SMART stands for "Self-Management and Recovery Training." It is a secular alternative to 12-step programs and relies on cognitive behavioral therapy. Their 4-Point Program focuses on building and maintaining motivation; coping with urges; managing thoughts, feelings, and behaviors; and living a balanced life. Based in Mentor, Ohio, they have online meetings and chat rooms and over three hundred face-to-face meetings around the world.

Women for Sobriety, Inc.: http://womenforsobriety.org; 215-536-8026. An abstinence-focused self-help program for women struggling with alcohol and drug addiction. Their program is based on positive thinking, manifesting your own happiness, interactive discussion, meditation, and good nutrition. Based in Quakertown, Pennsylvania, WFS hosts nearly seventy meetings in the United States and Canada and also has online peer support.

Glossary

ADD: Attention deficit disorder. People with ADD struggle to maintain focus on tasks, are easily distracted, tend to daydream, and often have difficulty with organization and following through. ADD and ADHD (see below) are conditions that affect over 5 percent of children worldwide[1] and up to 18 percent of children in the US.[2]

ADHD: Attention deficit hyperactivity disorder. In addition to the attention issues of those with ADD, people with ADHD are very active and impulsive. They can't sit still or relax. A thorough medical and psychological evaluation is usually necessary to diagnose ADHD. In order to make a diagnosis, doctors look for symptoms of restlessness, hyperactivity, and inability to concentrate that last six months and occur in more than one setting.

adrenal fatigue: A term applied to a host of symptoms, including exhaustion, nervousness, body aches, and sleep disturbances that are thought to be caused by chronic physical and emotional stress. If your adrenal glands are overproducing hormones, either in response to actual or perceived stress or because they are being stimulated by something like caffeine, they cease to work in their natural cycle to effectively control your hormones. When the normal daily rhythm of cortisol production by the adrenal glands becomes compromised, you can experience excessive fatigue, sleep issues, mood and concentration issues as well as hair loss, unexplained weight loss, lightheadedness, and low blood pressure.

adrenal glands: Two tiny almond-shaped glands that secrete hormones, which you can think of as chemical messengers. The adrenal glands sit at the top of your kidneys. Small and mighty, they are responsible for three important hormones in the body: adrenaline, aldosterone, and cortisol. Adrenaline (also known as epinephrine) is what produces your fight-or-flight response when in danger. Aldosterone is important in sodium regulation and blood-pressure control. Cortisol is a major stress hormone that helps maintain body temperature, blood sugar, and a healthy immune system. Dehydroepiandrosterone (DHEA), a precursor of estrogen and testosterone, is also produced by the adrenal glands.

ALS: Amyotrophic lateral sclerosis, also known as Lou Gehrig's disease, a neurological disease that affects nerve cells in the brain and spinal cord. As the nerves that would trigger your muscles to fire harden and die, you lose voluntary muscle movement. Most people with this debilitating and degenerative disease die within three to five years of being diagnosed, though some—including the pastor Evy

McDonald[3] and the physicist Stephen Hawking—have gone on to live long productive lives.

bath salts: A slang term in the drug world having nothing to do with Epsom salts or bathing crystals. It refers to synthetic stimulants that are chemically akin to cocaine, amphetamines, and MDMA and seem to produce a similar high. These are synthetic cathinones chemically related to the naturally occurring stimulant (called cathinone) found in the khat plant, which grows in East Africa and southern Arabia. Bath salts are cheap substitutes for methamphetamine and cocaine. Side effects include increased sociability, increased sex drive, hallucinations, nosebleeds, paranoia, panic attacks, and death.

benzodiazepines: A class of legal prescription medications used to treat anxiety, panic attacks, seizures, convulsions, sleep problems, and insomnia. Benzodiazepines include alprazolam (Xanax), lorazepam (Ativan), clonazepam (Klonopin), diazepam (Valium), and temazepam (Restoril). They work by enhancing the effects of the major inhibitory neurotransmitter gamma-aminobutyric acid (GABA), which decreases brain activity. Used illegally in larger than therapeutic doses, "benzos," as they are often called, can be highly addictive. Though doctors today seem to be a little more hesitant about prescribing them, over 125 million prescriptions for benzos were written in 2011.[4]

black-tar heroin: A form of heroin that is sticky like tar or hard like coal and may be dark orange or brown in color. It is less pure and generally less expensive than the more purified white-powder heroin. It is usually dissolved in water over a heated spoon and filtered before injecting or snorting.

brain fog: A condition in which the mind is just not sharp, it's difficult to focus, and even simple instructions seem impossible to understand. In the extreme you may feel disoriented and confused. Most people going through withdrawal from drugs or alcohol will experience brain fog, which can also be caused or exacerbated by underlying illness.

cannabinoid receptors: Receptors located throughout the body that are activated by cannabinoids, both those produced by the body and those introduced into the body, to produce physiological changes involved in appetite, pain sensation, mood, memory, and even the immune system.

cannabis: The genus designation for a plant group that has two main subtypes: *Cannabis sativa* and *Cannabis indica*. Cannabis plants were traditionally used for their hemp fiber, nutritious seeds, and THC-rich flowers; the psychoactive drug THC has medical and recreational uses.

CAT scan or CT scan: A computerized axial tomography (CAT) or computerized tomography (CT) scan formed by taking the information from several X-ray images inside the body and using a computer to convert them into a three-dimensional, detailed image. CAT scans are very helpful when looking at soft tissues in the body like the brain or the abdomen.

cathinone: A substance, also known as benzoylethanamine or beta-keto-amphetamine, found in the plant *Catha edulis* (khat or qat). It acts as a stimulant much like amphetamines; bath salts are a synthetic version.

CBD: Cannabidiol, the nonaddictive, nonpsychoactive part of the cannabis plant, which is now believed to help with anxiety, inflammation, and seizures as well as nausea and vomiting.

cocaine: An illegal stimulant made from the leaves of the coca plant, which is native to South America. Most people snort a white cocaine powder, though some will smoke a crystal form (freebase) to get a more intense high.

crystal meth: The common street form of the drug methamphetamine, a white crystalline substance that people inhale through the nose, smoke, or inject. It gives you an intense euphoria, alertness, confidence, and energy. This drug is one of the most effective at raising dopamine levels, giving users such an intense euphoria that it can be highly addictive. It takes away your appetite for food. Some users will go for days without eating or sleeping, exhausting their body's dopamine stores. A couple years on meth can age you a decade or more.

DNA: Deoxyribonucleic acid, the genetic material we inherit from our parents. It is located in the nucleus of almost every cell in our body. Our DNA is made up of four nucleotide bases: adenine (A), cytosine (C), guanine (G), and thymine (T). It is the sequence of these bases, which pair up to make the classic staircase double helix, that is then arranged into chromosomes that determine what information is available for everything that happens in the body.

Ecstasy: A synthetic drug, also known as MDMA (3,4-methylenedioxymetham-phetamine), similar to the stimulant methamphetamine and the hallucinogen mescaline. It enhances physical sensitivity and pleasure, but at high doses it can dangerously increase body temperature (hyperthermia), which can cause kidney failure and death.[5]

endocrine disruptors: Chemicals like pesticides, flame retardants, and other substances that mimic actual hormones in our body, either shutting down or increasing the production of any number of our natural hormones. Endocrine disruptors can result in early onset of puberty, extreme fatigue, low testosterone, which affects energy and libido in both men and women, and other negative health effects.

fentanyl: A fast-acting narcotic used in anesthesia for pain after surgery or medical procedures. Fentanyl is one hundred times the strength of morphine and fifty times the strength of heroin. Sadly, there are now synthetic versions of fentanyl hitting the streets of America, such as carfentanil, with a potency ten thousand times that of morphine. Overdose deaths in the US are often related to abuse of fentanyl or heroin that has had fentanyl added to it.

fibromyalgia: A condition of chronic and sometimes debilitating pain mostly in the muscles and joints. People who suffer from fibromyalgia typically experience fatigue, sleep problems, memory problems, and mood issues. Often patients are sensitive to touch, smell, sound, and light and exhibit headaches, upset stomach, and exhaustion. Doctors do not know what causes fibromyalgia. However, genes, infections, exposure to toxins, and emotional and physical trauma may trigger the disease.

Frankenfood: Genetically modified food that is as scary as Frankenstein's monster's appearance. (In Mary Shelley's famous 1818 novel, *Frankenstein*, an ambitious scientist creates a monster, hideous to behold.) This term is sometimes used to refer to any highly processed edible foodlike substances that have bright colors and synthetic flavors made in a laboratory. Although genetic modification is not necessarily negative, there are no long-term safety studies on the practice of inserting genes from different species into food for human consumption. There is a growing body of scientific evidence that shows that modifying food to make it resistant to pesticides can have negative consequences for humans.

friend of Bill W.: A code phrase alcoholics sometimes use to identify each other. Bill Wilson was the cofounder of Alcoholics Anonymous. If you see the sign "Friends of Bill W." at a conference or on a cruise, this actually means "AA meeting happening here."

functional medicine: A medical approach that focuses on identifying and addressing the root cause of each person's physiological condition or disease. Rather than focusing on the diagnosis and treatment of symptoms, an approach that dominates medical care today, functional medicine goes back to genetic vulnerability, environmental exposures, and life stresses from the womb onward. It looks at major transitions and lifestyle choices that have contributed to each person's present health condition.

GABA: Gamma-aminobutyric acid, a neurotransmitter in the brain and the nervous system. As a neurotransmitter it is involved in communication between cells. GABA plays an important role in behavior, cravings, focus, and the body's ability to handle stress. GABA is thought to be calming, and when levels are low, you may suffer from insomnia, anxiety, or depression. Prescription benzodiazepines like diazepam (Valium) and lorazepam (Ativan) bind to the same receptors as GABA and mimic GABA's natural calming effects. Medications used to treat insomnia, like zolpidem (Ambien) and eszopiclone (Lunesta), improve the ability of GABA to bind to GABA receptors in the brain. GABA can also refer to supplements with mild but similar activity in the brain.

gluten: A mixture of two proteins, prolamins and glutelins, found in wheat, barley, rye, and most oats and also in spelt, khorasan, emmer, einkorn, and triticale. Gluten is like glue in baking, holding the baked product (bread, pasta, etc.) together. About 1 percent of the population has celiac disease, when eating gluten triggers the immune system to attack your own body. About 6 percent of the population is considered gluten sensitive, experiencing symptoms like upset stomach, eczema, or brain fog when gluten is consumed. My clinical experience, based on testing I've done in the last two decades, suggests that these numbers are far too low. I have found that about 50 percent of Americans are gluten sensitive.

gluten-free: Containing no gluten. Many foods in their natural state, like fruits and vegetables, meat, dairy, and nuts, are gluten-free. Some grains like rice, corn, and buckwheat are also gluten-free. Those with celiac disease and those highly sensitive to gluten must avoid all grains with gluten, even those grains milled where gluten-containing grains were processed.

glutethimide: A hypnotic sedative that is only used for research today. Introduced in 1954 as a safe alternative to barbiturates to treat insomnia, it is addictive and can induce severe withdrawal symptoms. Doriden, Elrodorm, Noxyron, and Glimid were names of this compound sold in the past.

glyphosate: N-(phosphonomethyl)glycine, an herbicide and crop desiccant. Discovered by a Swiss chemist in the 1950s and then developed into an herbicide by Monsanto in the 1970s,[6] it kills most weeds and is marketed as Roundup. It inhibits a plant enzyme needed for the synthesis of the amino acids tyrosine, tryptophan, and phenylalanine. Monsanto has developed seeds that are glyphosate tolerant, so that it can be sprayed on fields of these crops, killing all the weeds that would compete with the crop. Most corn, soy, and cotton in the US is Roundup Ready![7] There has been a three-hundredfold increase in use of glyphosate in the US since the 1970s.[8] The World Health Organization's International Agency for Research on Cancer classified glyphosate as "probably carcinogenic in humans" in 2015.[9] One study found: "Since 1974 in the U.S., over 1.6 billion kilograms of glyphosate active ingredient have been applied, or 19% of estimated global use of glyphosate (8.6 billion kilograms)."[10]

harm reduction: A treatment model in which opioid addicts are given a large enough dose of opioid medication (like methadone) in a controlled setting, so that they will get no additional benefit from further use. These patients will no longer use IV heroin and share needles, because they would get no further benefit; thus harm to society and danger to the patient is reduced. The tradeoff is that these patients are in bondage forever to their opioid addiction, which is not without side effects, such as suppression of the pituitary and all the hormone challenges that follow.

hemp: A variety of the *Cannabis sativa* plant. It is grown specifically for many industrial uses, like making rope, fabrics, fiberboard, and paper. Seeds are used to make hemp oil and hemp milk. Most hemp varieties have very little THC and may have CBD, but are not typically cultivated for CBD content.

integrative medicine: A way of practicing medicine that puts the patient at the center, addressing physical, emotional, mental, social, spiritual, and environmental influences that impact a person's health. Most integrative medicine practitioners use a variety of approaches typically including nutritional and herbal medicine and incorporating chiropractic, massage, and acupuncture along with evidenced-based approaches from mainstream allopathic, naturopathic, and homeopathic modalities.

medical marijuana: Marijuana that was recommended by a doctor in the treatment of a medical condition. We know marijuana stimulates appetite and is very helpful for those who just can't eat, for example, because of the side effects of chemotherapy. Marijuana is anti-inflammatory and has antiseizure properties. People suffering from severe chronic pain or in the last days of life often request and are treated with medical marijuana. Generally, states legalize medical marijuana first, followed by recreational marijuana.

meth: Short for methamphetamine, a synthetic drug with more rapid and lasting effects than amphetamine. While initially legally prescribed for narcolepsy (daytime sleepiness), it is now almost entirely an illegal stimulant. See also "crystal meth."

Molly: Another name for MDMA (3,4-methylenedioxymethamphetamine) or Ecstasy. It is a synthetic drug chemically similar to stimulants and hallucinogens that affect dopamine, norepinephrine, and serotonin. When taken in capsules, it is often not even MDMA, but may be bath salts.

neurotransmitter: A natural substance made in the body that is released at the end of a nerve into the synapse (the space between two connecting nerves) to transfer an impulse or signal to another nerve fiber, muscle fiber, or some other receptor. Neurotransmitters are essential for the communication that occurs between the billions of nerve cells in our brains.

normie: In AA and the addiction world, one who doesn't have craving for alcohol or drugs, can take a few sips and leave a half-full glass of alcohol on the table without finishing it, and is usually either a nondrinker or a rare light drinker. The term often also implies that "they just don't understand." Normies might be heard saying, "Why don't you just stop?" or as my mom said to me, "Why do you have to drown yourself?" To many normies, those who drink too much simply lack self-control.

osteopath: A physician who has the same number of years of training as a conventional medical doctor and takes the same board exams, but in addition has training in bodywork and spinal manipulation. Osteopaths are fully licensed physicians who can practice in all areas of medicine. The letters DO following a name stand for "Doctor of Osteopathy."

partially hydrogenated fat: An unsaturated fatty acid that has gone through the process of having hydrogen added. This term can be used interchangeably with "trans fat" (see below).

peyote: A hallucinogenic drug containing mescaline that comes from the cactus *Lophophora williamsii*, which grows in the southwestern US and Mexico. It has been traditionally used in some Native American religious ceremonies. The psychoactive effects often include hallucinations (visual or auditory effects).

phlebotomist: A person trained to draw blood from veins for testing in a medical setting. The act of inserting a needle into a vein and drawing blood up into a syringe is called venipuncture.

phytonutrients: Specific, highly beneficial, health-promoting natural chemicals that come from plants, especially fruits and vegetables. Examples include carotenoids (found in carrots), lycopene (found in tomatoes), and resveratrol (found in red grapes) as well as phytosterols (found in most plants).

pituitary function: The action of the pituitary gland in producing hormones that stimulate other organs or glands to make other hormones. Hormones are chemical signals that have their effect at a distant location in the body, usually moving through the bloodstream. The key hormones from the pituitary are:
> Adrenocorticotropin (ACTH)
> Antidiuretic hormone (ADH)
> Follicle-stimulating hormone (FSH)
> Human growth hormone (HGH)
> Luteinizing hormone (LH)
> Melanocyte-stimulating hormone (MSH)
> Oxytocin
> Prolactin (PRL)
> Thyroid-stimulating hormone (TSH)

These hormones are involved in growth, blood pressure, stress and pain relief, the body's energy and heat production (metabolism), the balance of electrolytes (salts), thyroid gland function, male and female sex organ functions, lactation (production of breast milk), uterine contractions in childbirth, and kidney function.

pituitary gland: A tiny master endocrine gland, the size of a pea, which sits near the bottom of the hypothalamus at the base of the brain. The pituitary has a surprising number of hormones under its control (*see* pituitary function) that send signals to other endocrine tissue.

primary care provider (PCP): A health-care practitioner who oversees your general health and, according to some insurance plans, the person you must see before seeing a specialist. These medical providers (who can be doctors, nurse practitioners, or physician assistants) can care for most common medical problems. They are generally involved in your care for a long time and used to be known as "the family doctor."

psychoactive: A substance, either legal or illegal, that acts on the brain, changing perception, mood, consciousness, or behavior.

schizophrenia: A label used by doctors (mostly by psychiatrists) for patients who have psychotic symptoms like hallucinations and hearing voices. People suffering from schizophrenia are often paranoid—showing fear beyond the situation at hand—and have distorted perceptions, beliefs, and behaviors. They have trouble starting anything new, expressing emotion, finding pleasure, and sometimes even speaking. They may be confused and sometimes have bizarre behavior or movements. It is hard for them to pay attention, concentrate, and remember things. These symptoms can come and go.

sex hormones: Estrogen, progesterone, and testosterone, which are produced by our ovaries (women), testes (men), and adrenal glands. Sex hormones are important for normal development and function of reproductive organs (ovaries and uterus, testes and penis) and are the driving force at puberty and in pregnancy.

SNPs: Single-nucleotide polymorphisms, variations in single nucleotides (think of a single letter change) at a specific position in your DNA or RNA sequence. Nucleotides are the building blocks of DNA or RNA. There are just four of them in your DNA, adenine, cytosine, guanine, and thymine. With RNA, thymine is replaced by uracil. We each have about 10 million SNPs.[11] An example of an SNP would be that, at a particular position in the human genome where for most people the C nucleotide appears, in some individuals there is an A there. This means that there is an SNP at this specific position. This variation can have positive or negative health consequences. SNPs may allow us to adapt to environmental changes. Variations in these sequences of nucleotides can alter enzyme functions in the body, among other things.

THC: Tetrahydrocannabinol, the chemical responsible for most of marijuana's psychological effects, especially the euphoria it produces in some. It acts on the same receptors in our brain that natural cannabinoids act on. Activating the cannabinoid receptors with THC affects thinking, memory, pleasure, coordination, perceptions of hunger, and time perception.

thyroid disorder: Malfunction of the thyroid gland in which it is either overactive, as in the early stages of Hashimoto's disease, or underactive and no longer secreting enough thyroid hormone. In either situation you experience a host of unpleasant health consequences. Most thyroid disorders are highly treatable.

thyroid gland: The small gland at the base of the front of the neck that regulates growth and development, the rate of metabolism, heart rate, blood pressure, and body temperature.

toxin: Any poisonous substance produced by bacteria, animals, or plants. In this book and often in general conversation, the term "toxin" refers to anything that is harmful to the normal function of the body. Notable toxins include poisons like arsenic, heavy metals like mercury, and anything that negatively affects normal endocrine, brain, or other body functions.

trans fat: A trans-fatty acid, a fat made from liquid oils through a chemical process of adding hydrogen. This increases the food's shelf life and stability, but also makes it harmful to human health.

withdrawal: The symptoms that occur when you can no longer engage in your addiction, whether that is to drugs, alcohol, or certain behaviors. Withdrawal symptoms are both physical and psychological. They vary in severity depending on the addiction and are often unpleasant, even debilitating, for a short time. Everyone experiences withdrawal symptoms differently, depending on the drug in question, how long you have used it, and how much you were using. Withdrawal symptoms from opioids, for example, often include anxiety, sweating, vomiting, diarrhea, runny nose, chills, and leg or muscle spasms. Withdrawal symptoms from alcohol can include confusion, hallucinations, delirium tremens, seizures, and even death. When withdrawing from anything that brought pleasure, most recovering addicts will experience depression, anxiety, fatigue, brain fog, feelings of purposelessness, and a lack of motivation.

Notes

Introduction

1   Nicholas Carr, "How Smartphones Hijack Our Minds," *Wall Street Journal*, October 6, 2017, https://www.wsj.com/articles/how-smartphones-hijack-our-minds-1507307811.

2   "The Surgeon General's Priorities," *US Department of Health and Human Services*, accessed December 4, 2017, https://www.surgeongeneral.gov/priorities/index.html.

3   In 2015, 52,404 people died of drug overdoses, according to the CDC; 37,757 died in car crashes, according to the National Safety Council.

4   "Drug Overdose Deaths in the United States Continue to Increase in 2015," *Centers for Disease Control and Prevention*, last updated August 30, 2017, https://www.cdc.gov/drugoverdose/epidemic /index.html.

5   "Key Substance Use and Mental Health Indicators in the United States: Results from the 2015 National Survey on Drug Use and Health," HHS Publication No. SMA 16-4984, NSDUH Series H-51 (Rockville, MD: Center for Behavioral Health Statistics and Quality, 2016), accessed December 4, 2017, http://www.samhsa.gov/data/.

6   Larry A. Kroutil, "Prescription Drug Use and Misuse in the United States: Results from the 2015 National Survey on Drug Use and Health," *NSDUH Data Review* (September 2016), accessed December 4, 2017, https://www.samhsa.gov/data/sites/default/files/NSDUH-FFR2-2015/NSDUH -FFR2-2015.htm.

7   "Opioid Overdose: Understanding the Epidemic," *Centers for Disease Control and Prevention*, August 30, 2017, https://www.cdc.gov/drugoverdose/epidemic/index.html.

8   "The Surgeon General's Priorities."

9   Josh Katz, "Drug Deaths in America Are Rising Faster Than Ever," *New York Times*, June 5, 2017, https://www.nytimes.com/interactive/2017/06/05/upshot/opioid-epidemic-drug-overdose-deaths -are-rising-faster-than-ever.html.

10 German Lopez, "In One Year, Drug Overdoses Killed More Americans than the Entire Vietnam War Did," *Vox*, June 8, 2017, https://www.vox.com/policy-and-politics/2017/6/6/15743986/opioid -epidemic-overdose-deaths-2016.

11 "Alcohol Facts and Statistics," National Institute of Alcohol Abuse and Alcoholism, updated June 2017, https://www.niaaa.nih.gov/alcohol-health/overview-alcohol-consumption/alcohol-facts -and-statistics.

12 "Alcohol and Public Health: Alcohol-Related Disease Impact (ARDI): Average for United States 2006–2010, Alcohol-Attributable Deaths Due to Excessive Alcohol Use," *Centers for Disease Control and Prevention*, 2013, accessed December 4, 2017, https://nccd.cdc.gov/DPH_ARDI/Default /Report.aspx?T=AAM&P=f6d7eda7-036e-4553-9968-9b17ffad620e&R=d7a9b303-48e9-4440 -bf47-070a4827e1fd&M=8E1C5233-5640-4EE8-9247-1ECA7DA325B9&F=&D=.

13 There were more than 63,600 drug-overdose deaths in 2016. Holly Hedegaard et al., *Drug Overdose Deaths in the United States, 1999–2016*, NCHS Data Brief No. 294 (Hyattsville, MD: National Center for Health Statistics, 2017).

14 There were 40,200 motor vehicle deaths in 2016. National Safety Council, "NSC Motor Vehicle Fatality Estimates," accessed January 25, 2018, www.nsc.org/NewsDocuments/2017/12-month -estimates.pdf.

15 Candice L. Odgers et al., "Is It Important to Prevent Early Exposure to Drugs and Alcohol Among Adolescents?" *Psychological Science* 19 (2008): 1037–44, doi: 10.1111/j.1467-9280.2008.02196.x.

Chapter 1: Where Are You on the Addiction Spectrum?

1 Andrew Seaman, "More Than a Third of US Adults Prescribed Opioids in 2015," *Health News*, July 31, 2017, https://www.reuters.com/article/us-health-opioids-prescriptions/more-than-a-third-of-us-adults-prescribed-opioids-in-2015-idUSKBN1AG2K6; Beth Han et al., "Prescription Opioid Use, Misuse, and Use Disorders in U.S. Adults: 2015 National Survey on Drug Use and Health," September 3, 2017, http://annals.org/aim/article-abstract/2646632/prescription-opioid-use-misuse-use-disorders-u-s-adults-2015; "Prescription Opioid Overdose Data," *Centers for Disease Control and Prevention*, August 1, 2017, https://www.cdc.gov/drugoverdose/data/overdose.html.

2 Martin H. Teicher et al., "Childhood Maltreatment Is Associated with Reduced Volume in the Hippocampal Subfields CA3, Dentate Gyrus, and Subiculum," *PNAS* 109 (2012): E563–72, doi: 10.1073/pnas.1115396109; S. Wilson et al., "Problematic Alcohol Use and Reduced Hippocampal Volume: A Meta-Analytic Review," October 2017, https://www.cambridge.org/core/journals/psychological-medicine/article/problematic-alcohol-use-and-reduced-hippocampal-volume-a-metaanalytic-review/CF8CD1B418243DB4D9513F0EA301A6B7.

3 Severin Haug et al., "Predictors of Onset of Cannabis and Other Drug Use in Male Young Adults: Results from a Longitudinal Study," *BMC Public Health* 14 (2014): 1202, doi: 10.11 86/14 71-2458 -14-1202; James Hall, "Children Whose Parents Divorce 'More Likely' to Become Binge Drinkers," *The Telegraph*, August 28, 2011, http://www.telegraph.co.uk/news/uknews/8728398/Children-whose-parents-divorce-more-likely-to-become-binge-drinkers.html.

4 K. Beesdo et al., "Anxiety and Anxiety Disorders in Children and Adolescents: Developmental Issues and Implications for DSM-V," *Psychiatric Clinics of North America* 32 (2009): 483–524, doi: 10.1016/j.psc.2009.06.002.

5 Barbara J. McMorris et al., "Influence of Family Factors and Supervised Alcohol Use on Adolescent Alcohol Use and Harms: Similarities Between Youth in Different Alcohol Policy Contexts," *Journal of Studies on Alcohol and Drugs* 72 (2011): 418–28, https://www.ncbi.nlm.nih.gov/pmc/articles/PMC3084357/.

6 Rachel Lipari et al., "Risk and Protective Factors and Initiation of Substance Use: Results from the 2014 National Survey on Drug Use and Health," *NSDUH Data Review* (October 2015), NSDUH -DR-FRR4-2014.pdf.

7 State Reports from the 2016 NSDUH, "2015–2016 NSDUH State Prevalence Estimates," *Substance Abuse and Mental Health Services Administration*, last updated December 7, 2017, https://www.samhsa.gov/samhsa-data-outcomes-quality/major-data-collections/state-reports-NSDUH-2016.

8 2010 Statistical Abstract: State Rankings, "Resident Population, 2009," United States Census Bureau, last updated September 3, 2015, https://www.census.gov/library/publications/2009/compendia/statab/129ed/rankings.htm.

9 "13-Year-Old Boy Dies of Suspected Heroin Overdose," *CBS News*, April 4, 2017, http://www.cbsnews.com/news/nathan-wylie-13-year-old-boy-dies-of-suspected-heroin-overdose/.

10 "Mom's Post Goes Viral After Daughter Nearly Dies of Alcohol Poisoning," *Boston25News*, last updated September 7, 2016, http://www.fox25boston.com/news/moms-post-goes-viral-after-daughter-nearly-dies-on-alcohol-poisoning/435111091.

11 Ron Savage, "Warren Teen Dead in Heroin Overdose; Adult Neighbors Charged," *Fox2*, last updated January 27, 2017, http://www.fox2detroit.com/news/local-news/232034710-story.

12 David Parnell, "What Is Methamphetamine?" *Facing the Dragon*, accessed January 19, 2018, http://www.facingthedragon.org/whatismeth.htm.

13 Brandon was quoting chap. 3, "More About Alcoholism," in *Alcoholics Anonymous: The Story of How Many Thousands of Men and Women Have Recovered from Alcoholism*, 3rd rev. ed. (New York: Alcoholics Anonymous World Services, 1976), 43.

Chapter 2: Myths and Facts About Addiction

1 Elizabeth Reisinger Walker and Benjamin G. Druss, "Cumulative Burden of Comorbid Mental Disorders, Substance Use Disorders, Chronic Medical Conditions, and Poverty on Health Among Adults in the U.S.A.," *Psychology, Health and Medicine* 22 (2017): 727–35, doi.org/10.1080/135485 06.2016.1227855.

2   "Cancer Stat Facts: Cancer of Any Site," *National Cancer Institute*, accessed January 19, 2018, https://seer.cancer.gov/statfacts/html/all.html.

3   "The Brain-Gut Connection," *Johns Hopkins Medicine*, accessed January 19, 2018, https://www .hopkinsmedicine.org/health/healthy_aging/healthy_body/the-brain-gut-connection.

4   G. Vighi et al, "Allergy and the Gastrointestinal System," *Clinical and Experimental Immunology* 153 Supp. 1 (2008): 3–6, doi: 10.1111/j.1365-2249.2008.03713.x.

5   "ASAM Releases New Definition of Addiction," *ASAM News* 26 (2011): 1; "Definition of Addiction," *American Society of Addiction Medicine*, adopted April 19, 2011, accessed January 19, 2018, https://www.asam.org/resources/definition-of-addiction.

6   James White and G. David Batty, "Intelligence Across Childhood in Relation to Illegal Drug Use in Adulthood: 1970 British Cohort Study," *Journal of Epidemiology and Community Health*, November 14, 2011, doi: 10.1136/jech-2011-200252. See also James White, Catharine R. Gale, and David Batty, "Intelligence Quotient in Childhood and the Risk of Illegal Drug Use in Middle Age: The 1958 National Child Development Survey," *Annals of Epidemiology* 22/9 (September 2012): 654–57.

7   M. F. Fouad et al., "Ethanol Production by Selected Intestinal Microorganisms and Lactic Acid Bacteria Growing Under Different Nutritional Conditions," *Frontiers in Microbiology* 7 (2016): 47, doi: 10.3389/fmicb.2016.00047.

8   Andrew Lee Butters, "Is Yemen Chewing Itself to Death?" *Time*, August 25, 2009, http://content .time.com/time/world/article/0,8599,1917685,00.html.

9   Andrew Weil, MD, and Winifred Rosen, *From Chocolate to Morphine*, rev. ed. (New York: Houghton Mifflin, 2004), 29.

10   "Fact Sheets: Underage Drinking," *Centers for Disease Control and Prevention*, last updated October 20, 2016, http://www.cdc.gov/alcohol/fact-sheets/underage-drinking.htm.

11   "Principles of Adolescent Substance Use Disorder Treatment: A Research-Based Guide," *National Institute on Drug Abuse*, last updated January 2014, https://www.drugabuse.gov/publications /principles-adolescent-substance-use-disorder-treatment-research-based-guide/frequently-asked -questions/it-possible-teens-to-become-addicted-to-marijuana.

12   Danielle M. Dick and Arpana Agrawal, "The Genetics of Alcohol and Other Drug Dependence," *Alcohol Research and Health* 31 (2008): 111–18, https://pubs.niaaa.nih.gov/publications/arh312 /111-118.pdf.

Chapter 3: How Medical Doctors, Pharmaceutical Companies, the Food Industry, and Our Stressed-out Lives Push Us Toward Addiction

1   Cheryl Corley, "Autopsy Report: Prince Died of an Accidental Overdose," *NPR Morning Edition*, June 3, 2016, https://www.npr.org/2016/06/03/480564725/autopsy-report-prince-died-of -accidental-overdose.

2   Drug Enforcement Administration, "DEA Issues Nationwide Alert on Fentanyl as Threat to Health and Public Safety," news release, March 18, 2015, https://www.dea.gov/divisions/hq/2015 /hq031815.shtml.

3   "How Dangerous Is Fentanyl?" YouTube video, 00:48, from CNN, published May 10, 2016, https://www.youtube.com/watch?v=AAfFBQNuZ3U.

4   "Epidural and Spinal Anesthesia Use During Labor: 27-state Reporting Area, 2008," *National Vital Statistics Report* 59/05, 14 pp. (PHS) 2011-1120, *Centers for Disease Control and Prevention*, accessed December 8, 2017, https://www.cdc.gov/nchs/products/nvsr.htm.

5   "Fentanyl Citrate Injection, USP," *Food and Drug Administration*, accessed December 4, 2017, https://www.accessdata.fda.gov/drugsatfda_docs/label/2013/016619s034lbl.pdf.

6   The idea that fentanyl rapidly crosses the placenta is confirmed by the manufacturer's information. According to the manufacturer: "Fentanyl readily passes across the placenta to the fetus; therefore, Duragesic® is not recommended for analgesia during labor and delivery." https://www .accessdata.fda.gov/drugsatfda_docs/label/2005/19813s039lbl.pdf.

7   Louana George, personal communication.

8   A. B. Ransjö-Arvidson et al., "Maternal Analgesia During Labor Disturbs Newborn Behavior: Effects on Breastfeeding, Temperature, and Crying," *Birth* 28 (2001): 5–12, http://www.ncbi.nlm .nih.gov/pubmed/11264622.

9   Jan Riordan et al., "The Effect of Labor Pain Relief Medication on Neonatal Suckling and Breastfeeding Duration," *Journal of Human Lactation* 16 (2000): 7–12, doi: 10.1177/08903344 0001600103.

10 Marsha Walker, "Do Labor Medications Affect Breastfeeding?" *Journal of Human Lactation* 13 (1997): 131–37, doi: 10.1177/089033449701300214.

11 Marisa N. Spann, "Morphological Features of the Neonatal Brain Following Exposure to Regional Anesthesia During Labor and Delivery," *Magnetic Resonance Imaging* 33 (2015): 213–21, https://doi .org/10.1016/j.mri.2014.08.033.

12 Gregory Smith, personal communication.

13 Louana George, personal communication.

14 "Number of Children and Adolescents Taking Psychiatric Drugs in the U.S.," *Citizens Commission on Human Rights International*, accessed December 4, 2017, https://www.cchrint.org/psychiatric -drugs/children-on-psychiatric-drugs.

15 Kathleen Ries Merikangas et al., "Lifetime Prevalence of Mental Disorders in U.S. Adolescents: Results from the National Comorbidity Survey Replication–Adolescent Supplement (NCS-A)," *Journal of the American Academy of Child and Adolescent Psychiatry* 49 (2010): 980–89, doi: http:// dx.doi.org/10.1016/j.jaac.2010.05.017.

16 E. D. Kantor et al., "Trends in Prescription Drug Use Among Adults in the United States from 1999–2012," *Journal of the American Medical Association* 17 (2015): 1818–31, doi: 10.1001/jama .2015.13766.

17 Anna Lembke, *Drug Dealer, MD* (Baltimore: Johns Hopkins University Press, 2016), 25.

18 "Reducing Opioid Overdose and Misuse," *Oregon Health Authority*, accessed December 6, 2017, http://www.oregon.gov/oha/ph/preventionwellness/substanceuse/opioids/Pages/index.aspx.

19 "Oregon Had the 28th Highest Rate of Injury Deaths in U.S.," *Trust for America's Health*, news release, June 17, 2015, http://healthyamericans.org/reports/injuryprevention15/release .php?stateid=OR.

20 Hailey Branson-Potts, "Doctor Allegedly Prescribed Narcotics After Examining Dog X-Ray," *Los Angeles Times*, July 2, 2015, http://beta.latimes.com/local/lanow/la-me-ln-doctor-dog-x-ray -arrested-20150701-story.html.

21 Dave Bartkowiak Jr., "Dearborn 'Pill Mill' Raid: Doctor, Clinic Worker Arraigned on Drug Charges," *Click on Detroit*, updated August 18, 2017, https://www.clickondetroit.com/news /dearborn-pill-mill-raid-doctor-clinic-worker-arraigned-on-drug-charges.

22 Robert Lowes, "93-Year-Old 'Pill Mill' Physician Gets 10 Years in Prison," Medscape, August 14, 2017, http://www.medscape.com/viewarticle/884241#vp_4.

23 Ben Popken, "Industry Insiders Estimate EpiPen Costs No More Than $30," *NBC News*, September 6, 2016, https://www.nbcnews.com/business/consumer/industry-insiders-estimate -epipen-costs-no-more-30-n642091.

24 Amy M. Branum and Susan L. Lukacs, "Food Allergy Among U.S. Children: Trends in Prevalence and Hospitalizations," NCHS Data Brief No.10, *Centers for Disease Control and Prevention*, October 2008, https://www.cdc.gov/nchs/products/databriefs/db10.htm. More recent reports also confirm this CDC data. See, for instance, Ruchi Gupta, MD, interview by Robin Young, *Here & Now, NPR*, "Severe Allergic Reactions to Food Are Increasing, in Adults as Well as Children," August 24, 2017, http://www.wbur.org/hereandnow/2017/08/24/severe-food-allergies.

25 Nathan Bomey, "Mylan CEO Defends Price Boosts for Lifesaving EpiPen," *USA Today*, September 21, 2016, https://www.usatoday.com/story/money/2016/09/21/mylan-ceo-heather -bresch-epipen-congress-house-testimony/90773250/.

26 Popken, "Industry Insiders."

27 Amber Phillips, "How a Senator's Daughter Became CEO of the Company at the Center of the EpiPen Controversy," *Washington Post*, August 24, 2016, https://www.washingtonpost.com/news

/the-fix/wp/2016/08/24/how-a-senators-daughter-became-ceo-of-the-company-at-the-center-of
-the-epipen-controversy/?utm_term=.45bae59a0db2.

28 Jayne O'Donnell, "Family Matters: EpiPens Had High-Level Help Getting into Schools," *USA Today*, September 20, 2016, https://www.usatoday.com/story/news/politics/2016/09/20/family
-matters-epipens-had-help-getting-schools-manchin-bresch/90435218/.

29 Lauren Thomas, "EpiPen Maker Mylan Stock Jumps on Earnings Beat," CNBC, March 1, 2017,
https://www.cnbc.com/2017/03/01/epipen-maker-mylan-stock-jumps-on-earnings-beat.html.

30 Aaron M. Kessler, "Report: Drug Company Faked Cancer Patients to Sell Drug," *CNN*,
September 6, 2017, http://www.cnn.com/2017/09/06/politics/insys-cancer-drug-company
-faked-cancer-patients-to-sell-drug/index.html.

31 For more specifics on how the tobacco industry manipulated science, I recommend you read the
American Journal of Public Health's report, which outlines how the industry engineered science
to meet its own ends: https://www.ncbi.nlm.nih.gov/pmc/articles/PMC3490543/. See also "The
Financing of Drug Trials by Pharmaceutical Companies and Its Consequences," https://www
.ncbi.nlm.nih.gov/pmc/articles/PMC2868984/.

32 Stephanie Mencimer, "Did Drinking Give Me Breast Cancer?" *Mother Jones*, May/June 2018,
https://www.motherjones.com/politics/2018/04/did-drinking-give-me-breast-cancer.

33 Jurgen Rehm and Kevin Shield, "Alcohol Consumption," World Health Organization's International Agency for Research on Cancer, https://www.iarc.fr/en/media-centre/iarcnews/2016
/WCR_2014_Chapter_2-3.pdf.

34 The current government guidelines for your daily serving of vegetables can be found at https://
health.gov/dietaryguidelines/dga2000/document/build.htm.

35 Valerie Strauss, "Rats Find Oreos as Addictive as Cocaine: An Unusual College Research Project,"
Washington Post, October 18, 2013, https://www.washingtonpost.com/news/answer-sheet/wp
/2013/10/18/rats-find-oreos-as-addictive-as-cocaine-an-unusual-college-research-project/?utm
_term=.9607e389c999.

Chapter 4: How to Keep Opioids from Destroying Your Life

1 David Sheff, *Beautiful Boy: A Father's Journey Through His Son's Addiction* (New York: Mariner,
2009).

2 "Top Opium Poppy Producing Countries," *World Atlas*, last updated April 25, 2017, https://www
.worldatlas.com/articles/top-opium-poppy-producing-countries.html.

3 Central Intelligence Agency, "Field Listing: Illicit Drugs," *The World Factbook*, accessed January 24,
2018, https://www.cia.gov/library/publications/the-world-factbook/fields/2086.html.

4 Thadeus Greenson, "Fort Bragg Councilman Was Shot at Opium Grow; Draws Light to World
of Opium Poppies," *Eureka Times-Standard*, August 31, 2011, http://www.times-standard.com
/article/zz/20110831/NEWS/110839856.

5 Corky Siemaszko, "$500 Million Opium Poppy Field Discovered in North Carolina," *NBC News*,
May 26, 2017, https://www.nbcnews.com/storyline/americas-heroin-epidemic/500-million
-opium-poppy-field-discovered-north-carolina-n764801.

6 Jonathan Kaminsky, "U.S. Authorities Bust Opium Poppy Farm in Washington State," *Reuters*,
July 11, 2013, https://www.reuters.com/article/us-usa-drugs-poppies/u-s-authorities-bust-opium
-poppy-farm-in-washington-state-idUSBRE96B01920130712.

7 "Opioid (Narcotic) Pain Medications," *WebMD*, accessed January 24, 2018, https://www.webmd
.com/pain-management/guide/narcotic-pain-medications#1.

8 "Drug Abuse Warning Network, 2011: National Estimates of Drug-Related Emergency Depart-
ment Visits," HHS Publication No. (SMA) 13-4760, DAWN Series D-39, *Substance Abuse and
Mental Health Services Administration*, 2013, https://www.samhsa.gov/data/sites/default/files
/DAWN2k11ED/DAWN2k11ED/DAWN2k11ED.pdf.

9 "Opioid Overdose: Understanding the Epidemic," *Centers for Disease Control and Prevention*,
August 30, 2017, https://www.cdc.gov/drugoverdose/epidemic/index.html.

10 Shachar Peled, "Fentanyl Seized by Law Enforcement Doubled in 2016, DEA Says," *CNN*, May 19,
2017, https://www.cnn.com/2017/05/19/health/fentanyl-surge/index.html.

11 "Drug Fact Sheets: Fentanyl," *US Drug Enforcement Administration*, accessed January 25, 2018, https://www.dea.gov/druginfo/concern_fentanyl.shtml.

12 "Research Update on Fentanyl Outbreaks in the Dayton, Ohio Area," *Boonshoft School of Medicine at Wright State University*, updated April 28, 2017, https://ndews.umd.edu/sites /ndews.umd.edu/files/update-on-fentanyl-outbreaks-in-dayton-ohio-ou-r21-da042757-05-02 -2017.pdf.

13 M. Noble et al., "Opioids for Long-Term Treatment of Noncancer Pain," *Cochrane*, January 20, 2010, http://www.cochrane.org/CD006605/SYMPT_opioids-long-term-treatment-noncancer -pain; Maia Szalavitz, "Opioid Addiction Is a Huge Problem, but Pain Prescriptions Are Not the Cause," MIND guest blog, *Scientific American*, May 10, 2016, https://blogs.scientificamerican .com/mind-guest-blog/opioid-addiction-is-a-huge-problem-but-pain-prescriptions-are-not-the -cause/.

14 Emily O. Dumas and Gary M. Pollack, "Opioid Tolerance Development: A Pharmacokinetic/Phar-macodynamic Perspective," *AAPS Journal* 10 (2008): 537–51, doi: 10.1208/s12248-008-9056-1.

15 Benjamin J. Morasco et al., "Higher Prescription Opioid Dose Is Associated with Worse Patient-Reported Pain Outcomes and More Health Care Utilization," *Journal of Pain* 18 (2017): 437–45, http://www.jpain.org/article/S1526-5900(16)30356-X/fulltext.

16 "Timeline of Selected FDA Activities and Significant Events Addressing Opioid Misuse and Abuse," *US Food and Drug Administration*, last updated January 26, 2018, https://www.fda.gov /Drugs/DrugSafety/InformationbyDrugClass/ucm338566.htm.

17 Art Van Zee, "The Promotion and Marketing of OxyContin: Commercial Triumph, Public Health Tragedy," *American Journal of Public Health* 99 (2009): 221–27, doi: 10.2105/AJPH .2007.131714.

18 "Results from the 2008 National Survey on Drug Use and Health: National Findings," NSDUH Series H-36, HHS Publication No. SMA 09-4434, *Substance Abuse and Mental Health Services Administration* (2009), 58, http://www.dpft.org/resources/NSDUHresults2008.pdf.

19 Abby Alpert et al., "Supply-Side Drug Policy in the Presence of Substitutes: Evidence from the Introduction of Abuse-Deterrent Opioids," NBER Working Paper No. 23031, *National Bureau of Economic Research* (2017), http://www.nber.org/papers/w23031.

20 Maria L. La Ganga and Terence Monmaney, "Doctor Found Liable in Suit Over Pain," *LA Times*, June 15, 2001, http://articles.latimes.com/2001/jun/15/news/mn-10726.

21 "Prescription Painkiller Overdoses," *Centers for Disease Control and Prevention*, last updated July 3, 2012, https://www.cdc.gov/vitalsigns/methadoneoverdoses/index.html.

22 N. Tasevska et al., "Sugars in Diet and Risk of Cancer in the NIH-AARP Diet and Health Study," *International Journal of Cancer* 130 (2012): 159–69, doi: 10.1002/ijc.25990.

23 Vijay R. Varma et al., "Re-evaluating the Effect of Age on Physical Activity Over the Lifespan," *Journal of Preventative Medicine* 101 (2017): 102–8, https://doi.org/10.1016/j.ypmed.2017 .05.030.

24 Lizhou Liu et al., "Acupuncture for Low Back Pain: An Overview of Systematic Reviews," *Evidence-Based Complementary and Alternative Medicine* (2015): 328196, doi: 10.1155/2015 /328196.

25 D. Carr and J. Lythgoe, "Use of Acupuncture During Labour," *The Practising Midwife* 17 (2014): 10, 12–15, https://www.ncbi.nlm.nih.gov/pubmed/24873111; L. Mårtensson and G. Wallin, "Use of Acupuncture and Sterile Water Injection for Labor Pain: A Survey in Sweden," *Birth* 33 (2006): 289–96, https://www.ncbi.nlm.nih.gov/pubmed/17150067; E. Schytt et al., "Incompleteness of Swedish Local Clinical Guidelines for Acupuncture Treatment During Childbirth," *Acta Obstetricia et Gynecologica Scandinavica* 90/1 (2011): 77–82, https://www.ncbi.nlm.nih.gov /pubmed/21275919.

26 H. Cramer et al., "A Systematic Review and Meta-Analysis of Yoga for Low Back Pain," *Clinical Journal of Pain* 29 (2013): 450–60, doi: 10.1097/AJP.0b013e31825e1492.

27 U.S. Department of Health and Human Services (HHS), Office of the Surgeon General, *Facing Addiction in America: The Surgeon General's Report on Alcohol, Drugs, and Health* (Washington, DC: HHS, 2016), 2-2, https://addiction.surgeongeneral.gov/.

28 Y. I. Hser et al., "A 33-Year Follow-Up of Narcotics Addicts," *Archives of General Psychiatry* 58 (2001): 503–8, https://www.ncbi.nlm.nih.gov/pubmed/11343531.

Chapter 5: Braking Bad: Overcoming Your Addiction to Meth and Other Stimulants

1 Jane A. Buxton and Naomi A. Dove, "The Burden and Management of Crystal Meth Use," *Canadian Medical Association Journal* 178/12 (June 3, 2008): 1537–39, https://www.ncbi.nlm.nih.gov /pmc/articles/PMC2396355/.

2 Jan Dirk Blom, *A Dictionary of Hallucinations* (New York: Springer, 2010), 175.

3 D. Doyle, "Adolf Hitler's Medical Care," *Journal of the Royal College of Physicians of Edinburgh* 35 (2005): 75–82, http://www.rcpe.ac.uk/journal/issue/journal_35_1/Hitler's_medical_care.pdf.

4 Nicolas Rasmussen, "America's First Amphetamine Epidemic 1929–1971," *American Journal of Public Health* 98/6 (June 2008): 974–85, https://www.ncbi.nlm.nih.gov/pmc/articles/PMC2377281/.

5 "Author Says Hitler Was 'Blitzed' on Cocaine and Opiates During the War," interview with Norman Ohler, *NPR's Fresh Air*, March 7, 2017, https://www.npr.org/sections/health-shots/2017 /03/07/518986612/author-says-hitler-was-blitzed-on-cocaine-and-opiates-during-the-war; Rasmussen, "America's First Amphetamine Epidemic."

6 Kathryn Doyle, "Drug Use High Among Commercial Truck Drivers: Study," *Reuters*, October 25, 2013, https://www.reuters.com/article/us-drug-truckdrivers/drug-use-high-among-commercial -truck-drivers-study-idUSBRE99O0T520131025.

7 Elaine A. Moore, *The Amphetamine Debate: The Use of Adderall, Ritalin and Related Drugs for Behavior Modification, Neuroenhancement and Anti-Aging Purposes* (Jefferson, NC: McFarland, 2011), 136.

8 Peter M. Miller, ed., *Biological Research on Addiction: Comprehensive Addictive Behaviors and Disorders*, vol. 2 (London: Academic Press, 2013), 580.

9 Moore, *Amphetamine Debate*, 136.

10 Phillip Smith, "When Meth Was Medicine: Big Pharma Amphetamine Ads from the Days of Better Living Through Chemistry," *AlterNet*, October 16, 2016, https://www.alternet.org/drugs /when-meth-medicine-big-pharma-amphetamine-ads.

11 Erin Blakemore, "A Speedy History of America's Addiction to Amphetamine," *Smithsonian.com*, October 27, 2017, https://www.smithsonianmag.com/history/speedy-history-americas-addiction -amphetamine-180966989/; Rasmussen, "America's First Amphetamine Epidemic."

12 "Methamphetamine: History, Pharmacology, and Prevalence," *MethOIDE*, accessed February 11, 2018, http://methoide.fcm.arizona.edu/infocenter/index.cfm?stid=167.

13 "What Is the Scope of Methamphetamine Abuse in the United States?" *National Institute on Drug Abuse*, last updated September 2013, https://www.drugabuse.gov/publications/research-reports /methamphetamine/what-scope-methamphetamine-abuse-in-united-states.

14 Oregon-Idaho HIDTA Program, *Program Year 2018: Drug-Threat Assessment and Counter-Drug Strategy* (Salem, OR: Oregon-Idaho HIDTA Program, 2018), 6, http://oridhidta.org/reports/.

15 *World Drug Report 2017* (Vienna, Austria: United Nations Office on Drugs and Crime, 2017), https://www.unodc.org/wdr2017/field/WDR_2017_presentation_lauch_version.pdf.

16 J. Biederman et al., "Does Attention-Deficit Hyperactivity Disorder Impact the Developmental Course of Drug and Alcohol Abuse and Dependence?" *Biological Psychiatry* 44 (1998): 269–73, https://www.ncbi.nlm.nih.gov/pubmed/9715358.

17 Gabor Maté, *In the Realm of Hungry Ghosts: Close Encounters with Addiction* (Berkeley, CA: North Atlantic Books, 2010), 439.

18 C. Jaffe et al., "A Comparison of Methamphetamine-Dependent Inpatients with and Without Childhood Attention Deficit Hyperactivity Disorder Symptomatology," *Journal of Addictive Diseases* 24 (2005): 133–52, http://www.tandfonline.com/doi/abs/10.1300/J069v24n03_11.

19 M. Billiard, "Narcolepsy: Current Treatment Options and Future Approaches," *Neuropsychiatric Disease and Treatment* 4 (2008): 557–66, https://www.ncbi.nlm.nih.gov/pmc/articles/PMC2526380/.

20 "Prescribed Stimulant Use for ADHD Continues to Rise Steadily," *National Institute of Mental Health*, news release, September 28, 2011, https://www.nimh.nih.gov/news/science-news/2011/prescribed-stimulant-use-for-adhd-continues-to-rise-steadily.shtml.

21 "What Is ADHD?" *American Psychiatric Association*, reviewed July 2017, accessed February 11, 2018, https://www.psychiatry.org/patients-families/adhd/what-is-adhd; Alan Schwarz, "The Selling of Attention Deficit Disorder," *New York Times*, December 14, 2013, http://www.nytimes.com/2013/12/15/health/the-selling-of-attention-deficit-disorder.html?pagewanted=all.

22 Schwarz, "Selling of Attention Deficit Disorder."

23 "Attention-Deficit/Hyperactivity Disorder (ADHD): Data & Statistics," *Centers for Disease Control and Prevention*, last updated January 24, 2018, https://www.cdc.gov/ncbddd/adhd/data.html.

24 Alan Schwarz, "Drowned in a Stream of Prescriptions," *New York Times*, February 2, 2013, http://www.nytimes.com/2013/02/03/us/concerns-about-adhd-practices-and-amphetamine-addiction.html.

25 Anthony Samsel and Stephanie Seneff, "Glyphosate, Pathways to Modern Diseases II: Celiac Sprue and Gluten Intolerance," *Interdisciplinary Toxicology* 6 (2013): 159–84, https://www.ncbi.nlm.nih.gov/pmc/articles/PMC3945755/.

26 Keith R. Fluegge and Kyle R. Fluegge, "Glyphosate Use Predicts ADHD Hospital Discharges in the Healthcare Cost and Utilization Project Net (HCUPnet): A Two-Way Fixed-Effects Analysis," *PLOSOne*, August 19, 2015, http://journals.plos.org/plosone/article?id=10.1371/journal.pone.0133525.

27 Schwarz, "Selling of Attention Deficit Disorder."

28 T. E. Wilens et al., "Does Stimulant Therapy of Attention-Deficit/Hyperactivity Disorder Beget Later Substance Abuse? A Meta-Analytic Review of the Literature," *Pediatrics* 111 (2003): 179–85, https://www.ncbi.nlm.nih.gov/pubmed/12509574.

29 N. D. Volkow, "Long-Term Safety of Stimulant Use for ADHD: Findings from Nonhuman Primates [Commentary]," *Neuropsychopharmacology* 37 (2012): 2551–52, http://www.nature.com/npp/journal/v37/n12/full/npp2012127a.html; Elizabeth Harstad et al., "Attention-Deficit/Hyperactivity Disorder and Substance Abuse," *Pediatrics* 134 (2014): e293–301, doi: 10.1542/peds.2014-0992.

30 These experiments were published in a series of papers, including Bruce K. Alexander et al., "The Effect of Housing and Gender on Morphine Self-Administration in Rats," *Psychopharmacology* 58 (1978): 175–79, https://link.springer.com/article/10.1007/BF00426903#page-1; Tom Stafford, "Drug Addiction: The Complex Truth," *BBC Future*, September 10, 2013, http://www.bbc.com/future/story/20130910-drug-addiction-the-complex-truth; and Bruce Alexander et al., "Effect of Early and Later Colony Housing on Oral Ingestion of Morphine in Rats," *Psychopharmacology, Biochemistry, and Behavior* 15 (1981): 571–76.

31 Stafford, "Drug Addiction"; Bruce K. Alexander, "Addiction: The View from Rat Park (2010)," *Brucekalexander.com*, accessed February 12, 2018, http://www.brucekalexander.com/articles-speeches/rat-park/148-addiction-the-view-from-rat-park.

32 Bruce K. Alexander et al., "The Effect of Housing and Gender on Morphine Self-Administration in Rats," *Psychopharmacology* 58 (1978): 175–79, https://link.springer.com/article/10.1007/BF00426903#page-1; Stafford, "Drug Addiction."

33 S. E. Jacob and S. Stechschulte, "Formaldehyde, Aspartame, and Migraines: A Possible Connection," *Dermatitis* 19 (2008): E10–1, https://www.ncbi.nlm.nih.gov/pubmed/18627677.

34 Woodrow Monte, *While Science Sleeps* (CreateSpace, 2011).

35 Jason Lloyd-Price, Galeb Abu-Ali, and Curtis Huttenhower, "The Healthy Human Microbiome," *Genome Medicine* 8 (2016): 51, https://www.ncbi.nlm.nih.gov/pmc/articles/PMC4848870/.

36 "Microbiome," *PubMed Health Glossary*, https://www.ncbi.nlm.nih.gov/pubmedhealth/PMHT0025077/.

37 Luke K. Ursell et al., "Defining the Human Microbiome," *Nutrition Reviews* 70, Suppl 1 (August 2012): S38–S44, https://www.ncbi.nlm.nih.gov/pmc/articles/PMC3426293/.

38 B. Kowalewska-Kantecka, "Breastfeeding—An Important Element of Health Promotion," *Developmental Period Medicine* 20 (2016): 354–57, https://www.ncbi.nlm.nih.gov/pubmed/28391255; Fredrik Bäckhed et al., "Dynamics and Stabilization of the Human Gut Microbiome during the

First Year of Life," *Cell Host and Microbe* 17/5 (May 13, 2015): 690-703, http://www.cell.com/cell-host-microbe/fulltext/S1931-3128(15)00162-6.

39 M. M. Zaiss and N. L. Harris, "Interactions Between the Intestinal Microbiome and Helminth Parasites," *Parasite Immunology* 38/1 (January 2016): 5–11, https://www.ncbi.nlm.nih.gov/pmc/articles/PMC5019230/.

40 Fumio Watanabe et al., "Vitamin B$_{12}$-Containing Plant Food Sources for Vegetarians," *Nutrients* 6/5 (May 2014): 1861–73, https://www.ncbi.nlm.nih.gov/pmc/articles/PMC4042564/.

Chapter 6: Your Brain on Alcohol

1   Gabor Maté, *In the Realm of Hungry Ghosts: Close Encounters with Addiction* (Berkeley, CA: North Atlantic Books, 2010), 155.

2   "Excessive Alcohol Use: Preventing a Leading Risk for Death, Disease, and Injury at a Glance 2016," *Centers for Disease Control and Prevention*, last updated December 31, 2015, https://www.cdc.gov/chronicdisease/resources/publications/aag/alcohol.htm.

3   "Results from the 2016 National Survey on Drug Use and Health: Detailed Tables," *Substance Abuse and Mental Health Services Administration* (2017), 852, table 2.53B, https://www.samhsa.gov/data/sites/default/files/NSDUH-DetTabs-2016/NSDUH-DetTabs-2016.pdf.

4   Caren Lissner, "Are Women Increasingly at Risk of Addiction?" *Washington Post*, February 26, 2017, https://www.washingtonpost.com/national/health-science/are-women-increasingly-at-risk-of-addiction/2017/02/24/dfa5b98c-d2ba-11e6-9cb0-54ab630851e8_story.html?utm_term=.bfd792b25be5.

5   "Introducing Little Black Dress Vodka: Designed by Women, for Women," PR Newswire, February 29, 2012, https://www.prnewswire.com/news-releases/introducing-little-black-dress-vodka-designed-by-women-for-women-140863123.html.

6   "Johnnie Walker Black Label: The Jane Walker Edition," accessed April 27, 2018, https://www.johnniewalker.com/en-us/our-whisky/limited-editions/jane-walker.

7   Sarah Mart and Norman Giesbrecht, "Red flags on Pinkwashed Drinks: Contradictions and Dangers in Marketing Alcohol to Prevent Cancer," *Addiction* 110, no. 10 (October 2015), https://onlinelibrary.wiley.com/doi/abs/10.1111/add.13035.

8   "Women and Alcohol," *National Institute on Alcohol Abuse and Alcoholism*, updated June 2017, https://pubs.niaaa.nih.gov/publications/womensfact/womensfact.htm.

9   Stephanie Mencimer, "Did Drinking Give Me Breast Cancer?"

10 "Results from the 2016 National Survey," 820, table 2.37B.

11 Robert W. S. Coulter et al., "Differences in Alcohol Use and Alcohol-Related Problems between Transgender- and Nontransgender-identified Young Adults," *Drug and Alcohol Dependence* 154 (2015): 251–59, doi: 10.1016/j.drugalcdep.2015.07.006; Lisa R. Miller and Eric Anthony Grollman, "The Social Costs of Gender Nonconformity for Transgender Adults: Implications for Discrimination and Health," *Sociological Forum* 30 (2015): 809–31, doi: 10.1111/socf.12193.

12 Peter Smith, "A Sip from an Ancient Sumerian Drinking Song," *Smithsonian.com*, June 18, 2012, https://www.smithsonianmag.com/arts-culture/a-sip-from-an-ancient-sumerian-drinking-song-125002995/.

13 Joshua J. Mark, "Beer in the Ancient World," *Ancient History Encyclopedia*, March 2, 2011, https://www.ancient.eu/article/223/beer-in-the-ancient-world/; Iain Gately, *Drink: A Cultural History of Alcohol* (New York: Gotham Books, 2008).

14 Brian A. Nummer, "Historical Origins of Food Preservation," *National Center for Home Food Preservation*, May 2002, http://nchfp.uga.edu/publications/nchfp/factsheets/food_pres_hist.html.

15 John T. Sullivan, "Surgery Before Anesthesia," *Massachusetts General Hospital*, last modified May 11, 2005, https://neurosurgery.mgh.harvard.edu/history/beforeth.htm.

16 T. S. Saleem and S. D. Basha, "Red Wine: A Drink to Your Heart," *Journal of Cardiovascular Disease Research* 1 (2010): 171–76, doi: 10.4103/0975-3583.74259, https://www.ncbi.nlm.nih.gov/pmc/articles/PMC3023893/; Y. Gepner et al., "Effects of Initiating Moderate Alcohol Intake on Cardiometabolic Risk in Adults with Type 2 Diabetes: A 2-Year Randomized, Controlled Trial," *Annals of Internal Medicine* 163 (2015): 569–79, doi: 10.7326/M14-1650.

17   T. D. Fuller, "Moderate Alcohol Consumption and the Risk of Mortality," *Demography* 48 (August 2011): 1105–25, doi: 10.1007/s13524-011-0035-2; Michael Joseph, "Alcohol and Longevity: Does Drinking Increase Lifespan?" *Nutrition Advance*, March 6, 2017, https://nutritionadvance.com /alcoholic-beverages-longevity-lifespan/.

18   "Alcohol Use and Your Health," *Centers for Disease Control and Prevention*, last updated January 3, 2018, https://www.cdc.gov/alcohol/fact-sheets/alcohol-use.htm.

19   Maurizio Pompili et al., "Suicidal Behavior and Alcohol Abuse," *International Journal of Environmental Research and Public Health* 7 (2010): 1392–1431, doi: 10.3390/ijerph7041392.

20   "Alcohol Use and Your Health."

21   M. R. Piano and S. A. Phillips, "Alcoholic Cardiomyopathy: Pathophysiologic Insights," *Cardiovascular Toxicology* 14 (2014): 291–308, doi: 10.1007/s12012-014-9252-4.

22   S. C. Larsson et al., "Alcohol Consumption and Risk of Atrial Fibrillation: A Prospective Study and Dose-Response Meta-Analysis," *Journal of the American College of Cardiology* 64 (2014): 281–89, doi: 10.1016/j.jacc.2014.03.048.

23   C. Zhang et al., "Alcohol Intake and Risk of Stroke: A Dose-Response Meta-Analysis of Prospective Studies," *International Journal of Cardiology* 174 (2014): 669–77, doi: 10.1016/j.ijcard.2014.04.225.

24   R. Carnevale and C. Nocella, "Alcohol and Cardiovascular Disease: Still Unresolved Underlying Mechanisms," *Vascular Pharmacology* 57 (2012): 69–71, doi: 10.1016/j.vph.2012.06.005.

25   N. Hu et al., "Contribution of ALDH2 Polymorphism to Alcoholism-Associated Hypertension," *Recent Patents on Endocrine, Metabolic, and Immune Drug Discovery* 8 (2014): 180–85, https:// www.ncbi.nlm.nih.gov/pubmed/25354396.

26   G. Traversy and J. P Chaput, "Alcohol Consumption and Obesity: An Update," *Current Obesity Reports* 4 (2015): 122–30, doi: 10.1007/s13679-014-0129-4.

27   A. K. Singal et al., "Alcoholic Hepatitis: Current Challenges and Future Directions," *Clinical Gastroenterology and Hepatology* 12 (2014): 555–64, doi: 10.1016/j.cgh.2013.06.013.

28   S. Grad et al., "The Effect of Alcohol on Gastrointestinal Motility," *Reviews on Recent Clinical Trials* 11 (2016): 191–95, https://www.ncbi.nlm.nih.gov/pubmed/27527893.

29   M. Herreros-Villanueva et al., "Alcohol Consumption on Pancreatic Diseases," *World Journal of Gastroenterology* 19 (2013): 638–47, doi: 10.3748/wjg.v19.i5.638.

30   "Alcohol and Cancer Risk," *National Cancer Institute*, reviewed June 24, 2013, https://www.cancer .gov/about-cancer/causes-prevention/risk/alcohol/alcohol-fact-sheet.

31   Peter R. Martin et al., "The Role of Thiamine Deficiency in Alcoholic Brain Disease," *Alcohol Research and Health* 27 (2003): 134–42, https://pubs.niaaa.nih.gov/publications/arh27-2/134-142.htm.

32   Haihong Liu et al., "Frontal and Cingulate Gray Matter Volume Reduction in Heroin Dependence: Optimized Voxel-Based Morphometry," *Psychiatry and Clinical Neurosciences* 63 (2009): 563–68, doi:10.1111/j.1440-1819.2009.01989.x.

33   Erica N. Grodin et al., "Deficits in Cortical, Diencephalic, and Midbrain Gray Matter in Alcoholism Measured by VBM: Effects of Co-Morbid Substance Abuse," *NeuroImage: Clinical* 2 (2013): 469–76, doi: 10.1016/j.nicl.2013.03.013.

34   B. Bencherif et al., "Mu-opioid Receptor Binding Measured by [11C] Carfentanil Positron Emission Tomography Is Related to Craving and Mood in Alcohol Dependence," *Biological Psychiatry* 55 (2004): 255–62, https://www.ncbi.nlm.nih.gov/pubmed/?term=%E2%80%9CMu-opioid +Receptor+Binding+Measured+by+Positron+Emission+Tomography+is+Related+to+Craving +and+Mood+in+Alcohol+Dependence.

35   A. L. Pitel et al., "Face-Name Association Learning and Brain Structural Substrates in Alcoholism," *Alcoholism: Clinical and Experimental Research* 36 (2012): 1171–9, doi:10.1111/j.1530-0277 .2011.01731.x; S. J. Nixon et al., "Behavioral Dysfunction and Cognitive Efficiency in Male and Female Alcoholics," *Alcoholism: Clinical and Experimental Research* 19 (1995): 577–81, https:// www.ncbi.nlm.nih.gov/pubmed/7573777.

36   Alkermes, "Vivitrol Prescribing Information," https://www.vivitrol.com/content/pdfs/prescribing -information.pdf.

37   D. Church et al., "The Effect of Emotional Freedom Techniques on Stress Biochemistry: A Randomized Controlled Trial," *Journal of Nervous and Mental Disease* 200 (2012): 891–96, doi: 10.1097/NMD.0b013e31826b9fc1.

38 Stefan Voorspoels et al., "Analysis of Selected Phthalates in Food Samples," Coalition for Safer Food Processing and Packaging, *Ecology Center* 2017/SCT/R/1071, June 2017, accessed on February 8, 2018, http://www.kleanupkraft.org/PhthalatesLabReport.pdf.

39 "Our unpublished study indicates that the Vitamin B_{12} contents significantly differ among various commercially available Chlorella tablets (from zero to several hundred μg of Vitamin B_{12} per 100 g dry weight); we do not have any information on why such a huge variation occurs. Thus, vegetarians who consume Chlorella tablets as a source of Vitamin B_{12} should check the nutrition labeling of Chlorella products to confirm their Vitamin B_{12} contents." Fumio Watanabe et al., "Vitamin B_{12}-Containing Plant Food Sources for Vegetarians," *Nutrients* 6/5 (May 2014): 1861–73, https://www.ncbi.nlm.nih.gov/pmc/articles/PMC4042564/.

40 "Don't Double Up on Acetaminophen," *U.S. Food and Drug Administration*, last updated January 26, 2018, https://www.fda.gov/ForConsumers/ConsumerUpdates/ucm336581.htm.

41 "Drug Record: Acetaminophen," *LiverTox*, last updated January 18, 2018, https://livertox.nlm.nih.gov/Acetaminophen.htm; E. Yoon et al., "Acetaminophen-Induced Hepatotoxicity: A Comprehensive Update," *Journal of Clinical and Translational Hepatology* 4 (2016): 131–42, doi: 10.14218/JCTH.2015.00052.

42 W. Parker et al., "The Role of Oxidative Stress, Inflammation and Acetaminophen Exposure from Birth to Early Childhood in the Induction of Autism," *Journal of International Medical Research* 45 (2017): 407–38, doi: 10.1177/0300060517693423.

43 J. M. Louise et al., "Coffee and Herbal Tea Consumption Is Associated with Lower Liver Stiffness in the General Population: The Rotterdam Study," *Journal of Hepatology* 67 (2017): 339–48, http://www.journal-of-hepatology.eu/article/S0168-8278(17)30147-2/fulltext.

44 S. Casas-Grajales and P. Muriel, "Antioxidants in Liver Health," *World Journal of Gastrointestinal Pharmacology and Therapeutics* 6 (2015): 59–72, doi: 10.4292/wjgpt.v6.i3.59.

Chapter 7: The Cannabis Conundrum: Gateway Drug or Wonder Weed?

1   Perry G. Fine and Mark J. Rosenfeld, "The Endocannabinoid System, Cannabinoids, and Pain," *Rambam Maimonides Medical Journal* 4 (2013): e0022, https://www.ncbi.nlm.nih.gov/pmc/articles/PMC3820295.

2   John M. McPartland et al., "Care and Feeding of the Endocannabinoid System: A Systematic Review of Potential Clinical Interventions that Upregulate the Endocannabinoid System," *PLOS One* 9 (2104): e89566, https://www.ncbi.nlm.nih.gov/pmc/articles/PMC3951193.

3   Zerrin Atakan, "Cannabis, a Complex Plant: Different Compounds and Different Effects on Individuals," *Therapeutic Advances in Psychopharmacology* 2 (2012): 241–54, https://www.ncbi.nlm.nih.gov/pmc/articles/PMC3736954/.

4   "Drug Scheduling," *US Drug Enforcement Administration*, accessed December 7, 2017, https://www.dea.gov/druginfo/ds.shtml.

5   "Marijuana Overview: Legalization," *National Conference of State Legislatures*, August 30, 2017, http://www.ncsl.org/research/civil-and-criminal-justice/marijuana-overview.aspx.

6   Robin M. Murray et al, "Traditional Marijuana, High-Potency Cannabis and Synthetic Cannabinoids: Increasing Risk for Psychosis," *World Psychiatry* 15 (2016): 195–204, doi: 10.1002/wps.20341.

7   Robert C. Clarke and Mark D. Merlin, *Cannabis: Evolution and Ethnobotany*, reprint ed. (Berkeley, CA: University of California Press, 2016).

8   "One in Eight U.S. Adults Say They Smoke Marijuana," *Gallup News*, August 8, 2016, http://news.gallup.com/poll/194195/adults-say-smoke-marijuana.aspx.

9   "History of Washington State Marijuana Laws," *National Conference of State Legislators*, accessed December 8, 2017, www.ncsl.org/documents/summit/summit2015/.../wa_mj_law_history.pdf.

10 "2016 Washington State Healthy Youth Survey," *Washington State Department of Health*, accessed December 8, 2017, https://www.doh.wa.gov/Portals/1/Documents/8350/160-NonDOH-DB-MJ.pdf.

11 Deborah S. Hasin et al., "Prevalence of Marijuana Use Disorders in the United States Between 2001–2002 and 2012–2013," *JAMA Psychiatry* 72 (2015): 1235–42, doi:10.1001/jamapsychiatry.2015.1858.

12 "Is Marijuana Addictive?" *National Institute on Drug Abuse*, updated August 2017, https://www
.drugabuse.gov/publications/research-reports/marijuana/marijuana-addictive; The ASAM Review
Course in Addiction Medicine, July 27–29, 2017, Dallas, Texas.

13 "Principles of Adolescent Substance Use Disorder Treatment: A Research-Based Guide," *National
Institute on Drug Abuse*, updated January 2014, https://www.drugabuse.gov/publications/principles
-adolescent-substance-use-disorder-treatment-research-based-guide/frequently-asked-questions
/it-possible-teens-to-become-addicted-to-marijuana.

14 "NIDA Review Summarizes Research on Marijuana's Negative Health Effects," *National Institutes
of Health*, June 14, 2014, https://www.nih.gov/news-events/news-releases/nida-review-summarizes
-research-marijuanas-negative-health-effects.

15 "Legalizing Marijuana and the New Science of Weed," news release, *American Chemistry Society*,
March 23, 2015, https://www.acs.org/content/acs/en/pressroom/newsreleases/2015/march
/legalizing-marijuana-and-the-new-science-of-weed-video.html.

16 "Legalizing Marijuana and the New Science of Weed"; "Colorado Marijuana Study Finds Legal
Weed Contains Potent THC Levels," *NBC News*, March 23, 2015, https://www.nbcnews.com
/storyline/legal-pot/legal-weed-surprisingly-strong-dirty-tests-find-n327811.

17 "Colorado Marijuana Study."

18 Margaret E. Sears and Stephen J. Genuis, "Environmental Determinants of Chronic Disease and
Medical Approaches: Recognition, Avoidance, Supportive Therapy, and Detoxification," *Journal of
Environmental and Public Health* 2012 (2012): 356798, doi: http://dx.doi.org/10.1155/2012/356798.

19 Joseph Pizzorno, "What Should We Tell Our Patients About Marijuana (Cannabis indica and Cannabis sativa)?" *Integrative Medicine* 15 (2016): 8–12, https://edu.emersonecologics.com/2017/10/17
/what-should-we-tell-our-patients-about-marijuana-cannabis-indica-and-cannabis-sativa/.

20 "What Should We Tell Our Patients?"

21 Neil MacGillivray, "Sir William Brooke O'Shaughnessy (1808–1889), MD, FRS, LRCS Ed: Chemical Pathologist, Pharmacologist, and Pioneer in Electric Telegraphy," *Journal of Medical Biography*
25 (2017), http://journals.sagepub.com/doi/abs/10.1177/0967772015596276; W. B. O'Shaughnessy, "On the Preparations of the Indian Hemp, or Gunjah (Cannabis Indica)," *Provincial Medical
Journal* no. 123.J (1843): 363–69.

22 "Marijuana Timeline," *PBS.org*, accessed December 9, 2017, https://www.pbs.org/wgbh/pages
/frontline/shows/dope/etc/cron.html.

23 Nora D. Volkow, "The Biology and Potential Therapeutic Effects of Cannabidiol," (testimony,
before Senate Caucus on International Narcotics Control, Cannabidiol: Barriers to Research and
Potential Medical Benefits, Hart Senate Office Building, Washington, DC, June 24, 2015), https://
www.drugabuse.gov/about-nida/legislative-activities/testimony-to-congress/2016/biology-potential
-therapeutic-effects-cannabidiol.

24 Orrin Devinsky et al., "Cannabidiol in Patients with Treatment-Resistant Epilepsy: An Open-Label
Interventional Trial," *Lancet* 15/3 (March 2016): 270–78, http://www.thelancet.com/journals
/laneur/article/PIIS1474-4422(15)00379-8/abstract.

25 "60 Peer-Reviewed Studies on Medical Marijuana," *ProCon.org*, February 10, 2016, https://
medicalmarijuana.procon.org/view.resource.php?resourceID=000884.

26 A. Alhamoruni et al., "Pharmacological Effects of Cannabinoids on the Caco-2 Cell Culture Model
of Intestinal Permeability," *Journal of Pharmacology and Experimental Therapeutics*, 335/1 (October
2010): 92–102, http://jpet.aspetjournals.org/content/335/1/92?sid=c09c62d8-996e-4071-bbed
-ff8d46fca175.

27 Volkow, "The Biology and Potential Therapeutic Effects."

28 "Glaucoma and Marijuana Use," *National Eye Institute*, December 5, 2012, https://nei.nih.gov
/news/statements/marij.

29 Jacob Kaufman et al., "Medical Marijuana Utilization and Perceived Therapeutic Value in Patients
with ALS (P3.014)," *Neurology* 82 (10 Supplement) (2014): P3.014, http://n.neurology.org/content
/82/10_Supplement/P3.014.

30 C. W. Webb et al., "Therapeutic Benefits of Cannabis: A Patient Survey," *Hawai'i Journal of
Medicine and Public Health* 73 (2014): 109–11, https://www.ncbi.nlm.nih.gov/pubmed/24765558;

Sian Ferguson, "Can You Use Cannabis to Restore Your Natural Sleep Cycle?" February 20, 2018, https://www.healthline.com/health/medical-marijuana/cannabis-for-sleeping.

31 Volkow, "The Biology and Potential Therapeutic Effects"; Linda A. Parker et al., "Regulation of Nausea and Vomiting by Cannabinoids," *British Journal of Pharmacology* 163 (2011): 1411–22, doi: 10.1111/j.1476-5381.2010.01176.x.

32 Volkow, "The Biology and Potential Therapeutic Effects."

33 Parker, "Regulation of Nausea and Vomiting."

34 J. Guindon and A. G. Hohmann, "The Endocannabinoid System and Cancer: Therapeutic Implication," *British Journal of Pharmacology* 163 (2011): 1447–63, doi: 10.1111/j.1476-5381.2011.01327.x; Juan A. Ramos and Fernando J. Bianco, "The Role of Cannabinoids in Prostate Cancer: Basic Science Perspective and Potential Clinical Applications," *Indian Journal of Urology* 28/1 (January–March 2012): 9–14, https://www.ncbi.nlm.nih.gov/pmc/articles/PMC3339795/.

35 Andras Bilkei-Gorzo et al., "A Chronic Low Dose of fj9-Tetrahydrocannabinol (THC) Restores Cognitive Function in Old Mice," *Nature Medicine* 23 (2017): 782–87, doi:10.1038/nm.4311.

36 D. C. Hammell et al., "Transdermal Cannabidiol Reduces Inflammation and Pain-Related Behaviours in a Rat Model of Arthritis," *European Journal of Pain* 20/6 (July 2016): 936–48, https://www.ncbi.nlm.nih.gov/pmc/articles/PMC4851925/.

37 Mariangela Pucci et al., "Epigenetic Control of Skin Differentiation Genes by Phytocannabinoids," *British Journal of Pharmacology* 170/3 (October 2013): 581-91, http://onlinelibrary.wiley.com/doi/10.1111/bph.12309/abstract.

38 Anastasia S. Suraev et al., "An Australian Nationwide Survey on Medicinal Cannabis Use for Epilepsy: History of Antiepileptic Drug Treatment Predicts Medicinal Cannabis Use," *Epilepsy and Behavior* 70, Part B (May 2017): 334-40, http://www.sciencedirect.com/science/article/pii/S1525505017300732.

39 Orrin Devinsky et al., "Trial of Cannabidiol for Drug-Resistant Seizures in the Dravet Syndrome," *New England Journal of Medicine* 376 (2017): 2011–2020, doi: 10.1056/NEJMoa1611618.

40 Donald Abrams, "Cannabinoid-Opioid Interaction in Chronic Pain," *Clinical Pharmacology and Therapeutics* 90 (2011): 844–51, doi: 10.1038/clpt.2011.188.

41 Lucy J. Troup et al., "The Relationship Between Cannabis Use and Measures of Anxiety and Depression in a Sample of College Campus Cannabis Users and Non-Users Post State Legalization in Colorado," *PeerJ* 4 (2016): e2782, https://www.ncbi.nlm.nih.gov/pmc/articles/PMC5149055/.

42 Two studies funded by the British government found that mixtures of four dyes (and the food preservative sodium benzoate) impaired the behavior of even nonhyperactive children (Bateman, Warner et al. 2004; McCann, Barrett et al. 2007). As a result, the British government told the food industry to eliminate these dyes by the end of 2009. The European Parliament also passed a law requiring a warning notice on foods. For more information on this, read the Center for Science in the Public Interest's outstanding report, "Food Dyes, A Rainbow of Risks" (Washington, DC: Center for Science in the Public Interest, June 2010).

43 National Academies of Sciences, Engineering, and Medicine, *The Health Effects of Cannabis and Cannabinoids: The Current State of Evidence and Recommendations for Research* (Washington, DC: National Academies Press, 2017), chap. 10, "Prenatal, Perinatal, and Neonatal Exposure to Cannabis," https://www.ncbi.nlm.nih.gov/books/NBK425751/.

44 Kirsten Weir, "Marijuana and the Developing Brain," *Monitor on Psychology* 46 (2015): 48, http://www.apa.org/monitor/2015/11/marijuana-brain.aspx.

45 M. K. Dahlgren, "Marijuana Use Predicts Cognitive Performance on Tasks of Executive Function," *Journal of Studies on Alcohol and Drugs* 77 (2016): 298–308, https://www.ncbi.nlm.nih.gov/pubmed/26997188.

46 Alvin Powell, "Playing Catch-Up on Marijuana," *Harvard Gazette*, February 3, 2017, https://news.harvard.edu/gazette/story/2017/02/playing-catch-up-on-marijuana/.

47 Giovanni Battistella et al., "Long-Term Effects of Cannabis on Brain Structure," *Neuropsychopharmacology* 39 (2014): 2041–48, doi:10.1038/npp.2014.67; Madeline H. Meier et al., "Persistent Cannabis Users Show Neuropsychological Decline from Childhood to Midlife," *PNAS* 109 (2012): E2657–64, doi: 10.1073/pnas.1206820109.

48 Joanna S. Fowler, "PET Imaging Studies in Drug Abuse," *Journal of Toxicology: Clinical Toxicology* 36 (1998): 163–74, http://dx.doi.org/10.3109/15563659809028936; Francesca M. Filbe et al., "Long-term Effects of Marijuana Use on the Brain," *PNAS* 111/47 (November 25, 2014): 16913–18, https://www.ncbi.nlm.nih.gov/pmc/articles/PMC4250161/.

49 Matthew J. Smith et al., "Cannabis-Related Working Memory Deficits and Associated Subcortical Morphological Differences in Healthy Individuals and Schizophrenia Subjects," *Schizophrenia Bulletin* 40 (2014): 287–99, https://doi.org/10.1093/schbul/sbt176.

50 Matthew J. Smith et al., "Cannabis-Related Episodic Memory Deficits and Hippocampal Morphological Differences in Healthy Individuals and Schizophrenia Subjects," *Hippocampus* 25 (2015): 10.1002/hipo.22427.

51 Wayne Hall and Louisa Degenhardt, "Cannabis Use and the Risk of Developing a Psychotic Disorder," *World Psychiatry* 7 (2008): 68–71, https://www.ncbi.nlm.nih.gov/pmc/articles/PMC2424288/.

52 R. Radhakrishnan, S. T. Wilkinson, and D. C. D'Souza, "Gone to Pot: A Review of the Association Between Cannabis and Psychosis," *Front Psychiatry* 5 (2014): 54, doi: 10.3389/fpsyt.2014.00054, https://www.ncbi.nlm.nih.gov/pubmed/24904437.

53 Lena Palaniyappan et al., "Neural Primacy of the Salience Processing System in Schizophrenia," *Neuron* 79 (2013): 814–28, http://dx.doi.org/10.1016/j.neuron.2013.06.027.

54 H. Segal-Gavish et al., "BDNF Overexpression Prevents Cognitive Deficit Elicited by Adolescent Cannabis Exposure and Host Susceptibility Interaction," *Human Molecular Genetics* 26 (2017): 2462–71, doi: 10.1093/hmg/ddx139.

55 "Cannabis Use in Adolescence Linked to Schizophrenia," *Science Daily*, April 26, 2017, https://www.sciencedaily.com/releases/2017/04/170426124305.htm.

56 S. Dzodzomenyo, "Urine Toxicology Screen in Multiple Sleep Latency Test: The Correlation of Positive Tetrahydrocannabinol, Drug Negative Patients, and Narcolepsy," *Journal of Clinical Sleep Medicine* 11 (2015): 93–99, doi: 10.5664/jcsm.4448.

57 M. Bloomfield et al., "Dopaminergic Function in Cannabis Users and Its Relationship to Cannabis-Induced Psychotic Symptoms," *Biological Psychiatry*, June 29, 2013, http://dx.doi.org/10.1016/j.biopsych.2013.05.027.

58 Renee D. Goodwin et al., "Is Cannabis Use Associated with an Increased Risk of Onset and Persistence of Alcohol Use Disorders? A Three-Year Prospective Study Among Adults in the United States," *Drug and Alcohol Dependence* 161 (2016): 363–67, https://doi.org/10.1016/j.drugalcdep.2016.01.014.

59 Goodwin et al., "Is Cannabis Use Associated with an Increased Risk."

60 Megan E. Patrick, "High-intensity and Simultaneous Alcohol and Marijuana Use Among High School Seniors in the United States," *Substance Abuse* 38 (2017), http://www.tandfonline.com/doi/abs/10.1080/08897077.2017.1356421.

61 Shashwath A. Meda et al., "Longitudinal Influence of Alcohol and Marijuana Use on Academic Performance in College Students," *PLOS One* 12 (2017): e0172213, https://doi.org/10.1371/journal.pone.0172213.

62 "Tobacco," *World Health Organization*, updated May 2017, http://www.who.int/mediacentre/factsheets/fs339/en/.

63 "Smoking and Tobacco Use: Fast Facts," *Centers for Disease Control and Prevention*, updated November 16, 2017, https://www.cdc.gov/tobacco/data_statistics/fact_sheets/fast_facts/index.htm.

64 "Smoking and Tobacco Use."

65 "Current Cigarette Smoking Among Adults in the United States," *Centers for Disease Control and Prevention*, December 1, 2016, https://www.cdc.gov/tobacco/data_statistics/fact_sheets/adult_data/cig_smoking/index.htm.

66 "Trends in Current Cigarette Smoking Among High School Students and Adults, United States, 1965–2014," *Centers for Disease Control and Prevention*, updated March 30, 2016, https://www.cdc.gov/tobacco/data_statistics/tables/trends/cig_smoking/index.htm.

67 NIDA Blog Team, "Marijuana Withdrawal Is Real," *National Institute on Drug Abuse for Teens*, April 2, 2015, https://teens.drugabuse.gov/blog/post/marijuana-withdrawal-real.

68 E. Asevedo et al., "Systematic Review of N-acetylcysteine in the Treatment of Addictions," *Revista Brasileira Psiquiatria* 36 (2014): 168–75, https://www.ncbi.nlm.nih.gov/pubmed /24676047; Chad Kerksick and Darryn Willoughby, "The Antioxidant Role of Glutathione and N-Acetyl-Cysteine Supplements and Exercise-Induced Oxidative Stress," *Journal of the International Society of Sports Nutrition* 2/2 (2005): 38–44, https://www.ncbi.nlm.nih.gov/pmc /articles/PMC2129149/.

69 Bernard Schmitt et al., "Effects of N-acetylcysteine, Oral Glutathione (GSH) and a Novel Sublingual Form of GSH on Oxidative Stress Markers: A Comparative Crossover Study," *Redox Biology* (December 6, 2015): 198–205, https://www.ncbi.nlm.nih.gov/pmc/articles/PMC4536296/.

70 C. Saito, C. Zwingmann, and H. Jaeschke, "Novel Mechanisms of Protection Against Acetaminophen Hepatotoxicity in Mice by Glutathione and N-acetylcysteine," *Hepatology* 51/1 (January 2010): 246–54, https://www.ncbi.nlm.nih.gov/pubmed/19821517.

71 Tauseef Nabi et al., "Role of N-acetylcysteine Treatment in Non-Acetaminophen-Induced Acute Liver Failure: A Prospective Study," *Saudi Journal of Gastroenterology* 23/3 (May–June 2017): 169–75, https://www.ncbi.nlm.nih.gov/pmc/articles/PMC5470376/.

72 R. Scott Rappold, "Legalize Medical Marijuana, Doctors Say in Survey," *WebMD*, April 2, 2014, https://www.webmd.com/pain-management/news/20140225/webmd-marijuana-survey-web#1.

Chapter 8: Screens, Dopamine, and Recovering from Digital and Other Addictions

1 "Mobile Fact Sheet," Pew Research Center, February 5, 2018, http://www.pewinternet.org/fact -sheet/mobile/.

2 Vijay R. Varma et al., "Re-evaluating the Effect of Age on Physical Activity Over the Lifespan."

3 Vicky Rideout, *The Common Sense Census: Media Used by Tweens and Teens* (San Francisco: Common Sense Media, 2015), 13, https://www.commonsensemedia.org/research/the-common-sense -census-media-use-by-tweens-and-teens.

4 *The Nielsen Total Audience Report Q1 2017* (New York: Nielsen Company, 2017), 7, http://www .nielsen.com/us/en/insights/reports/2017/the-nielsen-total-audience-report-q1-2017.html.

5 *Nielsen Total Audience Report Q1 2017*.

6 A. M. Weinstein, "Computer and Video Game Addiction: A Comparison Between Game Users and Non-Game Users," *American Journal of Drug and Alcohol Abuse* 36/5 (September 2010): 268–76, https://www.ncbi.nlm.nih.gov/pubmed/20545602.

7 Min Liu and Jianghong Luo, "Relationship Between Peripheral Blood Dopamine Level and Internet Addiction Disorder in Adolescents: A Pilot Study," *International Journal of Clinical and Experimental Medicine* 8/6 (2015): 9943–48, https://www.ncbi.nlm.nih.gov/pmc/articles /PMC4538113/.

8 Tara Parker-Pope, "This Is Your Brain at the Mall: Why Shopping Makes You Feel So Good," *Wall Street Journal*, December 6, 2005, https://www.wsj.com/articles/SB113382650575214543.

9 Marta G. Novelle and Carlos Diéguez, "Food Addiction and Binge Eating: Lessons Learned from Animal Models," *Nutrients* 10/1 (January 2018): 71, https://www.ncbi.nlm.nih.gov/pmc/articles /PMC5793299/.

10 G. Damsma et al., "Sexual Behavior Increases Dopamine Transmission in the Nucleus Accumbens and Striatum of Male Rats: Comparison with Novelty and Locomotion," *Behavioral Neuroscience* 106/1 (February 1992): 181-91, https://www.ncbi.nlm.nih.gov/pubmed/1313243.

11 Todd Love et al., "Neuroscience of Internet Pornography Addiction: A Review and Update," *Behavioral Sciences* 5/3 (September 2015): 388–433, https://www.ncbi.nlm.nih.gov/pmc/articles /PMC4600144/.

12 M. Zack and C. X. Poulos, "Parallel Roles for Dopamine in Pathological Gambling and Psychostimulant Addiction," *Current Drug Abuse Reviews* 2/1 (January 2009): 11–25, https://www.ncbi .nlm.nih.gov/pubmed/19630734.

13 A. Weinstein and Y. Weinstein, "Exercise Addiction: Diagnosis, Bio-Psychological Mechanisms and Treatment Issues," *Current Pharmaceutical Design* 20/25 (2014): 4062-69, https://www.ncbi .nlm.nih.gov/pubmed/24001300; Marilyn Freimuth, Sandy Moniz, and Shari R. Kim, "Clarifying Exercise Addiction: Differential Diagnosis, Co-occurring Disorders, and Phases of Addiction," *International Journal of Environmental Research and Public Health* 8/10 (October 2011): 4069–81, https://www.ncbi.nlm.nih.gov/pmc/articles/PMC3210598/.

14 Rodrigo Narvaes and Rosa Maria Martins de Almeida, "Aggressive Behavior and Three Neu-rotransmitters: Dopamine, GABA, and Serotonin—A Review of the Last 10 Years," *Psychology & Neuroscience* 7/4 (2014): 601–7, http://psycnet.apa.org/fulltext/2014-56250-020.html; R. Yanowitch and E. F. Coccaro, "The Neurochemistry of Human Aggression," *Advances in Genetics* 75 (2011): 151–69, https://www.ncbi.nlm.nih.gov/pubmed/22078480.

15 J. P. Burkett and L. J. Young, "The Behavioral, Anatomical and Pharmacological Parallels Between Social Attachment, Love and Addiction," *Psychopharmacology* 224/1 (November 2012): 1–26, https://www.ncbi.nlm.nih.gov/pubmed/22885871.

16 Katherine Harmon, "Dopamine Determines Impulsive Behavior," *Scientific American*, July 29, 2010, https://www.scientificamerican.com/article/dopamine-impulsive-addiction/; "How Addic-tion Hijacks the Brain," *Harvard Health Publishing*, July 2011, https://www.health.harvard.edu /newsletter_article/how-addiction-hijacks-the-brain.

17 Peter Whybrow, "Why We Must Kick Our Addiction to Electronic Cocaine," *The Sun*, July 13, 2012, https://www.thesun.co.uk/archives/news/760579/why-we-must-kick-our-addiction-to -electronic-cocaine/; Nicholas Kardaras, "It's 'Digital Heroin': How Screens Turn Kids into Psychotic Junkies," *New York Post*, August 27, 2016, https://nypost.com/2016/08/27/its-digital -heroin-how-screens-turn-kids-into-psychotic-junkies/.

18 Seyed Amir Jazaeri and Mohammad Hussain Bin Habil, "Reviewing Two Types of Addiction— Pathological Gambling and Substance Use," *Indian Journal of Psychological Medicine* 34 (2012): 5–11, doi: 10.4103/0253-7176.96147; "October 2009 Hearings on Expanded Gambling in Massa-chusetts, Dr. Hans Breiter of Massachusetts General Hospital," YouTube video, published Novem-ber 5, 2009, accessed February 8, 2018, https://www.youtube.com/watch?v=1i_Iixu1PY4; M. N. Potenza, "The Neurobiology of Pathological Gambling," *Seminars in Clinical Neuropsychiatry* 6/3 (July 2001): 217–26, https://www.ncbi.nlm.nih.gov/pubmed/11447573.

19 Hilarie Cash, personal communication.

20 Brian A. Primack et al., "Use of Multiple Social Media Platforms and Symptoms of Depression and Anxiety: A Nationally Representative Study among U.S. Young Adults," *Computers in Human Behavior* 69 (2017): 1–9, https://doi.org/10.1016/j.chb.2016.11.013.

21 "More Sleep Would Make Us Happier, Healthier and Safer," *Psychology: Science in Action*, Ameri-can Psychological Association, accessed April 30, 2018, http://www.apa.org/action/resources /research-in-action/sleep-deprivation.aspx.

22 M. Hysing et al., "Sleep and Use of Electronic Devices in Adolescence: Results from a Large Population-Based Study," *BMJ Open* 5 (2015): e006748, doi: 10.1136/bmjopen-2014-006748.

23 A. A. Ginde et al., "Demographic Differences and Trends of Vitamin D Insufficiency in the US Population, 1988-2004," *Archives of Internal Medicine* 169 (2009): 626–32, doi:10.1001 /archinternmed.2008.604.

24 K. L. Knutson, "Does Inadequate Sleep Play a Role in Vulnerability to Obesity?" *American Journal of Human Biology* 24 (2012): 361–71, doi:10.1002/ajhb.22219.

25 Anusuya Chatterjee and Ross C. DeVol, *Waistlines of the World: The Effect of Information and Communications Technology on Obesity* (Santa Monica, CA: Milken Institute, 2012), http://www .milkeninstitute.org/publications/view/531.

26 C. S. Andreassen et al., "The Relationship Between Addictive Use of Social Media, Narcissism, and Self-Esteem: Findings from a Large National Survey," *Addictive Behaviors* 64 (2017): 287–93, https://doi.org/10.1016/j.addbeh.2016.03.006.

27 Daniela Ongaro, "Your Child's Phone and Tablet Could Be Harming Their Eyes, Expert Warns," *Daily Telegraph*, August 24, 2014, https://www.dailytelegraph.com.au/entertainment/arts/your -childs-phone-and-tablet-could-be-harming-their-eyes-expert-warns/news-story/c91174a8dcd55d0e 70f0836144a403c5; H. He et al., "Effect of Time Spent Outdoors at School on the Development of

Myopia Among Children in China: A Randomized Clinical Trial," *Journal of the American Medical Association* 314/11 (September 15, 2015): 1142–48, https://www.ncbi.nlm.nih.gov/pubmed/26372583.

28 J. Schüz, "Exposure to Extremely Low-Frequency Magnetic Fields and the Risk of Childhood Cancer: Update of the Epidemiological Evidence," *Progress in Biophysics & Molecular Biology* 107 (2011): 339–42, doi: 10.1016/j.pbiomolbio.2011.09.008; World Health Organization, International Agency for Research on Cancer, "Non-Ionizing Radiation, Part 1: Static and Extremely Low-Frequency (ELF) Electric and Magnetic Fields," *IARC Monographs on the Evaluation of Carcinogenic Risks to Humans* 80 (2002): https://www.ncbi.nlm.nih.gov/books/NBK390731/; J. Grellier, P. Ravazzani, and E. Cardis, "Potential Health Impacts of Residential Exposures to Extremely Low Frequency Magnetic Fields in Europe," *Environment International* 52 (January 2014): 55–63, https://www.ncbi.nlm.nih.gov/pubmed/24161447.

29 M. Havas, "Radiation from Wireless Technology Affects the Blood, the Heart, and the Autonomic Nervous System," *Reviews on Environmental Health* 28 (November 2013), https://www.ncbi.nlm.nih.gov/pubmed/24192494.

30 M. Nathaniel Mead, "Cancer: Strong Signal for Cell Phone Effects," *Environmental Health Perspectives* 116 (2008): A422, https://www.ncbi.nlm.nih.gov/pmc/articles/PMC2569116/; L. Hardell et al., "Pooled Analysis of Case-Control Studies on Malignant Brain Tumours and the Use of Mobile and Cordless Phones Including Living and Deceased Subjects," *International Journal of Oncology* 38 (2011): 1465–74, doi: 10.3892/ijo.2011.947.

31 William James, "The Gospel of Relaxation," *Scribners* (1899), 500, http://www.unz.org/Pub/Scribners-1899apr-00499.

32 Lige Leng, "The Relationship between Mobile Phone Use and Risk of Brain Tumor: A Systematic Review and Meta-Analysis of Trials in the Last Decade," *Chinese Neurosurgical Journal* 2 (2016), https://doi.org/10.1186/s41016-016-0059-y.

33 T. Koeman et al., "Occupational Extremely Low-Frequency Magnetic Field Exposure and Selected Cancer Outcomes in a Prospective Dutch Cohort," *Cancer Causes & Control* 25 (2014): 203–14, doi: 10.1007/s10552-013-0322-x, https://cnjournal.biomedcentral.com/articles/10.1186/s41016-016-0059-y; Grellier, Ravazzani, and Cardis, "Potential Health Impacts."

34 Martha Herbert and Cindy Sage, "Findings in Autism (ASD) Consistent with Electromagnetic Fields (EMF) and Radiofrequency Radiation (RFR)" (report prepared for the BioInitiative Working Group, 2012), 11–12, http://www.bioinitiative.org/report/wp-content/uploads/pdfs/sec20_2012_Findings_in_Autism_Consistent_with_EMF_and_RFR.pdf.

35 Lennart Hardell and Michael Carlberg, "Mobile Phone and Cordless Phone Use and the Risk for Glioma–Analysis of Pooled Case-Control Studies in Sweden, 1997–2003 and 2007–2009," *Pathophysiology* 22/1 (2015): 1–13, http://www.sciencedirect.com/science/article/pii/S0928468014000649.

36 Geoffrey Lean, "Mobile Phone Use 'Raises Children's Risk of Brain Cancer Fivefold,'" *Independent*, September 20, 2008, http://www.independent.co.uk/news/science/mobile-phone-use-raises-childrens-risk-of-brain-cancer-fivefold-937005.html.

37 Josh Cohen, "Why Is Midlife Such a Lonely Time?" *The Guardian*, July 14, 2015, https://www.theguardian.com/commentisfree/2015/jul/14/midlife-lonely-isolated-social-media; Stephen Marche, "Is Facebook Making Us Lonely?" *The Atlantic*, May 2012, https://www.theatlantic.com/magazine/archive/2012/05/is-facebook-making-us-lonely/308930/.

38 Phil Owen, "Do Video Games Make Depression Worse?" *Kotaku*, November 26, 2012, https://kotaku.com/5962636/do-video-games-make-depression-worse; Karen Trevorrow and Susan Moore, "The Association Between Loneliness, Social Isolation and Women's Electronic Gaming Machine Gambling," *Journal of Gambling Studies* 14/3 (December 1998): 263–84, https://link.springer.com/article/10.1023/A:1022057609568.

Chapter 9: Navigating the Medical Maze

1 D. Squires and C. Anderson, "U.S. Health Care from a Global Perspective," *The Commonwealth Fund*, October 8, 2015, http://www.commonwealthfund.org/publications/issue-briefs/2015/oct/us-health-care-from-a-global-perspective. For readers interested in a global perspective on health care, see Steven Brill, "Bitter Pill: Why Medical Bills Are Killing Us," *Time*, February 20, 2013, http://content.time.com/time/subscriber/article/0,33009,2136864,00.html.

2   E. C. Schneider et al., "Mirror, Mirror 2017: International Comparison Reflects Flaws and Opportunities for Better U.S. Health Care," *The Commonwealth Fund*, July 2017, http://www .commonwealthfund.org/publications/fund-reports/2017/jul/mirror-mirror-international -comparisons-2017; Melissa Etehad and Kyle Kim, "The U.S. Spends More on Healthcare Than Any Other Country—But Not with Better Health Outcomes," *Los Angeles Times*, July 18, 2017, http://www.latimes.com/nation/la-na-healthcare-comparison-20170715-htmlstory.html.

3   *Universal Declaration of Human Rights* (Paris: United Nations General Assembly, 1948), http:// www.un.org/en/universal-declaration-human-rights/.

Chapter 10: Dr. Paul's 13-Point Addiction Recovery Plan

1   Katrina Clarke, "Forest Bathing: A Practice with Roots in Japan Gains a Foothold in Canada," CBC, August 9, 2017, http://www.cbc.ca/life/wellness/forest-bathing-a-practice-with-roots-in -japan-gains-a-foothold-in-canada-1.4240492.

2   Anthony Samsel and Stephanie Seneff, "Glyphosate Pathways to Modern Diseases III: Manganese, Neurological Diseases, and Associated Pathologies," *Surgical Neurology International* 6 (2015): 45, https://www.ncbi.nlm.nih.gov/pmc/articles/PMC4392553/.

3   Mario Kratz et al., "The Relationship Between High-Fat Dairy Consumption and Obesity, Cardiovascular, and Metabolic Disease," *European Journal of Nutrition* 52 (2013): 1–24, https:// link.springer.com/article/10.1007%2Fs00394-012-0418-1.

4   Dariush Mozaffarian et al., "Circulating Biomarkers of Dairy Fat and Risk of Incident Diabetes Mellitus Among Men and Women in the United States in Two Large Prospective Cohorts," *Circulation* 133 (2016): 1645–54, https://doi.org/10.1161/CIRCULATIONAHA.115.018410.

5   Sangah Shin et al., "Association Between Milk Consumption and Metabolic Syndrome Among Korean Adults: Results from the Health Examinees Study," *Nutrients* 9/10 (October 8, 2017): E1102, http://www.mdpi.com/2072-6643/9/10/1102/pdf; Parvin Mirmiran et al., "High-fat Dairy Is Inversely Associated with the Risk of Hypertension in Adults: Tehran Lipid and Glucose Study," *International Dairy Journal* 43 (April 2015): 22–26, https://www.researchgate.net/publication /268691172_High-fat_dairy_is_inversely_associated_with_the_risk_of_hypertension_in_adults _Tehran_lipid_and_glucose_study; F. Raziani et al., "High Intake of Regular-Fat Cheese Compared with Reduced-Fat Cheese Does Not Affect LDL Cholesterol or Risk Markers of the Metabolic Syndrome: A Randomized Controlled Trial," *American Journal of Clinical Nutrition* 104 (2016): 973–81, https://www.ncbi.nlm.nih.gov/pubmed/27557654.

6   Dale E. Bredesen, *The End of Alzheimer's: The First Program to Prevent and Reverse Cognitive Decline* (New York: Avery, 2017), 140.

7   T. Inagaki et al., "Adverse Reactions to Zolpidem: Case Reports and a Review of the Literature," *Primary Care Companion to the Journal of Clinical Psychiatry* 12 (2010): doi: 10.4088/PCC .09r00849bro; D. F. Kripke et al., "Hypnotics' Association with Mortality or Cancer: A Matched Cohort Study," *BMJ Open* 2 (2012): e000850, doi: 10.1136/bmjopen-2012-000850.

8   Chelsea L. Robertson, "Effect of Exercise Training on Striatal Dopamine D2/D3 Receptors in Methamphetamine Users During Behavioral Treatment," *Neuropsychopharmacology* 41 (2016): 1629–36, doi:10.1038/npp.2015.331.

9   "Naloxone for Opioid Overdose: Life-Saving Science," *National Institute on Drug Abuse*, last updated March 2017, https://www.drugabuse.gov/publications/naloxone-opioid-overdose-life -saving-science/naloxone-opioid-overdose-life-saving-science.

Appendix 3: Essential Oils for Anxiety and Sleep

1   Mi-Yeon Cho et al., "Evidence of Aromatherapy on the Anxiety, Vital Signs, and Sleep Quality of Percutaneous Coronary Intervention Patients in Intensive Care Units," *Evidence-Based Complementary and Alternative Medicine* 2013 (2013): 381381, doi: 10.1155/2013/381381, https://www.ncbi .nlm.nih.gov/pmc/articles/PMC3588400/.

2   X. L. Wang et al., "Sesquiterpenoids from Myrrh Inhibit Androgen Receptor Expression and Function in Human Prostate Cancer Cells," *Acta Pharmacologica Sinica* 32 (2011): 338–44, doi: 10.1038/aps.2010.219.

3 Susan K. Hadley and Stephen M. Gaarder, "Treatment of Irritable Bowel Syndrome," *American Family Physician* 72 (2005): 2501–8, https://www.aafp.org/afp/2005/1215/p2501.html#afp 20051215p2501-b27.

4 H. Göbel et al., "Peppermint Oil in the Acute Treatment of Tension-Type Headache," *Schmerz* 30/3 (June 2016): 295-310, doi: 10.1007/s00482-016-0109-6, https://www.ncbi.nlm.nih.gov /pubmed/27106030.

5 J. D. Amsterdam et al., "Chamomile (Matricaria recutita) May Provide Antidepressant Activity in Anxious, Depressed Humans: An Exploratory Study," *Alternative Therapies in Health and Medicine* 18 (2012): 44–49, https://www.ncbi.nlm.nih.gov/pubmed/22894890.

6 S. Saiyudthong and C. A. Marsden, "Acute Effects of Bergamot Oil on Anxiety-Related Behaviour and Corticosterone Level in Rats," *Phytotherapy Research* 25 (2011): 858–62, doi: 10.1002/ptr.3325.

7 Safieh Mohebitabar et al., "Therapeutic Efficacy of Rose Oil: A Comprehensive Review of Clinical Evidence," *Avicenna Journal of Phytomedicine* 7 (2017): 206–13, https://www.ncbi.nlm.nih.gov /pmc/articles/PMC5511972/.

8 T. Hongratanaworakit and G. Buchbauer, "Relaxing Effect of Ylang Ylang Oil on Humans After Transdermal Absorption," *Phytotherapy Research* 20/9 (September 2006): 758–63, https://www .ncbi.nlm.nih.gov/pubmed/16807875.

9 Da-Jung Jung et al., "Effects of Ylang-Ylang Aroma on Blood Pressure and Heart Rate in Healthy Men," *Journal of Exercise Rehabilitation* 9/2 (April 2013): 250–55, https://www.ncbi.nlm.nih.gov /pmc/articles/PMC3836517/.

Glossary

1 G. Polanczyk et al., "The Worldwide Prevalence of ADHD: A Systematic Review and Metaregression Analysis," *American Journal of Psychiatry* 164 (2007): 942–48, https://www.ncbi.nlm.nih .gov/pubmed/17541055.

2 "State-based Prevalence Data of Parent Reported ADHD Diagnosis by a Health Care Provider," *Centers for Disease Control and Prevention*, last updated February 13, 2017, https://www.cdc.gov /ncbddd/adhd/prevalence.html.

3 Evy McDonald, "Another Perspective of ALS," *American Holistic Health Association*, accessed February 3, 2018, https://ahha.org/selfhelp-articles/another-perspective-of-als/.

4 "Benzodiazepines," *Drug Enforcement Administration*, 2013, https://www.deadiversion.usdoj.gov /drug_chem_info/benzo.pdf.

5 Feyza Bora, Fatih Yılmaz, and Taner Bora, "Ecstasy (MDMA) and Its Effects on Kidneys and Their Treatment: A Review," *Iranian Journal of Basic Medical Sciences* 19/11 (November 2016): 1151–58, https://www.ncbi.nlm.nih.gov/pmc/articles/PMC5126214/.

6 Charles M. Benbrook, "Trends in Glyphosate Herbicide Use in the United States and Globally," *Environmental Science Europe* 28/1 (2016): 3, https://www.ncbi.nlm.nih.gov/pmc/articles/PMC 5044953/.

7 William Neuman and Andrew Pollack, "Farmers Cope with Roundup-Resistant Weeds," *New York Times*, May 3, 2010, http://www.nytimes.com/2010/05/04/business/energy-environment/04weed .html?pagewanted=all.

8 Charles M. Benbrook, "Trends in Glyphosate Herbicide Use."

9 "Evaluation of Five Organophosphate Insecticides and Herbicides," *International Agency for Research on Cancer*, press release, March 20, 2015, https://www.iarc.fr/en/media-centre/iarcnews /pdf/MonographVolume112.pdf.

10 Charles M. Benbrook, "Trends in Glyphosate Herbicide Use."

11 "What Are Single Nucleotide Polymorphisms (SNPs)?" *Genetics Home Reference*, April 3, 2018, https://ghr.nlm.nih.gov/primer/genomicresearch/snp.

Index

milk thistle, 157
Mindfulness and the 12 Steps
  (Jacobs-Stewart), 263
Mind of Your Own, A (Brogan), 247
Minich, Deanna, 68
mirtazapine, 261
Morell, Theodor, 110
morphine, 4, 42, 44, 52, 65, 77, 78,
  79, 80, 97, 119, 304
MSG, 86, 87, 99
"My Dopamine Made Me Do It"
  (Seppala), 32
Mylan company, 60
Myth of the ADHD Child, The (Arm-
  strong), 117

N-acetylcysteine (NAC), 156, 157, 184–85
Nagayoshi, Nagai, 110
naloxone, 112, 286–88; carrying naloxone with you, 265–66; emergency
  overdose treatment, 287–88
naltrexone, 151–53, 236
Narcotics Anonymous, 2, 104, 241, 300
National Institute on Alcohol Abuse and
  Alcoholism, 61
nicotine, 180–83
Nimoy, Leonard, 39

obesity, 35, 110, 144, 204
old man and his hound, story of 34, 34
opioids, 1–5, 11, 77–107; are you at risk
  for addiction?, 81; carrying naloxone,
  265–66; Big Pharma and, 83, 84;
  cannabis and overdoses, 171; Diana's
  story, 56–58, 72; emergency overdose
  treatment, 287–88; fatalities and, 107,
  265; fentanyl in epidurals, 52–54,
  313n6; harm reduction approach,
  89–90, 306; how they work, 79, 98;
  initial prescriptions for, 4–5, 23; interventions and, 44–45; loss of libido,
  101; Maiya and, 1, 23, 44, 81–83, 85;
  Michael's story, 90–92, 149, 232;
  motivation to seek help, 87–89, 89;
  Nicky's story, 80–81; Pain Is a Vital
  Sign campaign, 84, 85; pain management and, 42, 44, 77, 81, 82–83, 98;
  patients describe the feeling, 98, 201;
  prescribed opioids, list of, 78–79; as a

public health crisis, 79–80; relapse, 2,
  30, 105–6, 106; street drugs, 79; term
  defined, 77–78; tolerance and, 82,
  83, 98; top opium poppy countries,
  78; types of, 78–79, 289; withdrawal
  from, 44, 95. *See also* fentanyl; heroin
opioids treatment plan, 92–97;
  buprenorphine, 92–93, 245; exercise,
  96; food, 94–95; message to the support team, 107; microbiome healing,
  96; quality sleep, 96; relapses and,
  105–6, 106; stress reduction, 95–96;
  supportive network for, 96–97; vitamin D, 95
opium, 39, 78, 79
oppositional personality, 27
O'Shaughnessy, William Brooke, 169
osteopath, 307
overdose: emergency treatment of,
  287–88. *See also* methadone; opioids
oxycodone, 30, 59, 77, 79; and acetaminophen, 79; and naloxone, 79
OxyContin, 79, 84

pain: accepting and feeling, 236–40;
  addiction spectrum and, 27; addressing the underlying cause, 98;
  cannabis for relief, 171, 189; fear of,
  82, 83–85; food solutions, 98–100;
  inflammation and, 97–98; integrative
  solutions, 97–99, 101–3; Jessica's
  story: finding the cause, 85–87;
  lifestyle changes for, 86–87, 99–101;
  medical establishment and, 84–85;
  opioids for, 42, 44, 77, 81, 82–83;
  opioid tolerance and, 82, 83, 98; Pain
  Is a Vital Sign campaign, 84, 85;
  prescribed, addictive drugs and, 30,
  44, 56–59, 98; quantifying, 19; relief
  to-do list, 239–40; self-medicating
  and, 8; stopping opioids and, 98, 238;
  turmeric for relief, 157
pain, emotional: integrative solutions
  for, 103–5; recovery journal, 104
Pain Is a Vital Sign campaign, 84, 85
PCP, 168
pediatricians: prescribing opioids, 85;
  prescribing stimulants, 115, 118; treatment of addiction by, 3

About the Authors

Paul Thomas, MD, ABAM, FAAP, is an integrative physician and addiction specialist with a thriving clinical practice in Portland, Oregon. He is the founder of Fair Start, an addiction clinic that has successfully treated over 500 opioid addicts since it opened in 2009. His YouTube channel has over 592,000 active and engaged subscribers and his most popular video has had upward of 31 million views. Dr. Paul received his medical degree from the Dartmouth Geisel School of Medicine and completed his pediatric residency at the University of California–San Diego. He is a diplomat of the American Board of Addiction Medicine and a board-certified pediatrician. He is the father of nine children (ages twenty-one to thirty-five), three biological and six adopted. Dr. Paul lives with his family in Portland, Oregon. Learn more about him at www.paulthomasmd.com.

Jennifer Margulis, PhD, is an award-winning science writer, Fulbright grantee, and sought-after speaker. She has worked as a journalist, media consultant, and health advocate for over fifteen years. Her articles have appeared in the *New York Times*, the *Washington Post*, *Smithsonian* magazine, *Ms.* magazine, *More* magazine, *O: The Oprah Magazine*, and dozens of other magazines, newspapers, and online sites. She received her BA from Cornell University, her MA from the University of California–Berkeley, and her PhD from Emory University. She also produces radio features for Jefferson Public Radio. Dr. Margulis has taught literature in inner-city Atlanta, appeared live on prime-time TV in France, and worked on a child survival campaign in Niger, West Africa. Originally from Boston, she lives with her husband and four children in southern Oregon. Learn more about her at www.jennifermargulis.net.